Constance Hammen

Depression Runs in Families

The Social Context of Risk and Resilience in Children of Depressed Mothers

Springer-Verlag
New York Berlin Heidelberg London
Paris Tokyo Hong Kong Barcelona

Constance Hammen
Department of Psychology
University of California
Los Angeles, CA 90024-1563
USA

Series Editor:
Lauren B. Alloy
Department of Psychology
Temple University
Philadelphia, PA 19122
USA

With five illustrations.

Library of Congress Cataloging-in-Publication Data
Hammen, Constance L.
Depression runs in families: The social context of risk and resilience in children of depressed mothers / Constance Hammen.
p. cm. — (Series in psychopathology)
Includes bibliographical references.
ISBN-13: 978-1-4684-6412-2 e-ISBN-13: 978-1-4684-6410-8
DOI: 10.1007/978-1-4684-6410-8

1. Children of depressed persons—Mental health. 2. Depression, Mental—Etiology. 3. Mother and child. 4. Depressed persons—Family relationships. I. Title. II. Series.
[DNLM: 1. Child of Impaired Parents. 2. Depressive Disorder. 3. Depressive Disorder—etiology. 4. Depressive Disorder—in infancy & childhood. 5. Family. 6. Parent–Child Relations. WM 171 H224d]
RC537.H3 1991
616.85′27—dc20
DNLM/DLC
for Library of Congress 90-10460

Printed on acid-free paper.

Typeset by Best-set Typesetter, Ltd., Hong Kong.

9 8 7 6 5 4 3 2 1

Series in Psychopathology

Series Editor
Lauren B. Alloy

Series in Psychopathology

Editor: Lauren B. Alloy

Published Volumes:
Depression Runs in Families: The Social Context of Risk and Resilience in Children of Depressed Mothers

Forthcoming:
Hopelessness Depression

Neurobehavioral Systems, Personality, and Psychopathology

Acknowledgments

The research project that this book is based on came to be called the UCLA Family Stress Project. It began in the early 1980s as an attempt to study the childhood origins of depression. It was the collaborative effort of many people. It would not have been undertaken at all without the instigation, enthusiasm, and planning of then–graduate students David Gordon and Carol Jaenicke. Later, when the original enthusiasm gave way to the sheer amazement at the magnitude of the task we had undertaken, Dorli Burge and Cheri Adrian made it continue. Involved at every level of both tedium and excitement as the project matured, they were there through the last of the follow-ups. Their extraordinary talent and dedication were essential to the project. The enormous psychic rewards of an academic profession are nowhere more apparent than in the opportunity to use the abilities entrusted to us to do meaningful work in the company of dedicated and enthusiastic students. It was a privilege for me to have this opportunity over the past few years.

Jean Kaufman played a major part in keeping the ship afloat and everyone in good humor. Libbi Burney Hamilton was a mainstay in the follow-up stages, just as Brian Zupan was in the earlier phases. Carolyn Anderson and Marilyn Conrad contributed their interest, support, and good ideas, and early on we were glad to have the help of Pam Kimsey, Aimee Ellicott, Maren Jones, and other graduate students at UCLA.

The countless administrative aspects of the study required the help of many, and over the years I was fortunate to have the assistance of Kelly Ellis, Memee Peggs, Tina Goodman-Brown, Robin Gilson, and Miki Carpenter. All of them have gone on to graduate studies in helping professions. There were many dedicated and talented undergraduates who played important roles in the project and who have now gone on to graduate programs and to their own projects. Although there are too many to mention all of them, a few deserve special recognition and good wishes for their own futures: Marie Martel, Nangel Lindberg, Lisa Harris, Naomi Oderberg, Michael Friedmann, Howard Fulfrost, Kirsten Fleming, and

Debbi Stackman. The assistance of all the others is also gratefully acknowledged.

Early in the project Donald Hiroto was helpful, and a grant to him from the Veterans Administration helped to get the study off the ground. Special thanks are owed to the William T. Grant Foundation for funding for most of the study. They showed faith in a newly forming developmental psychopathologist, and their support certainly opened new vistas in my career.

Finally, the families who consented to participate in this study must be acknowledged. Their immeasurable contribution, the courage to reveal their most vulnerable experiences and the women's undeniable concerns about making the best family lives possible, earned our respect and gratitude. Although this report offers little to the women and children in return for their efforts, the work affirms our concern for their struggles and for finding solutions.

Contents

1
Studies of Children of Depressed Parents

Depression runs in families.

This simple conclusion has a far from simple explanation or meaning. Some would argue that in its severe or chronic forms, depression is a disease whose underlying pathophysiology is genetically transmitted. Others would argue that depression arises in a psychosocial context, and that its intergenerational patterns reflect maladaptive interpersonal, situational, and intrapsychic processes that are played out in family life and child socialization. Still others would emphasize the transactional nature of multiple processes, encompassing both biological and psychosocial factors unfolding in the family context.

Not surprisingly, these three approaches to psychopathology represent competing perspectives on most forms of psychological disorder. The study of affective disorders offers an excellent opportunity to consider these models and their utility in explicating familial patterns of depression. There are several reasons for pursuing this goal in the context of depressive disorders: practical matters of the widespread incidence and pernicious consequences of mood disorders, and theoretical issues in which depression provides a lively forum for development of a variety of hypotheses.

Mood Disorders: A Major Public Health Problem

Nearly everyone experiences depression as part of living—it is a normal and usually brief reaction to the perils of existence, the failures, setbacks, disappointments, and losses that attend modern life. Depression can last a few hours, a few days, or even weeks, but for most individuals it is transitory and, however unpleasant it may feel, it does not impair functioning. Yet, for a substantial minority—and some would argue that this is a growing number—depression is a debilitating and even life-threatening disorder.

The constellation of mood and physical, behavioral, and psychological symptoms that comprise the syndrome of clinically significant depression has been found to occur to between 4 and 8% of the adult population (Karno et al., 1987). Earlier investigations using less stringent, reliable standards or including milder forms of depression estimated the rates to be even higher, up to 18% in various U.S. cities and Western nations (Boyd & Weissman, 1981). At any given moment, between 9 and 20% of the population will report some significant depression symptoms even if they do not meet formal diagnostic criteria for depression (e.g., Boyd & Weissman, 1981).

The syndrome of manic depression, now termed bipolar disorder, is more rare, estimated to affect less than 1% of the population (Boyd & Weissman, 1981; Robins et al., 1984). However, as criteria for identifying milder forms of bipolar disorder have improved, investigators have suggested that the rates of symptoms may be higher than originally suspected (Depue et al., 1981). Moreover, these mild or even subsyndromal forms of affective disorder may be early warning signs of later, full-scale major affective disorders.

The sheer numbers of people with affective disorders marks them as our most common psychiatric problem. Yet the great majority of individuals, especially those with major or chronic unipolar depression, do not seek treatment. But even beyond the magnitude of the problem, there are three striking features of mood disorders. One is impairment, a second is recurrence and chronicity, and the third is the apparently increasing rates and shifting demographic patterns.

Impairment of functioning due to moderate or severe affective disorder has a unique twist that separates such disorders from many other kinds of psychiatric conditions, all of which by definition involve impaired functioning. The low mood, apathy, lack of energy, loss of pleasure, negative outlook on the self and the future that typify depression, for instance, often seem "irrational" to others. Whereas psychotic or bizarre symptoms or behaviors of depression and mania may be detectable as illness, most of the less florid mood-related symptoms are often viewed as controllable. That is, people in this culture are typically held responsible for their own moods and expected to overcome dysphoric states by will, effort, and activity. Yet it is a major characteristic of clinical depression that mood affects the way people construe themselves and their worlds. Additionally, the bodily experiences of low energy, poor appetite, and sleep disturbances are part of the depression syndrome. Thus a depressed person may be entirely "capable" as a worker or parent but feel unable to perform the functions of these roles. An individual who is depressed may experience paralyzing doubts about her own worth as a person that exacerbate dysphoria and may heighten sensitivity to criticism or even lead to social withdrawal. Yet to an outsider, they may be unrealistic in terms of the person's skills, personal qualities, appearance, and desirability. Similarly, a man who has lost his job due to layoff may experience depression that affects his outlook, energy, and self-respect. When others can see that the job loss had nothing to do with his capability and urge him to take the obvious coping measures of seeking new work, he himself may feel that such measures are useless and overwhelming.

The pervasiveness of depressive symptoms is likely to spill over to all major role functions, including family relationships. To the extent that family members, however well-intentioned, cannot comprehend the negative outlook that colors all of the feelings and actions of the depressed person, there is likely to be tension or even open conflict that may exacerbate the depression (Coyne, Wortman, & Lehman, 1985; Coyne et al., 1987). A fairly typical pattern in major affective disorders may therefore involve not only impairment of role functioning but also conflict and/or overinvolvement with significant others. Moreover, the depressed individual is likely to feel even more depressed and guilty about her feelings and behaviors. The depressed woman may feel worse *because* she feels impatient and uncaring toward her children or doesn't want to go to work in the mornings, or the depressed man may feel worse *because* he is apathetic toward his wife or unenthusiastic about his job.

The second notable feature of major depression that has become increasingly apparent is that it is commonly recurrent. Bipolar disorders have always been defined as recurrent, with patterns of depression and mania or hypomania recurring in cycles typically unique to the individual but generally involving at least several major episodes in a lifetime (Goodwin & Jamison, 1984). However, it is increasingly apparent that many bipolar patients do not recover entirely between episodes but rather display significant rates of continuing symptoms and impairment of functioning (Clayton, 1984). Now we are learning that unipolar disorders are also likely to recur, with 50 to 85% of patients who seek treatment for an episode experiencing at least one additional episode (Clayton, 1984; Keller, 1985; Zis & Goodwin, 1979). It has been estimated that the mean number of lifetime episodes of major depression in affected individuals is five or six, based on naturalistic studies of clinic records (Angst, 1973). It has now been shown for a variety of age groups that the best predictor of depression is past depression (e.g., Clayton, 1984; Hammen, Mayol, deMayo, & Marks, 1986; Lewinsohn, Hoberman, & Rosenbaum, 1988).

Added to the recurrence of major depression is the chronicity problem. It has been estimated by Depue and Monroe (1986) that chronic depression occurs in at least 25% of depressed cases. Keller and colleagues found that approximately 20% of their sample of depressed patients failed to recover from an additional episode following initial response to treatment (Keller, Lavori, Endicott, Coryell, & Klerman, 1983). Keller et al. (1983) also found that about 25% of depressed patients they studied had a pattern they called "double depression," that is, major episodes superimposed on chronic dysthymic disorder. Even when they recover from the major episode, nearly 60% remained chronically symptomatic (Keller, 1988).

A final note about the natural history of affective disorders concerns demographic distributions and apparent changing patterns. It has been well established that women are at greater risk for major depression and significant depressive symptoms than men are, by a ratio of about 2:1 (Boyd & Weissman, 1981; Nolen-Hoeksema, 1987), although the explanation for the pattern is a matter of controversy. Now there is evidence that the gender gap may be narrowing, and that there may be increasing rates of affective disorders for young people in general (Klerman & Weissman, 1989). Klerman et al. (1985) and Gershon, Hamovit, Guroff, and Nurnberger (1987) have detected increased rates of both unipolar and bipolar disorders in the young relatives of ill patients. That is, higher rates of disorder in the younger relatives than in older relatives suggest that the age of onset of major affective disorders may be shifting downward, compared to earlier findings suggesting that unipolar disorders were largely of middle age onset. Epidemiological studies indicate that the rates of depressive disorders are highest in young adults (e.g., Robins et al., 1984).

These findings about the phenomenology and patterns of occurrence of affective disorders add up to several conclusions. First, because of their sheer high rates of prevalence, affective disorders touch many individuals and their families. Second, because family and interpersonal role functioning are highly likely to be impaired, unipolar and bipolar disorders are not just individual ailments but also afflict families. Third, because so many women are depressed, and especially if they are affected in young adult childbearing years, their depressions are likely to occur in the context of parenting roles. Fourth, a good number of individuals with major affective disorders will have recurrent or even chronic symptoms. Thus they and their families will come to experience depressive disorders as a significant portion of their lives. For all of these reasons it seems vital to expand our investigations of the impact of depressive disorders on individuals and their families.

The purpose of this book is to explore this issue, to pursue the various perspectives on the effects of parental affective disorders on children, and to present results from the UCLA Family Stress project. Based on the reported research available and on this project, which was designed to address some of the gaps in the research, the goal is to summarize what there is to know about the topic to date.

Above all, the goal of the book is to come to some conclusions about the meaning of the assertion "depression runs in families." After all, differences in the explanations of this truth suggest different implications for identification and treatment of high risk individuals. Shall we focus on medical interventions and genetic counseling? Should the child or the family be targeted for psychotherapy? What needs to be changed for children at risk if they are to cope with their vulnerabilities, and are these factors intrapsychic or situational? If the parent is effectively treated, will the children's risk for disorder diminish? How do we identify which children are at risk for depressive disorders, and at what ages? The list of questions could be greatly expanded.

Early High Risk Research

The assertion that depression runs in families is the major theme of this chapter. The appearance of research specifically designed to investigate the risk to children due to parental affective disorder has been relatively recent. Initially, indirect evidence appeared in the form of studies of children of schizophrenic patients, in which depression or affective disorders were often employed as a comparison group. A discussion of this early work is followed by separate reviews of offspring studies in unipolar and bipolar affective disorders. Each of these sections distinguishes between earlier research largely based on indirect information about children's functioning and the most recent research based on direct interview evaluations of children. The purpose is to give a flavor of the kinds of methods and results that have marked the field up to this point, to provide a context for describing the project that is the major focus of this book.

The development of the high risk paradigm of studying children of ill parents can be attributed largely to schizophrenia researchers. Originating mostly in the 1970s, several excellent investigations were launched to determine whether children of schizophrenic parents displayed early signs of impairment and what factors contributed to their dysfunction. The studies were for the most part very sophisticated. They typically tested current theories about the nature of schizophrenia vulnerability (such as cognitive- and information-processing debilities and social adjustment). The designs, which were longitudinal, included comparison groups consisting of other psychopathology to test the question of specificity of schizophrenia for children's risk. Of particular relevance to our current concerns, about a half dozen of them included comparison groups of parents with affective disorders. The Massachusetts Mental ealth Center longitudinal project employed a small comparison group of psychotic depressed mothers (Cohler, Grunebaum, Weiss, Hartmen, & Gallant, 1977; Gamer, Gallant, Grunebaum, & Cohler, 1977), and the Rochester Child and Family Study employed both psychotic depressed and nonpsychotic depressed comparison groups (Fisher & Kokes, 1983). The St. Louis High-Risk Study (Worland et al., 1984) and the Stony Brook High-Risk Study (Weintraub & Neale, 1984) both included hospitalized depressed groups comprised of unipolar and bipolar affective disorders. The Minnesota High-Risk Study (Rolf, 1972; Garmezy & Devine, 1984) and the Rochester Longitudinal Study (Sameroff, Barocas, & Seifer, 1984; Sameroff, Seifer, & Zax, 1982) included "neurotic" depressed comparison parents.

A comprehensive summary of the findings of these studies is beyond the scope of this review (see Watt, Anthony, Wynne, & Rolf, 1984). With respect to the issue of risk to children of parents with affective disorders, however, several trends are evident. Overall, most of the studies found evidence of comparable levels of impairment in children of schizophrenic and depressed parents (with exceptions depending on measure, timing, and comparison) compared with children of normal parents. Moreover, several of the studies, on some measures, found that children of depressed parents were even more impaired than their schizophrenia counterparts. One of the earliest collections of work concerning the impact of parental depression on children is drawn in large part from the schizophrenia high risk studies (Morrison, 1983).

Although schizophrenia studies are highly suggestive of risk to offspring of children of parents with affective disorders, their limitations preclude specification of the nature of the risk and its predictors. For instance, the studies did not have available any systematic diagnostic procedures for describing children's psychopathology, so that there are no diagnostic data on the youngsters to compare with current studies. Also, the characterization of parental depression is highly compromised by differences between DSM II and DSM III criteria for affective disorders. For example, many of the parents termed "psychotically depressed" turned out to be bipolar, rather than unipolar. "Neurotic depression" is a very heterogeneous category no longer used, and the Minnesota Study, for example, included mothers with anxiety disorders in the neurotically depressed group. Further, it has been speculated that some of the parents who were characterized as schizophrenic under the DSM II criteria might be considered depressed if evaluated by today's DSM III criteria, thus calling into question a fundamental distinction between groups. Other issues, such as the current mood status of depressed parents at the time of testing and variability in the demographic features of the sample, make it more difficult to draw firm conclusions about children's risk due to affective disorder of the parents.

Despite the limitations of these studies, they represent clear evidence that children of parents with major psychopathology may display a variety of cognitive, social, and academic dysfunctions. Further, they hint that such dysfunctions may be related more to the severity and chronicity of parental disturbance than to the specific diagnosis of the parent. In view of such findings, it is rather ironic that the earliest wave of offspring studies aimed at affective disorders rarely included a comparison group for evaluating the specificity of outcomes. Indeed, these early studies, to which we now turn, were less sophisticated in design than the schizophrenia studies.

Studies of Offspring of Unipolar Depressed Parents

Early Offspring Studies Without Direct Interviews

Two review articles provide comprehensive coverage of the first generation of studies of children of unipolar depressed parents. Orvaschel, Weissman, and Kidd (1980) presented results of five such studies available to them. Of the five, three were high risk schizophrenia comparison groups, as described previously. Only two, Weissman, Paykel, and Klerman (1972) and Welner, Welner, McCrary, and Leonard (1977), were specifically designed to compare children of depressed and normal parents. Weissman et al. focused on role functioning in depressed women, noting major social role impairment in parenting and family functioning. They also obtained maternal reports of children's functioning from 35 depressed women and 27 normal nondepressed women, observing disturbed functioning in 58% of the offspring of depressed women. Welner et al. designed a study unique in its inclusion of interviews of both children and parents in a sample of 29 depressed patients and 41 controls; however, their interviewers were not blind to parental status and did not yield contemporary DSM III diagnoses. They reported significantly higher rates of certain kinds of depressive symptoms in the offspring of depressed parents than in the control group children, and they noted that 7% of the former met diagnostic criteria for depressive diagnoses.

A few years later, Beardslee, Bemporad, Keller, and Klerman (1983) found a somewhat larger number of offspring studies of patients with affective disorders to review. However, most of the newly available studies were especially focused on children of parents with manic depression, and these are reviewed in a separate section. Two studies are noteworthy for inclusion of sufficient samples of unipolar depressed parents. Conners, Himmelhock, Goyette, Ulrich, and Neil (1979) collected parent reports of symptoms in children from a sample of 16 bipolar parents and 43 "other" (unipolar depressed); there was no normal comparison group. Using the standardized Conners Parent Questionnaire (CPQ; Conners, 1969), the authors found that parents reported significantly higher rates of symptoms in the offspring of unipolar compared to bipolar parents. Children of unipolar depressed parents were viewed as having more conduct problems, anxiety, impulsivity, and hyperkinesis (there was no factor on the scale that represented depressive symptoms as such).

Two additional studies were aimed not specifically at children of depressed parents but rather at children of parents with various psychiatric disturbances. El-Guebaly, Offord, Sullivan, and Lynch (1978) compared children of parents who were equally divided into groups of 30 each of alcoholic, unipolar depressed, and schizophrenic inpatients. Interviews of the patient's spouse, chart information, and standardized checklists completed by the spouse about the children were obtained. The overall findings indicate that 24% of the children scored in the range of clinically significant problems. However, there were no differences between the diagnostic groups. There was a tendency for boys to be viewed as more dysfunctional, especially if the ill parent was the father. The authors conclude that psychiatric disturbance in the parent in general imparts a risk to children for disorder. Rutter (1966) also reported symptoms and adjustment in children of diverse groups of psychiatrically ill parents, among whom were 43 depressed parents. Although the children of the latter group appeared to have wide-ranging symptoms and diagnoses, the focus of Rutter's work supports the hypothesis that stressful conditions, rather than the form of parental psychopathology itself, contribute to children's outcomes. Similar conclusions were reached by Cooper, Leach, Storer, and Tonge (1977) in their London study of children of 26 psychiatric patients, although the study does not specifically identify parental groups of depressed parents. A more recent version of the study conducted by Rutter and colleagues is discussed in greater detail in the section on research on offspring of parents with psychiatric diagnoses.

These early studies of children of depressed parents are flawed in many ways, owing in part to inadequate methods of characterizing diagnoses in children, small samples, or limited comparison groups. Although it is therefore impossible to draw conclusions about the magnitude, stability, and origins of children's risk for psychopathology if their parents have depressive disorders, it is nevertheless possible to find consistent evidence that the children experience a variety of dysfunction. In general, these conclusions apply to both girls and boys, and to children at different ages. Do similar results occur in the more recent studies that have had the advantage of improved diagnostic methods? This is the question to which we now turn.

Recent Research on Children of Unipolar Depressed Parents

Direct Interview Studies

There are relatively few direct interview studies of children of depressed parents, largely because improvements in the assessment and systematic diagnosis of affective disorders in children have occurred fairly recently. The studies that report children's outcomes in terms of DSM III diagnostic categories are summarized in Table 1.1.

Myrna Weissman and her colleagues have had an especially active ongoing project studying patterns of depression in families (e.g., Weissman, Gershon, et al., 1984; Weissman, Kidd, & Prusoff, 1982; Weissman & Paykel, 1974; Weissman, Prusoff, et al., 1984). The Weissman, Prusoff, et al., investigation was not itself a direct interview study, relying instead on parent reports. Nevertheless, it is noteworthy for its careful character-

TABLE 1.1. Direct diagnostic interview method studies of children of a unipolar depressed parent.

	Method		
Project	Parent sample	Child sample	Child assessment
Children at Risk for Affective Disorders Study at Massachusetts General Hospital (Keller et al., 1986; Beardslee et al., 1987)	37 unipolar depressed (3 fathers, 20 mothers, 14 both parents; 86% major depressive disorder, 14% minor depression or dysthymia)	33 males, 39 females Ages 6–19	DICA[b] with mother and child; Rochester Adaptive Behavior Inventory; DSM III criteria
Yale Family Study of Major Depression (Weissman, Gammon, et al., 1987)	56 unipolar depressed (22 fathers, 34 mothers)[a]	63 males, 62 females	K-SADS-E with mother and child in most cases; DSM III criteria
	35 normal (sex unspecified)	42 males, 53 females Ages 6–23	
University of Illinois project (Klein et al., 1988)	24 unipolar major depressed (5 fathers, 19 mothers)	27 males, 20 females	Modified SADS-L with child only; self-report Life Activities Inventory of Social Impairment; DSM III criteria
	19 rheumatological and orthopedic medical illness (8 fathers, 11 mothers)	25 males, 8 females	
	8 normal (sex unspecified)	25 males, 13 females Ages 14–22	
Western Psychiatric Institute project (Orvaschel et al., 1988)	34 unipolar recurrent major depression (8 fathers, 26 mothers)	32 males, 29 females	K-SADS-E with mother and child; Teacher Report Form—Child; Behavior Checklist; DSM III criteria
	29 normal (sex unspecified)	29 males, 17 females Ages 6–17	

[a] Estimation, sex unspecified.
[b] Diagnostic Interview of Children and Adolescents (Herjonic & Reich, 1982).

ization of the diagnoses and clinical histories of the parents, including 44 with hospitalization for major depression, 89 with nonhospitalized major depression, and 82 normals. The children between ages 6 and 18 were found to differ significantly by parent group. The children of depressed parents were three times more likely to have diagnosable disorders, with depression the most common disorder. The high risk children also had more school problems and were more frequently in treatment for their emotional difficulties. Recently, the Weissman group began direct interview evaluations of those offspring who were available and were still children. As indicated in Table 1.1, Weissman, Gammon, et al. (1987)

reported results of diagnostic evaluation of 125 children of a parent with major depressive disorder who had been treated at the Yale University Depression Research Unit and 95 children of normal comparison families, all between the ages of 6 and 23. The families were mostly middle and upper-middle class, educated beyond high school levels; the majority of families represented intact marriages. About 40% of the depressed parents were men. Children of a depressed parent were significantly more likely to have a lifetime diagnosis of major depression as well as substance abuse. They were also significantly more likely to have more multiple diagnoses (2.4, compared with 1.7 in the normal group). The offspring of depressed parents were also more likely to have been in treatment, including hospitalization, for psychological problems. Moreover, the age of onset of major depression was significantly younger for the high risk children than for children of normal parents who experienced depression. In a separate report on this sample, Weissman (1988) also noted that children of depressed parents were significantly more likely to have experienced a variety of health problems, injuries, and accidents.

Beardslee, Keller, and Klerman (1985) and Keller et al. (1986) also compared children in families of clinically depressed patients with those of normal community controls. One of the goals of the project was to investigate the effects of family characteristics on rates of disorder in offspring. Beardslee et al.'s initial report included only five normal comparison families but nevertheless found significantly higher rates of disorder in offspring of depressed parents than normals. Keller et al. found statistically significant associations between various measures of depressed parents' severity and chronicity of disorder and children's diagnoses and poor adaptation. This was especially pronounced when the depressed parent was the mother. The investigators also demonstrated that negative quality of the parents' relationship, including contacts with divorced biological parents of children, predicted more negative outcomes in the children. While the findings are seemingly clinically straightforward, this is the first study to empirically document the relationship between degree of impairment in the depressed parent and impairment in the child.

Orvaschel, Walsh-Allis, and Ye (1988) compared children of parents with recurrent unipolar depression with a normal community sample. As anticipated, offspring of unipolar parents experienced significantly more affective disorders, or any disorders. They also had more attention deficit disorder—a finding not uniformly observed in other studies. Children of unipolar parents were also more likely to have been treated for emotional and behavioral problems (33%). Further, parents with earlier age of onset of depression were more likely to have depressed children, a finding consistent with that of Keller et al. (1986) and Klein, Clark, Dansky, and Margolis (1988).

Klein et al. (1988) conducted an interview study unique for its inclusion of a medical comparison group and for the analysis of dysthymia in adolescent offspring of unipolar patients. Overall, the offspring groups differed significantly on affective disorders, with the unipolar depressed group reporting more major depression and dysthymia. Indeed, employing several different criteria for dysthymia, Klein et al. found that nearly one in six adolescent children of depressed parents experienced chronic low-grade depression. They argue that such a disorder must not be the result of the stress of parental illness as such, since the medical comparison group did not display evidence of dysthymia. Moreover, they found that parental illness characteristics such as chronicity, multiple affectively ill relatives, early onset, and multiple hospitalizations were associated with presence of dysthymia in children. On the other hand, the groups did not differ on the presence of nonaffective disorders. For these reasons, Klein and colleagues suggest that early onset dysthymia may represent an especially severe form of affective disorder with a genetic component. Moreover, because mild symptomatology may not lead to treatment and because there were high rates of social impairment in the dysthymic offspring, it is essential to consider such offspring at high risk, perhaps necessitating early intervention.

Welner and Garrison (1985) reported a direct interview study of 7- to 17-year-old offspring of parents with affective disorders. Although 67 children of 55 proband families were studied and compared to 48 children from 29 normal families, the numbers of parents with unipolar and bipolar disorders were not reported. Also, a category termed "complicated depression" was included but not defined. Overall, the authors found significantly higher rates of diagnoses in the proband offspring in all categories: affective, anxiety, attention deficit, and conduct disorders.

Studies Employing Nondiagnostic Evaluations of Children

Hirsch, Moos, and Reischl (1985) reported one of the first investigations of offspring of depressed parents that included a medically ill comparison group. The authors reasoned that stressful life events may be an important mediator of the risk to children, and children of affectively ill parents should therefore be compared with offspring whose parents also experience illness conditions. The sample consisted of adolescents between the ages of 12 and 18, with 16 in each group: parents in treatment for Research Diagnostic Criteria (RDC) major or minor unipolar depression, parents with rheumatoid arthritis, and normal parents. Youngsters were administered the Hopkins Symptom Checklist (SCL; Derogatis, Lipman, Rickels, Uhlenhuth, & Covi, 1974), a self-esteem scale (Rosenberg, 1965), a life events checklist, a scale of school satisfaction, and the Family Environment Scale (FES; Moos & Moos, 1981). Direct interviews were also conducted covering peer friendships and aspects of school and family life. In general, the authors found that children of depressed parents were the most impaired in terms of symptoms, self-esteem, and school satisfaction (although there were no group differences in family climate variables). However, the depressed and medical group youngsters did not differ from each other, and for both groups there was an association between stressful life events and symptoms. The authors conclude that the risk for dysfunction in adolescents may be attributed to parental disability rather than specific diagnosis. This conclusion differs from that of Lee and Gotlib (1989b; reported later), who observed that their medical group offspring differed significantly from the children of depressed mothers on most indices. Lee and Gotlib suggest that the differences in conclusions may stem from possible nondiagnosed psychopathology in the medically ill parents in the Hirsch et al. (1985) study. Note that Klein et al. (1988) also observed differences in the two groups' levels of affective disorder, but not nondepressive diagnoses. In general, the adolescent offspring of medically ill parents in the Klein study resembled offspring of normal parents.

Billings and Moos (1985a) reported the status of offspring at a 1-year follow-up from their previous report. In the earlier, cross-sectional study (Billings & Moos, 1983), questionnaire data on children and families indicated significantly higher levels of dysfunction in offspring of depressed parents compared to matched normal controls. In the 1985 report, Billings and Moos investigated the 1-year follow-up status of offspring in three groups: children of remitted depressed patients, children of nonremitted depressed patients, and children of normal control families. While children of currently depressed parents displayed the expected high rates of dysfunction compared to normal group children, the critical comparisons between the remitted and control groups were also significant. An index of dysfunction based on several measures of behavioral, emotional, and health problems indicated that 52.2% of nonremitted families had a disturbed child, with a rate of 26.5% in the remitted group and 9.5% in the normal group. On the whole, children of remitted depressed parents fared better than those of currently depressed parents but less well than normal children. The authors attribute this pattern to residual parental symptoms and continuing elevated levels of stress in the remitted families, and they also suggest that changes in the family milieu may occur more slowly than parental symptom changes. This hypothesis is supported by findings that both parent symptoms and child functioning are significantly related to family and environmental attributes.

Lee and Gotlib (1989b) recently reported a study that is noteworthy for its inclusion of both medically ill and nondepressed psychiatric, as well as normal comparison groups to test the hypothesis that negative outcomes in children are specific to depression in parents. However, the study is limited by lack of diagnostic evaluations of the children, which would provide comparable data to other recent offspring studies. The authors studied children of 16 currently unipolar depressed women (either dysthymic disorder or major depression), 10 nondepressed psychiatric women, 8 medically ill women (mostly with rheumatoid arthritis, who were not depressed and had no psychiatric treatment), and 27 nonpatient women. All children were between 7 and 13. Mothers and their children were reassessed 6 to 8 weeks after the initial evaluations. Children's adjustment was measured by maternal reports on the Child Behavior Check List (CBCL; Achenbach & Edelbrock, 1983), a well-validated scale of 118 items covering a variety of internalizing and externalizing behaviors. Also, interviewers completed the Child Assessment Schedule (CAS; Hodges, 1983), assessing children's functioning in different domains. Depressed mothers viewed their children as having more internalizing symptoms than did medical and normal mothers but did not differ from children of nondepressed psychiatric mothers. In a slightly larger sample based on the initial testing only, Lee and Gotlib (1989a) noted that two-thirds of the children of depressed mothers were seen by their parent has having internalizing symptoms in the clinical range. Similar findings were reported by interviewers; children of depressed mothers were seen as having more fears, physical complaints, and mood disturbance than children of normal mothers. However, for the most part they did not differ from psychiatric comparison children. Overall, the groups did not differ on externalizing problems on the CBCL or on acting out symptoms on the CAS (Lee & Gotlib, 1989a,b). The authors conclude that children's maladjustment is specific neither to maternal depression nor to general maternal disability in that children of medically ill mothers did not differ from children of normal mothers. Little information is available on the severity of the affective disorder in this sample in terms of past history of episodes and age of onset, and the depressed women's depression had decreased significantly in the six weeks between testings. Thus it is unclear whether the small unipolar sample is comparable to other studies of children of offspring with major affective disorder. Nevertheless, the results are compatible with the recurring observation of increased risk for symptoms, especially internalizing symptoms, in children of women with psychiatric disturbance.

An entirely different methodology for evaluating the symptoms of children of depressed mothers was reported by Breslau, Davis, and Prabucki (1988). An epidemiological sample was identified in Cleveland, consisting of 333 mother–child pairs on whom psychiatric interview information was available for both based on the Diagnostic Interview Schedule (Robins, Helzer, Croughan, & Ratcliff, 1981). The purpose of the study was to compare mother and child reports of child symptoms. The youngsters were between the ages of 8 and 23 (60% below age 18), and 55 of the mothers had received lifetime diagnoses of major depressive disorder. Children's symptoms were reported as scale scores rather than diagnoses, but they indicated that children of depressed women viewed themselves as having significantly more depressive symptoms than children of normal women. Maternal report ratings, on the other hand, depicted the children as having significantly more symptoms not only of depression but of all other categories (e.g., anxiety disorders, oppositional, antisocial, and inattention, impulsivity, and hyperactivity).

At the Laboratory of Developmental Psychology at NIMH, Radke-Yarrow and her colleagues have undertaken a series of direct observation studies of mothers with affective disorders and their infants and toddlers. In the initial reports, because of the children's young ages, diagnostic evaluations as such have not been reported, but the investigators have studied aspects of the children's functioning. Radke-Yarrow, Cummings, Kuczynski, and Chapman (1985), for example, reported incidence of types of attachment between 99 two- and three-year-old children and their mothers. They found significantly higher rates of insecure attachment in children of women with affective disorders than normal women. The effect was especially pronounced for women with bipolar affective illness, with 79% displaying typical or severe insecure attachment. The findings are noteworthy because attachment quality has been shown to be associated with children's adaptive functioning, such as competence with peers and adults, independence, and symptoms. Children with insecure attachment may acquire a negative view of themselves and the world that affects later development. Radke-Yarrow et al. speculate that maternal depression is associated with quality of interaction with the child, which in turn shapes attachment patterns. Thus mothers of insecurely attached children were observed to express more negative and less positive emotions when interacting with their children. Radke-Yarrow and Sherman (1990) wrote a later report focused on "high risk" offspring, defined as having both parents with affective disorder (not specifically defined or described) and high levels of environmental stress due to unusual family life and impaired parental behavior. The 50 children of 25 such families were compared with 36 children of 18 normal, intact families. Direct interviews of the child and maternal questionnaire reports indicated that 40% of the high risk children received DSM III diagnoses, compared with 11% of normal family offspring. The diagnoses spanned a wide range, from depressive disorders to conduct and attention deficit disorders. Many of the high risk children also experienced school and academic difficulties. A major focus of the report was on "survivorship," the qualities of the children at risk who seemed to function relatively well despite adversity; see Chapter 8 for a fuller discussion.

Preliminary results of an English study of 39 depressed and 21 control mothers of 2- to 3-year-olds also paint a picture of significant disturbance in the very young children of depressed women. Pound, Cox, Puckering, and Mills (1985) did not describe the methods of obtaining ratings of children's problems but reported marked levels of "substantive" problems in 44% of children of depressed women, compared to 19% of control children. Moreover, the rates were even higher (63%) for children whose mothers were characterized as having personality disorders and/or extensive previous history of depression. Pound and colleagues paint a bleak picture of severe stressful conditions, marital disharmony, and personal history of poor relationships with parents among the women defined as depressed. The influence of family and environmental factors on maternal functioning is very similar to the findings of Billings and Moos (e.g., 1985) on unipolar families. It is further interesting to note that in the Pound et al. study, none of the clinically depressed mothers was in psychiatric treatment. One implication is that the incidence and impact of parental affective disorders in low income groups may not be represented adequately in offspring studies that are based on recruitment from treatment facilities.

Conclusions and Implications of Studies of Unipolar Samples

Without exception, across an array of methodologies and samples, children of depressed parents are at increased risk for psychopathology and dysfunction. Despite the unanimity of this opinion, however, its meaning is far from clear. The magnitude of the excess of diagnoses varies greatly from one study to the next in the most diagnostically advanced studies, and the rates of disorder appear to be high for other diagnoses besides depression.

If there is one striking gap in the conclusions to be drawn, it is the inability to determine whether children's risk is unique to parental depression. The great majority of studies do not include any comparisons other than normal controls, obscuring an answer to the question of whether there is something particular about clinical depression that exacts a toll on youngsters. Some evidence is available from the studies that compared groups of different pathologies. Although these studies of schizophrenia, and in one case alcoholism, indicated few differences in children's outcomes, the investigations were generally conducted before reliable diagnostic procedures were available to adequately characterize child and adult psychopathology in terms we understand today. Three recent studies employed a medical illness control group but drew different conclusions about the specificity of adverse outcomes to parent depression.

The unresolved issue of specificity of parental depression to children's negative outcomes is part of the broader matter of what accounts for children's risk. The studies of unipolar parents and their offspring have differed enormously on the degree to which they have attempted to answer this question. The earliest studies, based on the high risk schizophrenia samples, generally did not include variables that would be considered relevant to depression vulnerability today. Only recently have the depression studies, designed specifically to examine risk in samples of affective disorders, begun to examine issues of variations in severity and other characteristics of parental disorder, the effects of stressful environments both within the family and in general functioning, or quality and patterns of parent-child relationships. Considerable additional work is needed to characterize the nature and contributors to children's risk—and thereby provide helpful information to families, mental health professionals, and the community.

Studies of Children of Bipolar Parents

Early Studies

Many of the original investigations of offspring of manic depressive parents were included in the comparison groups of the schizophrenia high risk studies of the 1970s—in some cases even lumped together with unipolar parents or psychotic depressed parents. Thus the early studies are difficult to evaluate with respect to the particular impact of bipolar parents.

Following the schizophrenia high risk offspring studies, several investigations were designed specifically to explore psychopathology in children of parents with major affective disorder. Greenhill and Shopsin (1979) interviewed a randomly selected outpatient population about their children's emotional and psychiatric symptoms. The parent group included 28 bipolar, 10 unipolar, and 2 schizoaffective patients, reporting on 85 offspring. The offspring ranged in age from 3 to 46, and information about them was collected from structured interviews of the parent and from the Conners Parent Questionnaire. The bipolar offspring were rated as having higher levels of symptom severity on the CPQ, and this was especially true for males. Also, it was noted that there was a sharp increase in severity scores after age 19. The authors report that one-third of the bipolar sample, one-quarter of the unipolar sample, and none of the schizoaffective samples of offspring were viewed by their parents as having significant disorders. These ranged broadly from fears to trouble with the law, and the investigators suggest that nonspecific mood-behavior disturbances may be a harbinger of later affective illness. There was no indication of manic depression in the sample, although three offspring were treated for schizophrenia or schizoaffective disorder.

In a later report that was a forerunner of the direct interview studies, Greenhill, Shopsin, and Temple (1980) reported on the 12 offspring of 7 patients (5 bipolar and 2 unipolar). The youngsters ranged in age from 7 to 17. Of the 9 bipolar offspring, 5 had diagnosable disorders, including 2 with major depression and 3 with conduct disorder. One of three unipolar offspring was diagnosed with attention deficit disorder. Overall, the authors noted that depressive symptoms with anhedonia predominating occurred in half of the sample.

Kuyler, Rosenthal, Igel, Dunner, and Fieve (1980) interviewed parents of a more homogeneous bipolar sample about their children. The sample included 49 children between the ages of 6 and 18 of 27 patients;

4 youngsters were considered to have an affective disorder (depression) and 18 had undiagnosed disorders considered likely to include personality disorders, adjustment reactions, and hyperkinetic disorders. It is noteworthy that the incidence of disorder was significantly higher in children whose parents were divorced. The authors also note that diagnosable depression did not occur in children younger than 13.

Waters, Marchenko, and Smiley (1983) reported on their Canadian sample of adult offspring of bipolar patients. They were able to directly interview 53 offspring of 17 manic depressive parents, and they reported that 31% met criteria for major affective disorder including bipolar and unipolar forms. Nine of the offspring were themselves bipolar, an additional 13% had "other affective disorder," including minor depression and dysthymia, and two had committed suicide. Eleven percent had other disorders that were nonaffective. There were also high rates of school difficulties.

A report by Mayo, O'Connell, and O'Brien (1979) should be mentioned, although it was not designed to study offspring of bipolar parents. Instead, in the course of investigating the functioning of families following patient treatment, they interviewed 22 children of 12 manic depressive patients. Forty-five percent of the children were considered to be at least moderately symptomatic. Although specific figures were not reported, the authors indicated that most of the children would be given diagnoses such as unsocialized aggressive reaction or overanxious reactions. Two would be classified with childhood depression. The investigators comment generally on the psychological impact of having a manic depressive parent and present their observations on common patterns of dysfunctional dynamics in the bipolar families they studied.

The work of the Stony Brook high risk project allowed the comparison of competence measures across samples of children of unipolar, bipolar, normal, and schizophrenic parents (Weintraub, Winters, & Neale, 1986). Thus the study is unique in the range of its comparison groups. The unipolar group included both major and minor depression. Altogether, there were 113 children of depressed parents, 73 of bipolar parents, 57 of schizophrenic parents, and 297 children of normal parents. (The initial group [Phase 1] included larger samples, but not all were available for various follow-up assessments or for specific outcomes [Weintraub, 1987].) Teachers' ratings across a variety of dimensions on the Devereux Elementary School Behavior Rating Scale indicated that the offspring of patients were viewed by their teachers as more deviant on factors of aggressive disruptiveness, cognitive competence, and social competence than children of normal parents. However, the diagnostic groups did not differ between themselves. Similarly, on peer ratings there were differences between normal group offspring and the patient group children but no differences between patient groups. The authors conclude that children of parents with affective disorders are seen by teachers as unable to meet demands of the school environment and poor achievers. Their peers see them as withdrawn, abrasive, and unhappy. Thus, rather than specific affective problems, the offspring of affectively disturbed parents display deviance across a range of academic, social, and emotional behaviors. The authors note that there was little evidence of clinically significant depression in the children, and they suggest that lowered competence may be a precursor of depression, in that failure experiences in school and socially might precede the development of depressive reactions. In a report of later follow-up evaluations of the children, Weintraub (1987) found that 43% of the unipolar offspring had affective disorders, compared to 25% of the control youngsters, and bipolar offspring had rates of disorders similar to the unipolar group.

As noted previously, recent studies of infants and toddlers of parents with affective disorder have been reported by NIM investigators. In a series of direct observation and parent interview studies of 7 male children of manic depressive parents, a variety of social and affective disturbances have been noted. For instance, Zahn-Waxler, McKnew, Cummings, Davenport, and Radke-Yarrow (1984) found significantly more symptoms in the offspring of bipolar parents than those of normal parents. The toddlers were more likely to show excessive shyness, hyperactivity, poor impulse control, and tantrums, as well as severe symptoms such as head banging, or unusual fears. Gaensbauer, Harmon, Cytryn, and McKnew (1984) found that this same group of infants studied longitudinally at ages 12, 15, and 18 months displayed impaired attachment to their mothers and generalized disturbances in affective regulation. Zahn-Waxler, Cummings, McKnew, and Radke-Yarrow (1984) observed the toddlers at age 30 months in interactions with playmates and with adults, and observed them to display a variety of difficulties with peers, including less sharing and helping and less social interaction. Also, they displayed preoccupation with the distress of others, especially during adults' hostile interactions. The investigators speculate that the difficulties in social interaction and emotion regulation may reflect their own parents' impairments and set the stage for vulnerability to develop depression. Zahn-Waxler et al. (1988) reported 4-year follow-up diagnostic information on the initial 7 sons of manic depressed parents and found various, and serious, disturbances. Only one child did not receive a diagnosis (but was later referred by his school for treatment for depression and separation anxiety). Not only did the offspring show a variety of internalizing and externalizing disorders, but they also showed less insight in empathy tasks and displayed particular sensitivity to conflict.

Finally, as noted previously, bipolar offspring in an extended sample of the NIMH project displayed insecure attachment to their mothers, compared with both unipolar and normal group children (Radke-Yarrow et al., 1985). These intensive, direct observation studies thus paint a picture of significant impairment, beginning at a very young age, in children of manic depressive parents. However, it needs to be noted that at least in the studies of the small group of young boys of manic depressive parents, 5 of the 7 co-parents had diagnoses of unipolar depression (Davenport, Zahn-Waxler, Adland, & Mayfield, 1984), so that the specific effects due to bipolar disorder cannot be discerned.

Recent Investigations with Direct Interview Methods

In the past few years several direct interview studies have been reported that have given rates of DSM III diagnoses in children of manic depressive parents. Table 1.2 presents the characteristics of the samples.

The Cytryn, McKnew, Bartko, Lamour, and Hamovit (1982) study is a later investigation using methods developed by McKnew, Cytryn, Efron, Gershon, and Bunney (1979) in their report of 30 children of 16 hospitalized patients, most manic depressive. The 1982 study attempted to improve on those methods by including blind interviewers as well as a normal control group. The researchers interviewed 19 school-age children of manic depressive parents and 21 normal comparison offspring. Two interviews were given, 4 months apart. Overall, there were significantly higher rates of disorder in the children of patients than in normals. The study concentrated on affective disorders in children, and as predicted, they observed elevated rates of major depression and dysthymic disorder. One difficulty with the study, however, is that although the parents are termed "manic depressive," the text refers to them more generally as hospitalized for "major affective disorder" and elsewhere alludes to bipolar, unipolar, or schizoaffective. Thus it is not clear if the sample contained a mixture of unipolar and bipolar index parents.

Decina et al. (1983) compared children of carefully specified bipolar parents with children of normals. They observed significantly higher rates of affective disorders in the children of bipolar parents than normal group offspring, noting that more than 50% of the children had diagnosable difficulties. Interestingly, they also noted the presence of a variety of subclinical symptoms in half of the nondiagnosed children of bipolar parents. Such behaviors included expansiveness, excitability, exhibitionism, need for constant attention and admiration, need for reassurance, and others suggestive of hyperthymic or depressive personality.

The study by Gershon et al. (1985) also investigated school-age children of bipolar and normal parents. Unlike most other reports, however, it failed to find differences between the groups in major or minor depression. However, the researchers did observe significantly higher rates of all diagnoses combined in the bipolar offspring group, suggesting higher risk for nonspecific disorders but not uniquely affective disorders. The authors note that they were surprised by the relatively high rates of diagnosable disorder in the normal comparison group and suggest that further

TABLE 1.2. Direct diagnostic interview method studies of children of a bipolar parent.

Project	Method		
	Parent sample	Child sample	Child assessment
Cytryn et al., 1982	13 hospitalized manic depressive (sex unspecified) 13 normal (sex unspecified)	10 males, 9 females 13 males, 8 females Ages 5–15	Structured interview with child: Weinberg; DSM III criteria for current and recent past
Decina et al., 1983	18 bipolar: 11 BP I, 7 BP II (7 fathers, 11 mothers) 14 normal (sex unspecified)	14 males, 17 females 8 males, 10 females Ages 7–14	Structured interview with child; parent questionnaires; DSM III criteria
Gershon et al., 1985	19 bipolar I (sex unspecified) 22 normal (sex unspecified)	12 males, 17 females 16 males, 21 females Ages 6–17	K-SADS-E with parent and child; DSM III criteria
Nurnberger et al., 1988	23 bipolar or schizoaffective (sex unspecified) 9 bipolar (both parents schizoaffective, or one ill parent and major disorder in extended family on other side (sex unspecified) 39 normal (sex unspecified)	15 males, 23 females 9 males, 6 females 18 males, 21 females Ages 15–25	SADS-L with child; Sensation Seeking Scale (Zuckerman, 1971); General Behavior Inventory (Depue et al., 1981)
Klein, Depue, and Slater, 1985	24 bipolar (11 fathers, 13 mothers) 14 nonaffective psychiatric outpatients (10 fathers, 4 mothers)	19 males, 18 females 13 males, 9 females Ages 15–21	SADS-L (modified to include subsyndromal affective disorders) with child

investigations with careful diagnostic methods are needed to see if such effects occur in other samples.

Klein, Depue, and Slater (1985) reported a study noteworthy for its methodological refinements, including a psychiatric, nonaffective comparison group, use of structured methods of identifying subsyndromal disorders including cyclothymia, and limitation of the offspring sample to 15- to 21-year-olds. The characteristics of the study are noted in Table 1.2. Overall, Klein et al. found significantly higher rates of affective disorders in the offspring sample (38%) than in the psychiatric comparison group (5%), although the two groups did not differ on rates of nonaffective diagnoses. In particular, the authors noted the relatively high rate of cyclothymia, thought to be an early marker of later bipolar disorder, in the offspring of bipolar parents. Of 16 diagnosable youngsters, 9 met criteria for cyclothymia. The authors conclude that since the psychiatric group did not display as much evidence of affective disorders as the manic depressive offspring group, the findings cannot be attributed to the distress of being raised by ill parents and are instead specifically associated with bipolar illness in the parent. However, it should be noted that the risk to children for disorder was significantly higher for bipolar mothers than for bipolar fathers. This result could reflect either sex-linked genetic or environmental transmission.

Nurnberger et al. (1988) recently reported preliminary findings from a study that is unique in several respects. It is longitudinal, and data are presented for the rates of appearance of new diagnoses in the offspring, who are between the ages of 15 and 25. The offspring were included in the study only if they did not initially display evidence of disorder. Groups were selected to compare offspring thought to be at increased genetic risk due to family loading for affective disorder, by comparing those with one ill parent and those with two ill parents or one ill parent and evidence of affective disorder in the extended family of the normal parent. Finally, the study attempted to identify markers of psychiatric risk, specifically the Sensation Seeking Scale (Zuckerman, 1971) and the General Behavior Inventory (Depue et al., 1981). The two instruments respectively are intended to assess emergent psychopathology in the form of need for stimulation, and subsyndromal depressive and hypomanic symptoms. Overall, the authors report that offspring of both groups of bipolar parents have twice the rate of disorder of normal comparisons, including five cases of "major affective disorder" and a variety of subsyndromal cases termed hyperthymic personality, depressive personality, and cyclothymia. Such results are reminiscent of the observation by Decina et al. (1983) of traits suggesting affective disturbances. In terms of the personality marker variables, Nurnberger et al. found that the total score and several subscales of the Sensation Seeking Scale differentiated the groups, with the suggestion of increased disinhibition in the high risk groups. Also, the latter scored higher on the hypomanic subscales of the General Behavior Inventory. The authors speculate that offspring of bipolar parents may be prone to respond to dysphoria with disinhibitory behavior (alcohol and drug consumption, sexual activities), and the combination of dysphoria and such responses may be a marker for major mood disorder.

Comparisons Between Unipolar and Bipolar Families

Although several of the early schizophrenia high risk and affective disorders offspring studies included both unipolar and bipolar parents, most studies did not compare outcomes of the two groups. The few exceptions present a mixed picture. For instance, the Stony Brook project found few differences between children of bipolar, unipolar, and schizophrenic parents as viewed by their teachers (Weintraub et al., 1986) or in terms of follow-up diagnoses (Weintraub, 1987). Nor did Welner and Garrison (1985) find differences between unipolar and bipolar offspring. However, Winters, Stone, Weintraub, and Neale (1981) found cognitive and attentional disturbances in performances of children of unipolar parents that resembled those of schizophrenic offspring, whereas bipolar offspring generally did not differ from children of normal parents. Conners et al. (1979) had reported that unipolar parents rated their children as more symptomatic than did bipolar parents on the Conners Parent Questionnaire. Greenhill and Shopsin (1979), however, had reported that bipolar parents rated their children as more symptomatic than did unipolar parents. It is possible that part of the discrepancy between the studies is due to the older ages of the offspring described by Greenhill and Shopsin. Finally, Radke-Yarrow and colleagues (1985) observed more severe attachment disturbances in the very young children of bipolar mothers compared with unipolar mothers, suggesting a poor prognosis for later social adjustment for these youngsters.

Conclusions and Implications of Studies of Bipolar Samples

Most of the same issues that clouded the conclusions about offspring of unipolar depressed patients also operate here: insufficiency of comparison groups, inconsistency in reported outcomes, and lack of information about the contributors to risk. For instance, none of the studies of bipolar offspring have examined characteristics of parental psychiatric history or fully explored various psychosocial factors that might increase risk of negative outcomes. Some excellent projects have been launched, but the conclusions to be drawn thus far are meager.

Other High Risk Samples

Children of Psychiatrically Ill Parents

Rutter and colleagues set out to identify the consequences of general parental psychiatric disorder on children, rather than test the effects of specific forms of disorder. Rutter and Quinton (1984) reported the results of a 4-year longitudinal study of children under age 15 who were the offspring of male or female psychiatric patients. The parent patient sample included those diagnosed with schizophrenia, manic depression, phobic anxiety state, alcoholism, or depression (the latter group comprising about half of the sample of 137). Patients were also classified by presence of "personality disorder," a descriptive designation for abnormal personality features and persistent social impairment for all of their adult life. Over half of the male patients and about one-quarter of the female patients were considered to have personality disorders. Since the patients were drawn from the Camberwell Psychiatric Register, a comparison sample of families was also drawn from the same neighborhood, a low income inner city borough of London. Because of the socioeconomic composition of the groups, most of the families experienced a variety of adverse conditions.

Children's status was evaluated from interviews of the mothers covering diagnostic information (although no standardized criteria for children were available at the time of the data collection in approximately 1966). Also, teachers completed questionnaires on all the children at yearly intervals. A variety of complex questions were addressed by Rutter and Quinton (1984), but only those pertaining to children's outcomes are noted here. Teacher questionnaires indicated an inconsistent pattern of significant differences between high risk and control children from year to year, although in all cases indicating higher rates of problems in the children of parents with psychiatric disturbance. The authors interpret this to reflect high rates of transient disorder in the comparison sample of children. However, when rates of persistent disturbance are compared (defined as deviant levels of scores for at least three of the four yearly assessments), the rate was nearly twice as high (32% for boys and 21% for girls) in the psychiatric parent sample. The parent interviews about children's symptoms in the high risk families indicated that about one-third of boys and one-quarter of the girls were initially diagnosable; 31% of boys and 12% of girls were judged to have persistent diagnosable disorders over the 4-year period. The most common problem reported was conduct disorder, especially for boys. However, Rutter and Quinton statistically controlled for level of family adversity according to an index based on psychosocial conditions, and they concluded that children of psychiatric patients did not show any increases in psychopathology when such factors are taken into account. They suggest that parental psychopathology is just one of several psychosocial risk factors that may impart risk in combination with one another. It should also be noted that presence of personality disorder in a parent was significantly associated with disturbance in children, especially conduct disorders, and children's problems were especially likely if the personality disorder was associated with parental hostility expressed in the family context.

Children of Alcoholic Parents

Many books have appeared in the past few years aimed at adult offspring of alcoholic parents, arguing for recognition of the pernicious effects of having been reared in such homes. Alcoholic parents are alleged to cause great harm to children's emotional and behavioral well-being, leading to major problems in interpersonal relationships, work satisfaction, and adjustment as well as personality difficulties in adulthood. Despite the plausibility of many of these claims, and the potential therapeutic value of the treatments based on such assumptions, in actuality there is only modest evidence of the negative consequences of parental alcoholism. To a great extent, the problem has been methodological. Only a relatively few studies have been based on representative and adequately diagnosed samples of alcoholics, examining cross sectional or longitudinal effects on children assessed with standardized instruments.

West and Prinz (1987) recently reviewed the literature, noting empirical shortcomings. On the basis of available studies of adequate design, they concluded that there is modest evidence of children's dysfunction associated with rearing by an alcoholic parent. The negative outcomes for children are particularly likely to include externalizing disorders such as hyperactivity and conduct disorder, school problems, substance abuse, and delinquency. There was less evidence of social impairment, depression, and anxiety, although some indications of such dysfunctions are noted. The authors conclude that the majority of children of alcoholic parents do not appear to suffer serious negative consequences, and the quest for individual differences in outcomes should be a high priority. West and Prinz suggest that alcoholism's effects are likely mediated by family disruption stemming from the alcoholism, but that critical features of such disruption have yet to be identified.

Children of Parents with Anxiety Disorders

As interest in anxiety disorders increases, studies of the familial patterns of such disorders are beginning to emerge. Turner, Beidel, and Costello (1987) compared 16 children of a parent with anxiety disorder, 14 children of a parent with dysthymic disorder, and 13 offspring of normal parents. The children were all between the ages of 7 and 12. The investigators found that children of patients with anxiety disorders were more anxious and fearful, had more school difficulties, and engaged in more solitary behaviors than children in the other two groups. Also, 7 of the 16 anxiety disorders offspring met criteria for diagnosable disorder—a much higher rate than any other group. They were twice as likely to have an anxiety disorder as the offspring of dysthymic parents and seven times more likely than children of normal parents. Rosenbaum et al. (1988) examined the offspring of parents with anxiety disorders using procedures developed by Kagan and colleagues (e.g., Kagan, Resnick, & Snidman, 1987) for identifying inhibited behavior. They found, as predicted, that more of the young children of anxious patients displayed behavioral inhibition in the laboratory sessions.

Since behavioral inhibition may be a precursor of anxiety disorders, both of these studies suggest that children of parents with anxiety disorders, like those with affective disorders, are at risk for psychopathology. This suggestive evidence needs to be pursued to determine the psychosocial, as well as possible genetic components of the risk, and to determine the specificity of patterns of outcomes in the different families.

Summary and Directions for Further Research

An array of studies of variable methodological merit yields firm evidence for the proposition that depression runs in families. But we are left with other questions: Do other problems besides depression also run in families, and do depression and other problems exist in families besides those with parental affective disorder? Are some kinds of families more likely to produce depression than others? *Why* is it that children of parents with affective disorders experience depression and other dysfunction?

Questions such as these prompted the development of the study that is a major focus of this book. Problems of limited methodologies raised questions about the reliability and generality of children's risk, and design inadequacies left open the question of the specificity of negative outcomes due to parental affective disorders. Additionally, the majority of the studies that consider children's risk for disorder have failed to examine the contributing variables that explain such outcomes and provide guidelines for helping families. In the next chapter, therefore, the methodological and conceptual decisions guiding the investigation as well as the procedures for the study that is the basis for this book are presented.

2
Methods of the Current Study

My students and I began planning for the current study some years ago at the stage identified in Chapter 1 when there were virtually no published direct interview studies of children of depressed parents. Only a handful each of indirect studies of unipolar and bipolar families existed, and these were greatly limited in scope and conclusions. All of the existing research indicated a clear need for additional study because of the apparent high rate of risk to children for psychopathology.

In this chapter, the methods and conceptual framework for what became the UCLA Family Stress Project are described. First, the limitations of the previous offspring studies are outlined, so that the choices of methods for the current study are placed in perspective. Next, the conceptual underpinnings of the investigation are discussed briefly, in order to provide a basis for understanding the selection of variables. Finally, the participants and procedures of the study are described.

Methodological Limits of Previous Research

Design Difficulties

Need for Comparison Groups

The typical affective disorders offspring study outlined in Chapter 1 consisted of a psychiatric parent group and a normal comparison group. In the initial, exploratory stages of research, this is a useful strategy, because it simplifies the design and facilitates finding negative outcomes in children if they do exist. Nevertheless, such designs shed little light on the sources of the children's difficulties.

As noted in the brief discussion of schizophrenia high risk studies, the investigators were well aware of the need for psychiatric comparison groups as a way to evaluate the specific impact of the disorder in question. The schizophrenia offspring researchers included a variety of comparisons, commonly depressed patients of different types, to determine whether schizophrenia as such, or psychopathology in general, contributed to children's risk for poor outcomes. The research was relatively uniform in reporting that children of depressed parents commonly fared as poorly as, and in some cases even worse than, children of schizophrenic parents (reviewed in Gotlib & Lee, 1990). It is ironic, therefore, that researchers of affective disorder took so long to include comparisons other than normal groups. Possibly the influence of genetic models of offspring risk accounted for the failure to include comparisons that might clarify the psychosocial risk factors. At any rate, it seems important to design studies to include controls for illness in general, and for psychopathology in general, so that the specific contribution of affective disorders in parents can be evaluated.

There has been progress in recent studies that include chronic medically ill parents (e.g., Hirsch et al., 1985; Klein et al., 1988; Lee & Gotlib, 1989a, b). Nevertheless, the coexistence of depressive symptoms in some of the medically ill subjects is a reality that needs to be taken into account. It is quite difficult, moreover, to find psychiatric comparison groups that do not also include substantial levels of depression, or that have comparable levels of symptoms and impairment as unipolar and bipolar patients. Klein et al. (1985) included a psychiatric comparison in their study of offspring of bipolar parents, but their psychiatric group may not have been as severely impaired as the bipolar families. Clearly, it is not a simple matter to find the appropriate comparison groups, but offspring research needs to be able to draw conclusions about the specificity of the impact of the disorder under investigation.

Need for Longitudinal Studies

With exceptions only currently beginning to appear, the affective disorders offspring research discussed in the first chapter typically has been cross-sectional. Although this was a useful beginning for a topic of investigation, it is now time to move on to longitudinal research for at least two reasons. One is that the continuity of the effects on children needs to be examined. Is there an effect only when the parent is acutely ill, or are there enduring effects; are there onsets over a period of time after exposure to parental pathology? Second, there is a much more reasonable basis for drawing causal conclusions if there is at least a known temporal order of phenomena. We can be more certain, for instance, that maternal depression is the cause, rather than the consequence, of a child's disturbance, if the maternal disorder is observed to occur first. Similarly, other psychosocial contributors can be observed to learn if they have a predictive relationship to children's behavior over a prospective course. On the other hand, longitudinal study does not imply that simple linear effects are the best model, and the mutual influence of family members on each other may need to be taken into account.

Issues in Subject Selection and Evaluation

Diagnostic Heterogeneity

Early offspring studies were hampered by limitations in diagnostic methods; even the schizophrenia high risk research found that changes in diagnostic practices between DSM II and DSM III led to different definitions of schizophrenia; in some cases, individuals once classified as schizophrenic or depressed were later seen as bipolar. Thus prior to the use of Research Diagnostic Criteria and their subsequent versions in the Schedule for Affective Disorders and Schizophrenia and the use of DSM III, parental illness may not have been reliably established. Even more troublesome was the failure of some of the earlier studies to differentiate between unipolar and bipolar samples or to report outcomes separately for the two groups (see review by Beardslee et al., 1983). Clearly there are major differences in the phenomenology and likely origins of the two disorders, so that it is essential to keep them distinct when analyzing their impact. Only a small number of studies have attempted to compare unipolar and bipolar families (e.g., Conners et al., 1979; Radke-Yarrow et al., 1985; Weintraub et al., 1986; Welner & Garrison, 1985) but have reached different conclusions. Thus unresolved issues make this a fruitful question for further investigation.

Clinical and Demographic Heterogeneity

With the exception of the large scale direct interview study of 125 unipolar offspring reported by Weissman, Gammon et al. (1987), most investigations have been relatively limited in size. This characteristic is especially likely to become a problem because of heterogeneity of genders of affectively ill parents and in the clinical features of the disorder. For instance, many of the offspring studies reviewed (and also see Tables 1.1 and 1.2) combine mothers and fathers and do not report children's outcomes separately by who was the affected parent. It would be both practically and theoretically informative to know whether children are at different risk for psychopathology depending on illness in the mother or the father. Also, there is a range of apparent severity of disorders, samples sometimes including both outpatient and inpatient samples, unipolar parents with either dysthymia or major depression, and other mixtures of features. It would be useful to have either relatively homogeneous samples or large enough samples to evaluate the effects of different patient subgroups (e.g., see Keller et al., 1986; Weissman et al., 1982). Moreover, some of the studies appear to have included evaluations of children while the parent was experiencing acute symptoms and possible hospitalization. Is is unclear whether the outcomes are in response to the family disruption or associated with the ill parent's typical functioning.

Heterogeneity of Children's Characteristics

The offspring studies of parents with affective disorders have included children at all ages, including the relatively recent studies of infants and toddlers (e.g., Radke-Yarrow et al., 1985; Zahn-Waxler, McKnew et al., 1984). Nevertheless, within samples that include too broad a range of ages it is possible that important developmental differences in incidence and expression of dysfunction in children might be missed. Therefore, somewhat homogeneous groups of children at different ages ought to be studied, or studies that include children across a range of ages should report outcomes by different age subgroups.

Limited Evaluations of Children's Diagnoses

As noted previously, a major achievement of the most recent offspring studies has been direct interviews of children, as well as their parents, to determine diagnostic status. Taking advantage of the relatively new methods of diagnosis available for children using structured interview formats (e.g, the Kiddie-SADS; Orvaschel, Puig-Antich, Chambers, Tabrizi, & Johnson, 1982; Puig-Antich, Chambers, & Tabrizi, 1983), the most recent studies therefore provide more reliable assessments than those of the past. Based on the observation that parents and children may report somewhat different information, it is important to include interviews from both sources (Puig-Antich et al., 1983; Weissman, Wickramaratne et al., 1987).

Selection of Additional Measures of Functioning and Mediational Factors

Multiple Areas of Functioning in Children

With a few exceptions, the majority of studies of offspring of parents with affective disorders have not reported other kinds of outcomes besides diagnoses. It is important to characterize not only what diagnostic criteria a child might meet, but also how she or he performs at school, in peer relationships, in terms of social competence and problem solving, and in terms of subjective experiences of the self, the world, and others. In addition to providing a multifaceted view of the child as a way of characterizing current functioning, such diverse variables might help to determine differences between vulnerable and invulnerable children. What precisely are the areas of dysfunction in children that are attributable to parental illness? If we can learn what gaps in competencies exist, we can not only understand better how diagnosable disorders come about but also consider what areas need to be treated or subjected to preventive interventions.

Moreover, it seems important to have information from various sources. In addition to the information provided by the mother, which itself might be open to biases, data should be collected from the child and from observers of the child outside the family. Thus teachers, peers, and trained observers can all provide useful perspectives for more fully understanding the child.

Need for Mediational Factors

One of the gravest gaps in the current research on high risk children of parents with affective disorders concerns explanatory factors—the "whys" and "hows" of risk. Risk factors associated with dysfunctional outcomes in children can operate at different levels. As Rutter and Quinton (1984) noted, parental characteristics can have direct effects on children (e.g., the psychiatric symptoms lead to abuse of the child); they can have indirect effects (e.g., psychiatric symptoms can impair parenting ability, which affects children's functioning); they can be correlates of the disorder that have effects on children's outcomes (e.g., stress and marital discord can be outcomes of parental illness that have effects on children).

With the important exception of Myrna Weissman and her colleagues, who early described the maternal relationships of depressed women with their children (e.g., Weissman & Paykel, 1974; Weissman et al., 1972), the majority of studies of offspring in affective disorders have not been guided by theoretical views on why or how children might suffer negative consequences. The genetic perspective has, of course, been implicit in many such studies. Yet most of the early works did not include collection of information that might shed light on nonbiological contributors to children's psychopathology. Since a major impetus of the present work was to extend contemporary studies of adult risk for depression into childhood, such theoretical perspectives played a major role in the design of the present work, and it is to those points of view that we now turn.

Theoretical Background: Risk for Depression

Initial planning and data collection for the UCLA Family Stress Project began in the early 1980s at a time when vigorous activity in the psychological study of adult depression was relatively recent. In prior years, psychopathologists had been investigating schizophrenia and anxiety, but little attention had been devoted to depression in psychology. Breakthroughs in diagnosis and in the pharmacological treatment of depressive disorders contributed to increased awareness of affective disorders. Also, Beck's (1967, 1976) cognitive theory of depression sparked an enormous interest in issues of psychological vulnerability. Subsequent studies of cognitive correlates of adult (and college student) depression provided limited tests of vulnerability hypotheses, however. There was an apparent need for studies testing causal hypotheses, and the study of childhood antecedents to depression offered one tempting path to pursue.

Review of the studies of children of depressed parents, as Chapter 1 indicates, suggested that such offspring might be a useful target for exploring the origins of certain kinds of depression, since such children were at apparent risk for disturbance. At the same time, conceptual and methodological limitations in the research on adult depression made it seem that the study of high risk children might offer a rich basis for exploring more multifaceted models of depression vulnerability. Therefore, against this background the current project was undertaken, with the goal of studying and integrating three possible mechanisms of depression vulnerability in the high risk children. These were dysfunctional cognitions, stressful life events, and dysfunctional family relations.

The Genetics of Affective Disorders

Contemporary research has amply documented the potential of genetic contributions to the risk for developing affective disorders (see report of the NIMH Workshop on Family and Genetic Studies of Affective Disorders; Blehar, Weissman, Gershon, & Hirschfeld, 1988). In the bipolar disorders the evidence is particularly strong, based both on family studies and genetic linkage investigations, although the findings imply diverse genetic pathways (e.g., Baron et al., 1987; Egeland et al., 1987; Gershon, 1990). In the unipolar depression research, family studies are especially convincing, illuminating a familial concentration of affective disorders (e.g., Weissman, Merikangas, et al., 1986). However, genetic marker studies are unlikely to provide critical information because of the heterogeneity of unipolar depressions and the probability of polygenic modes of transmission (Blehar et al., 1988).

Findings consistent with genetic transmission are far from convincing evidence that the nature of offspring risk has been accounted for, however. The NIMH workshop on genetics of affective disorders strongly recommended continued research on psychosocial factors in risk for disorders (Blehar et al., 1988). There are several reasons why vigorous psychosocial research ought to be pursued. First, in the absence of direct evidence of a genetically transmitted disease, we do not know what it is that may be transmitted, or how biological vulnerability might be activated. It is apparent from twin studies, for instance, that even genetically identical siblings may not be concordant, opening the door for consideration of psychological factors that might influence the experience and expression of affective disorders. Second, some of the most consistent data come from family studies, where genetic mechanisms are inferred, but which cannot rule out environmental explanations. Third, both unipolar and bipolar disorders are quite heterogeneous in their manifestations (e.g., Akiskal, Bitar, Puzantian, Rosenthal, & Walker, 1978; Akiskal, King, Rosenthal, Robinson, & Scott-Strauss, 1981; Depue et al., 1981), and it is likely that they are also mixed with respect to cause. We already know, for instance, that manic depressive disorder has been found to have different modes and loci of transmission in apparently different subgroups (Baron et al., 1987; Egeland et al., 1987). The well-known heterogeneity of nonbipolar depressive disorders (e.g., reviewed in Hammen, in press-b) strongly suggests multiple pathways of causation, possibly some biological, others psychological, and their interactions. Fourth, from a practical standpoint, no matter what causes the disorders, psychosocial factors that might be found to influence the course, severity, and response to treatment of affective disorders could have profound implications for identifying and treating vulnerable individuals.

For all of these reasons, the current study tackles several psychological and contextual approaches to children's risk. This strategy in no way minimizes the possible contribution of genetic (biological) influences. Improved methods of genetic investigations are welcomed, but the primary goal of this nongenetic study is to help address an obvious imbalance in past research.

Cognitive Contributions to High Risk Research

Aaron Beck's cognitive model of (unipolar) depression (1967, 1976) profoundly affected the way many psychopathologists have come to view depression. Grounded in an information-processing model, the cognitive perspective views depression as a disorder of thinking in which biased, negative views predominate and affect mood. Depressed people think in highly negative ways about themselves, their worlds, and the future. Such selective negativism contributes to the tendency to become depressed when even minor negative events occur and to intensify or perpetuate dysphoria and the related symptoms of the syndrome of depression. From this point of view, vulnerability to depression may arise from traumatic or depriving childhood experiences in which negativistic beliefs about the self and the world are acquired. Such deep underlying beliefs, or schemas, may give rise to depression when activated by events or thoughts. Beck's perspectives have undergone changes over time (reviewed in Hammen, 1985, 1988a). Research generated to test the views has moved away from cross-sectional, nonclinical, descriptive studies that were generally supportive (e.g., review by Hammen & Krantz, 1985) toward efforts to test the role of underlying cognitions as vulnerability factors for depression.

Toward that end, the research team working on the present study hypothesized that children of depressed mothers might show evidence of relatively negative schemas about themselves, and that such negative self-schemas might predict future development of depression when the children were observed over time. Furthermore, we speculated that they might acquire such negative self-concepts from observational learning by exposure to their mothers' own characteristic self-criticism and negative cognitions. Alternatively or additionally, they might acquire such negative self-cognitions through negative or maladaptive learning experiences in interactions with their mothers, or from experiences of failure or poor performance at school or with peers, and in dealing with stressful life events.

The attributional reformulation of the learned helplessness model (Abramson, Seligman, & Teasdale, 1978) is also a cognitive model emphasizing potential dysfunctions in the ways people think about themselves. Specifically, it hypothesizes that a negative attribution style is a vulnerability factor for depression; when people blame themselves for negative events, and view the causes as unchanging and general about themselves, they may become depressed. Measures of attribution style for adults (Seligman, Abramson, Semmel, & von Baeyer, 1979) and children (Seligman et al., 1984) have been developed; they have shown the predicted associations with depressed mood in at least some samples.

The present investigation included several measures of children's hypothesized dysfunctional cognitions and explored their predicted relationship with subsequent psychopathology as well as their correlates. A fuller discussion of the specific hypotheses and findings is presented in Chapter 4, and the methods employed are described later in this chapter.

Stressful Life Events and Depression

A second area of research that has generated large quantities of data in contemporary studies of adult depression concerns stressful life events. Reviews of research have indicated significant statistical associations between occurrence of stressful life events and depressive symptoms in community samples and in clinical populations (e.g., Billings & Moos, 1982; Lloyd, 1980; Paykel, 1979; Thoits, 1983). The relationship between stressors and course of disorder has been implicated in bipolar illness as well (Ambelas, 1979; Bidzinska, 1984; Ellicott, Hammen, Gitlin, Brown, & Jamison, 1990; Kennedy, Thompson, Stancer, Roy, & Persad, 1983). However, there is considerable room for improvement in the predictive relationship between affective disorders and stress, and, as argued more fully elsewhere (Hammen, 1988a), both methodological and conceptual developments are needed.

Methodologically, questionnaire methods of assessment of stressful events and their significance, which were relied on in the past, often obscure the meaning of events for individuals and may fail to fully characterize the nature of stressful circumstances. Not only is this a problem for research on adults, but for children the problem may be exacerbated by the failure of this method to take into account their stage of development and the meaning of particular events at different ages. An important methodological development has been the contextual threat interview assessment of stressful events, described by Brown and colleagues (e.g., Brown & Harris, 1978). Individuals are interviewed not only about event occurrence, but also about the circumstances surrounding the event so that its significance can be gauged in individual cases. There were no similar procedures for children; thus it was necessary to develop such interviews. The interviews and their scoring are labor-intensive but capable of yielding rich information about the events in context, so that their threat can be more objectively rated and their circumstances more fully understood.

An additional methodological shortcoming in stress research has been the overemphasis on episodic stressors to the relative neglect of chronic, ongoing strains that might exert an impact on mood. Such chronic stressors might also mediate the impact of episodic stressors. Brown's work provides one model for assessing what he terms "ongoing difficulties"; Pearlin and colleagues (Pearlin, Menaghan, Lieberman, & Mullan, 1981) present another method. In the current study, a new procedure was developed, somewhat modeled after that of Pearlin et al. in terms of scaling areas of strain by behavioral anchor points. The procedures for both episodic and chronic stress assessment are described later.

Conceptual shortcomings in stress research on depression center on limited explanatory mechanisms. Formerly, the major point of view was that stressful events required change, and change required adaptive capabilities that might overwhelm the individual's biological mechanisms of adaptation. However, subsequent empirical results have corrected this generalization, indicating that it is not any change but negative events generally, and often social exits in particular, that are associated with depression (e.g, Paykel, 1979). The concept of meaning subsequently became central, permitting a fruitful integration with cognitive perspectives. Now it is commonly believed that it is the interpretation of stressors that mediates their stressfulness; what might be a major catastrophe for one person might be a stimulating challenge for another. Other cognitive and environmental variables, such as coping capabilities and social resources, should also be included in efforts to understand why one person becomes depressed following a negative event and another does not (e.g., Billings, Cronkite, & Moos, 1983; Brown & Harris, 1978; Lazarus & Folkman, 1984; Thoits, 1983).

It was predicted in the present investigation that stressful events and chronic stressors would contribute to children's negative outcomes. The general proposition was tested in two ways. First, the design called for a comparison group in which women were chronically medically ill, postulating that illness may have its effects on children because of the strain it puts on the parents and family. Thus a nonpsychiatric comparison for illness-related stress could help to separate children's risk due specifically to affective disorder, while comparisons of the illness groups with the normal group could clarify the magnitude of outcomes due to illness stress. Second, several measures of episodic and chronic stress were included to evaluate differences within groups and to relate children's outcomes to magnitude of stressful conditions. The hypotheses and results are discussed more fully in Chapter 5.

Effects of Dysfunctional Relationships

Some of the earliest offspring research, as well as the most recent, has emphasized dysfunctional relationships, specifically parent–child relations, in the etiology of depression. For instance, retrospective reports by depressed adults found negative and critical interactions between depressed individuals and their parents compared to nondepressed people (see review by Burbach & Borduin, 1986; Holmes & Robins, 1987; Perris et al., 1986). Research on depressed children and adolescents has implicated dysfunctional interpersonal relationships (McKnew & Cytryn, 1973; Puig-Antich et al., 1985a, b). Also, Weissman and colleagues (Weissman & Paykel, 1974; Weissman et al., 1972) noted the apparent disruptions in interpersonal and parental functioning in depressed women, even in periods of recovery. Certainly, developmental psychopathologists have emphasized parent–child relations as crucial predictive factors in children's adjustment (e.g, Hetherington & Martin, 1979; Maccoby & Martin, 1983). Growing interest in interpersonal functioning in adult depressives has focused on relationship difficulties and dysfunctional patterns of coping with depression in family contexts (review by Barnett & Gotlib, 1988; Coyne, Kahn, & Gotlib, 1987).

At the time the present study was undertaken, however, there were no existing reports of direct assessment of parent–child interactions in families with affective disorder. The retrospective or indirect report methods were highly suggestive of difficulties in this area, but direct observations were needed to rule out the possible confounding effects of negative reports by depressed individuals. Therefore, in the present study assessments of interaction quality were undertaken, as described later, and the hypotheses and results are reported more fully in Chapter 6.

Methods of the Study: Families and Their Characteristics

Eligibility and Recruitment

Affective Disorders

The goal was to obtain women with affective disorders and comparison groups of chronically medically ill women and women without medical or psychiatric conditions. The affective disorders groups included women who were in treatment. Women were the subjects of recruitment for two reasons. One is that they constitute the larger parent group with children, as affective disorders are typically associated with considerable marital and family instability and more of the women would live with their children. Another reason is that we believed that an investigation of psychosocial factors in families required that we not lump together fathers and mothers, as many previous offspring studies have done. Instead, we wanted to study the effects of one kind of relationship, that of mother and child, and believed that maternal relations with children are likely to be the most central in children's lives. This does not mean that paternal affective disorders are unimportant or that children's relationships with fathers are inconsequential. It simply reflects a practical decision.

Women currently in treatment were recruited, because the treatment source was a way to identify women with significant affective disorders. Specifically, in this way we avoided recruiting families based on children's disorder or treatment status, so as not to bias the study in favor of finding psychopathology in children. However, to avoid confounding the effects of maternal disorder with the acute distress families might feel if the mother has just been hospitalized or was in the throes of an episode, women did not participate in the study until at least 3 months after beginning treatment.

Additional requirements for the women with affective disorders were that they had to have recurrent episodes and that the episodes dated either from before the child's birth or in infancy.The goal of the first requirement was to exclude individuals who might have relatively minor outpatient depressions that might have little implication for the woman's typical functioning. Some past offspring studies included both mild and severe cases, but we wished to consider only major affective disorders that might be representative of clinically significant disorder. Moreover, our intention was to study women whose affective illness impinged on the child from birth or infancy. Thus women were excluded if they began to have recurring episodes of depression that developed later in the child's life. Additionally, the affective disorder had to be the primary psychiatric condition. Women with current substance abuse, schizophrenia, or organic psychiatric conditions were excluded. Women were not screened with respect to Axis II personality disorders, as these are not covered fully in the SADS interview. Also, women whose diagnoses were sufficiently ambiguous that they were not clearly primary unipolar or bipolar disorders were excluded. Women were not specifically required to have been hospitalized for psychiatric treatment at some point, although most had been, as will be described. Finally, it should be noted that although the resulting sample is representative of major unipolar and bipolar disorder, some of the most severe cases are probably not represented. For instance, a few women were excluded because their psychiatric difficulties were so pronounced that they had lost or relinquished custody of their children in divorce proceedings and they had little contact with their children.

To obtain women with affective disorders meeting the criteria noted, and who had at least one child between the ages of 8 and 16, staff members of the UCLA Affective Disorder Clinic or Neuropsychiatric Institute hospital, the UCLA Psychology Clinic, and several community agencies were asked to identify potential subjects. If the subjects were located, the agency staff person asked them to give consent for one of our project staff members to contact them for screening. In addition, several psychiatrists and psychotherapists in private practice who were known to see patients with affective disorders were also asked to participate, and one or two individuals were recruited from self-help groups for patients with affective disorders. In the final sample there were 16 women with recurrent unipolar depression, with 22 children in the appropriate age range, and 14 bipolar women with their 18 children.

Chronic Medical Illness Comparison

The selection of the chronic medical illness comparison required identifying a disease that had a course and level of impairment comparable to that of unipolar and bipolar affective disorders. Thus we wanted to avoid an immediately life-threatening illness but include one that involved periods of relatively well functioning, intermittent symptoms and acute exacerbations possibly requiring hospitalization. Finally, we wanted to include medical illnesses that would have an onset before the child's birth or during his or her infancy. For all of these reasons, we chose insulin-dependent diabetes with juvenile onset and severe early onset rheumatoid arthritis. Women with these conditions were recruited from a diabetes registry, from newsletters of organizations and self-help groups, and from specialty medical practices. Women were screened to eliminate those with recurrent major depression or significant psychiatric disorders. However, several of the women had experienced a single previous episode of major depression, or minor depressions, or intermittent dysthymia. Most such diagnoses would likely be termed adjustment disorder with depressed mood as in the DSM III nomenclature. We believed that elimination of women who had no previous depression would have resulted in a sample unrepresentative of women with chronic medical illnesses. In some of the analyses to be reported, the current and past histories of depressive symptoms were taken into account. Three of the children included in the study were adopted at birth, owing to significant medical complications associated with birth in some insulin-dependent diabetic women. The study included 14 medically ill women and their 18 children between ages 8 and 16. Of these women, 11 had juvenile onset diabetes and the other 3 suffered from rheumatoid arthritis.

Normal Comparison

The normal comparison group was selected to match the demographic characteristics of the children in the other groups. Families were recruited through the schools for the most part, including the same schools as patient families or schools selected because of their demographic composition. An array of public and private schools was represented. When parents indicated willingness to be contacted for participation, they were initially screened to eliminate those in treatment for psychological matters and those with significant medical problems. Women were selected for participation if they had no history or current evidence of significant psychiatric problems or treatment. Some of the families included were experiencing stressful circumstances such as divorce or financial difficulties, and an effort was made to include single-parent families. The final sample included 24 women with their 38 children.

Exclusionary Criteria for the Children

As noted, no families were selected because the child was the identified patient in treatment (although after selection of the families it became known that some of the children were currently or recently in psychological treatment). Also, children were omitted if they had significant chronic health problems. This resulted in exclusion of three siblings of participants.

Demographic Characteristics of the Families

Race

Table 2.1 presents the demographic characteristics of the families. The participants were mostly Caucasian, and the groups did not differ significantly overall in distributions of white and nonwhite participants. However, the unipolar and normal groups contained the most nonwhite families and were similar to each other in overall proportions.

Marital Status

As Table 2.1 indicates, there was considerable variability in the marital status of the women. The majority of women with affective disorders were currently divorced or separated, compared with the medical and normal comparison groups. The effect was statistically significant, $\chi^2(1, n = 68) = 9.50, p < .01$. This result is typical of persons with affective disorders, who are known to have relatively high rates of divorce and marital disruption (e.g, Barnett & Gotlib, 1988).

Socioeconomic Status

Socioeconomic status based on Hollingshead Two-Factor (occupation and education) scores indicated that the groups in the final sample differed significantly, $F(3, 64) = 3.79, p < .01$. As the table indicates, the unipolar group had more women represented in the lower categories than did the other groups. This effect was due largely to women on public assistance because of psychiatric disability (and being single heads-of-household). Since we believe that economic and occupational difficulties associated with affective disorder are potentially significant sources of stress in the

TABLE 2.1. Demographic characteristics of mothers/families.

Variable	Unipolar	Bipolar	Medical	Normal	Overall
	Group				
Number of families	16	14	14	24	68
Race					
Percent white	68	93	100	71	81
Percent nonwhite	32	7	0	29	19
Marital status					
Percent married or cohabitating	25	43	71	75	56
Percent divorced or separated	75	57	29	25	44
Socioeconomic category[a]					
Percent I–III	56	93	100	92	85
Percent IV–V	44	7	0	8	15
Maternal education					
Percent more than 1 year of college	69	79	93	79	79
Percent high school or less	31	21	7	21	21
Mean maternal age	38.4	37.9	40.2	37.1	38.2
Mean chronic stress[b]	2.9	3.3	3.4	3.7	3.4

[a] Based on Hollingshead ratings.
[b] Higher scores represent lower levels of stress.

families, many subsequent analyses evaluated the specific effects of chronic stressors, of which socioeconomic status is an indicator.

OTHER CHARACTERISTICS OF WOMEN IN THE STUDY

As Table 2.1 indicates, the majority of the women were relatively well educated, with at least some college training. The groups did not differ in the distribution of educational attainment. Also, maternal age did not differ across the groups, with most women in their late thirties.

Clinical Characteristics of the Mothers

UNIPOLAR WOMEN

The unipolar women reported a mean of 11 lifetime episodes of major depression ($SD = 8.7$), and 6 women reported that they had had "too many to count." About half of the women in this group experienced "double depressions" of chronic or intermittent dysthymia punctuated by acute episodes of major depression. Ten of the women had been hospitalized at least once for treatment of depression, with an average of 1.7 ($SD = 1.6$) hospitalizations for the group as a whole. The mean age of onset of depression was 18.2 years ($SD = 7.8$), with the majority reporting onset in childhood or adolescence. At the time of the initial contact with the study, the mean Beck Depression Inventory (BDI) score was 20.4 ($SD = 11.8$).

Bipolar Women

The women in this group reported a mean of 7.2 diagnosable episodes of mania or depression (SD = 5.1), and one person said she had experienced "too many to count." Only one woman had not been hospitalized for psychiatric treatment, and the group reported a mean of 2.3 hospitalizations (SD = 2.0) overall. A little more than half of the women in this group would probably be characterized as bipolar I with both major depressions and manic episodes, with the others viewed as bipolar II (depression and hypomania). Age of onset was 21.4 years (SD = 9.2), with half reporting childhood or adolescent beginning of symptoms. At the time of first evaluation for the study, the women's mean Beck Depression Inventory score was 15.9 (SD = 16.7).

Comparison Groups

The medically ill women had been hospitalized a mean of 5.8 times for medical treatment (SD = 8.6). Their mean age of onset of medical illness was 17.4 years (SD = 11.1). At the initial evaluation for the study, medically ill women had a mean BDI score of 6.6 (SD = 6.0). The normal comparison women had a mean BDI of 4.4 (SD = 3.9). Eight of the women in the medical group (57%) had experienced depression that would likely be termed DSM IIIR adjustment disorder with depressed mood or periods of minor depression at some point in the past. Five of the women in the normal comparison group experienced similar depressions. The majority of the remaining women had no more than brief, subclinical depression in the past.

For certain analyses that attempt to take into account the role of depression as such on children's outcomes, a 7-point scale was devised so that all participants' past depressive experiences could be scored. On this scale, a 7 represented more than one hospitalization and several episodes of major depression, 4 indicated one major depression or dysthymia without impairment, and 1 represented no depression at all; intermediate scores were anchored with gradations between these values. All women in the unipolar and bipolar groups were rated at 6 or 7 and these groups did not differ. The mean rating of medically ill women was 3.2 (SD = 1.6), and the normal women averaged 2.6 (SD = 1.1). As intended, the difference between the affective and comparison groups was highly significant, $t(64) = 15.35$, $p < .0001$.

Age and Sex of the Children

Table 2.2 presents children's ages and genders by maternal diagnosis group. Overall, there were 96 children in the age range of 8 to 16 who were directly studied. No more than two children per family were included if there were several in the age range. Forty families had one child and 28

TABLE 2.2. Sex and age of children included in study.

Sex	Group: Unipolar	Bipolar	Medical	Normal	Total
Boys					
n	10	8	9	19	46
Mean age	13 yr, 7 mo	13 yr, 1 mo	12 yr, 10 mo	12 yr, 5 mo	12 yr, 10 mo
SD	2 yr, 6 mo	2 yr, 5 mo	2 yr, 10 mo	2 yr, 2 mo	2 yr, 5 mo
Girls					
n	12	10	9	19	50
Mean age	11 yr, 9 mo	14 yr, 1 mo	13 yr, 0 mo	11 yr, 1 mo	12 yr, 2 mo
SD	2 yr, 2 mo	3 yr, 0 mo	2 yr, 10 mo	2 yr, 11 mo	2 yr, 8 mo
Totals					
n	22	18	18	38	96
Mean age	12 yr, 7 mo	13 yr, 8 mo	12 yr, 11 mo	11 yr, 9 mo	12 yr, 6 mo
SD	2 yr, 8 mo	2 yr, 9 mo	2 yr, 9 mo	2 yr, 2 mo	2 yr, 8 mo

Note: Sex: $\chi^2(3, 96) < 1$, ns. Age: adolescent (age 13 or older) versus preadolescent, $\chi^2(3, 96) = 4.69$, ns., $F(3, 92) = 2.45$, $p > .05$.

families had two children between 8 and 16. There were 46 boys and 50 girls, very equally distributed within the maternal groups. Also, the groups did not differ overall in children's ages.

Because some families contributed two children, certain statistical analyses that assume independent observations would not be valid. Therefore, where appropriate, the analyses were conducted on one child per family, based on random selection in families with two children.

Procedures of the Study

Once each mother had been recruited for the study, information was obtained in two sessions. In the first, she was scheduled for an individual session by herself, to complete a confirmatory diagnostic evaluation, and to provide information of various kinds about herself and her family. Typically within the next 2 to 4 weeks, the woman and her child(ren) were seen together. At the family session, diagnostic information was obtained directly from each child, and the children also completed several questionnaires and procedures. Separately, the mother completed additional questionnaires. Then the mother and each child completed two brief interaction tasks that were videotaped. Table 2.3 presents a list of the procedures completed, and when they were scheduled.

Families were also contacted at 6-month intervals up to a total of 3 years. At each follow-up, the interviewer collected most of the required information by telephone in separate contacts with the mother and each child. Telephone interviews were used because of the enormous and prohibitive logistical difficulties of arranging face-to-face meetings. Following

TABLE 2.3. Research instruments and procedures.

	Data source		
Evaluation	Mother	Child	School
Initial	SADS-L, current K-SADS: lifetime, current MMPI Short Form Beck Depression Inventory Social Adjustment Scale Chronic Stress interview Child Behavior Check List Family History RDC interview Parent Perception Inventory	K-SADS: lifetime, current Childhood Depression Inventory Peabody Picture Vocabulary Test Piers–Harris Children's Self-Concept Scale Levels of processing self-schema task Children's Attributional Style Questionnaire Parent Perception Inventory	School records Teacher report Conners Teacher Report Form or Teacher Child Behavior Check List
	Interaction task: Conflict Discussion Interaction task: Achievement		
Follow-up	SADS: change K-SADS: change in child Stressful Life Events interview Self and child events Child Behavior Check List Beck Depression Inventory	K-SADS: change Stressful Life Events interview-self Sources of Support interview Child Depression Inventory	School records Conners Teacher Report Form or Teacher Child Behavior Check List (each spring)

each interview, the mother and child(ren) were mailed questionnaires to be completed and returned by mail.

Families were paid for each contact, with separate payments of the mother and each child.

Methods and Instruments

EVALUATION OF THE MOTHER

Personal Psychiatric Status and Mood

The Schedule for Affective Disorders and Schizophrenia-Lifetime version (SADS-L; Endicott & Spitzer, 1979) was used to obtain diagnostic information about past and current functioning in the areas covered by the SADS. The SADS is based on the Research Diagnostic Criteria, but with modifications it was used to obtain DSM III Axis I diagnoses as well. Interviewers were advanced clinical psychology graduate students or psychologists on the project staff with extensive training in the use of the

SADS. During training and the initial phases of the study, a reliability analysis based on 32 cases yielded a kappa coefficient of 1.00 for current and .92 for past diagnoses. Additionally, the principal investigator independently diagnosed each mother from tapes of interviews. Agency diagnostic, treatment, and history information was obtained for women with affective disorders, and in any case of discrepancies, the research team made decisions based on all available data.

Participants also completed the Beck Depression Inventory (BDI; Beck, Ward, Mendelson, Mock, & Erbaugh, 1961), a self-report questionnaire that measures severity of depressive symptoms. The BDI is widely used and numerous studies have established its reliability and validity for symptom assessment (Beck, Steer, & Garbin, 1988).

Women additionally completed a short form of the Minnesota Multiphasic Personality Inventory (MMPI; Overall, Higgins, & DeSchweinitz, 1976), which we used primarily to confirm the nonpsychiatric status of women in the normal comparison group. No participant in the latter group had a clinically elevated profile (standardized T-scores were less than 70).

Assessment of Psychopathology in Relatives

The mother was interviewed using the Family History-Research Diagnostic Criteria method (Andreasen, Endicott, Spitzer, & Winokur, 1977) to identify psychopathology in her first-degree relatives (parents and siblings). Information was also obtained from the mother about the child's biological father, current step-father if any, and paternal relatives if known.

Level of Functioning and Chronic Stressful Conditions

Women's level of functioning was assessed with the self-report form of the Social Adjustment Scale (Weissman & Bothwell, 1976). The scale assesses women's levels of functioning in several areas, including occupational, relationships with immediate family and children, extended family, and recreational. Its psychometric properties are adequate, and they are reported in Weissman, Sholomkas, and John (1981; Weissman & Bothwell, 1976).

There are different but not entirely satisfactory methods available for assessing ongoing strains. The notion of chronic strains or stress is conceptually distinct from social adjustment, although it may overlap with women's level of functioning, just as social adjustment is meant to be distinct from symptom level although it overlaps with it. We employed elements of Brown's approach (Brown & Harris, 1978), in that level of chronic stress was assessed independent of the woman's own reactions about her situation. And like Pearlin and colleagues (1981), we attempted to measure various role areas, including marital/social, employment, finances, relationships with children, relationships with extended family, and personal and family health. Difficulties had to have persisted for at least 6 months, and an interview probed each role area. Ratings were based on a behaviorally specific 5-point scale for each role area. For instance, a 5 indicated exceptionally positive circumstances, 4 was relatively strain-free, down to 1, which represented extremely adverse circumstances. As an example, in the financial area, 5 indicated more than enough money and no budgeting required, 4 indicated comfortable circumstances with a need for some budgeting but ample money for basics and leisure with some available for savings; 3 indicated enough money for essentials with careful planning required and not much available for leisure; 2 indicated meager conditions with just enough for basic food and housing; 1 indicated hardship, poverty, insufficient housing, food, or health care.

Reliability between independent raters was based on a sample of 34 cases. The overall reliability coefficient for the average rating across areas was .97, with a range of .93 for finances to .99 for health of self (all values highly significant, $p < .001$). Test–retest reliability was established for a separate set of 44 unipolar and bipolar patients, over a period ranging from 6 to 20 months. Reliabilities ranged between .58 and .74 for the subscales, which may be considered adequate since the levels of chronic strains are expected to show some changes over time as circumstances altered. Finally, validity was established by comparisons of scale scores to comparable Social Adjustment Scale values and to socioeconomic status, women's ratings of marital satisfaction, and level of employment. In all cases, positive and significant correlations with independent indicators support the concurrent and construct validity of the scale. Additional details are reported in Hammen, Adrian, et al. (1987). The means of the four groups of women are reported in Table 2.1.

Evaluation of Children

Children's Symptoms and Functioning

Children's diagnostic status was evaluated by separate direct interviews with the mother and the child, using the Kiddie-SADS semistructured interview (Chambers et al., 1985; Orvaschel et al., 1982; Puig-Antich et al., 1983). The schedule yields RDC-based diagnoses for children, and with minor modifications it gives DSM III diagnoses. The lifetime version was administered initially to obtain details of past diagnoses. It is known that children and mothers have access to, and differentially report, somewhat different information about the child, and therefore it is recommended that information from both sources be used to make diagnostic decisions (e.g., Puig-Antich et al., 1983; Weissman, Wickramaratne, 1987).

The children's interviewers were extensively trained clinical psychology graduate students or project staff psychologists and were blind to maternal diagnostic status. Diagnostic reliability was evaluated on a subsample of 35 children who were rated independently from audiotapes by a second judge. The independent ratings yielded a kappa coefficient of .84 ($p < .001$) on current diagnoses and 96% exact agreement on scale ratings of symptom severity. The research team pooled information from both the mother and child to arrive at final diagnostic decisions. When information was available from mental health professionals if the child was in treatment, it was reviewed as well.

Children also completed the Children's Depression Inventory (CDI; Kovacs, 1981), a self-report scale of severity of depressive symptoms. The CDI has been shown to have moderately good test–retest reliability and the ability to discriminate children with major depressive disorders from nondepressed children (Kazdin & Petti, 1982; Saylor, Finch, Spirito, & Bennett, 1984).

A verbal IQ estimate was obtained from the Peabody Picture Vocabulary Test-Revised (Dunn & Dunn, 1981). This is an interviewer-administered test of verbal ability that has been widely normed and standardized. It does not require reading or writing, and children express their understanding of a vocabulary work by pointing to the drawing that best represents its meaning.

Mothers completed the Child Behavior Checklist (CBCL; Achenbach, 1978; Achenbach & Edelbrock, 1983) for each child. The questionnaire yields overall scores for Behavior Problems and Social Competence, as well as overall scores of Internalizing and Externalizing disorders. The CBCL has been extensively normed, separately for boys and girls, and for children at different age levels. The scale has high test–retest reliability and has been shown to discriminate between clinic-referred and non-referred children (Achenbach & Edelbrock, 1983; see also Achenbach, McConaughy, & Howell, 1987).

Additional information about children's school performance and academic functioning was obtained where possible from the school. Initial evaluations were typically obtained within 6 months of entry into the project by contacting the child's teacher (or homeroom teacher if several were available). Without disclosure of the purpose of the child's participation, teachers were requested to evaluate the child's behaviors in the classroom and provide information about academic functioning. Grade reports were also requested. In the early stages of the study the best available instrument for teacher use was the Conners Teacher Rating Scale (Conners, 1969), a 39-item scale designed to measure the presence and severity of childhood behavior disorders. Conners reported high levels of test–retest reliability on subscores of the scale and demonstrated its ability to discriminate between normal and diagnosed children. Later, when a teacher version of the Child Behavior Check List became available, it was employed (Edelbrock & Achenbach, 1984). The Teacher Report Form of the CBCL has been well validated, and unlike the Conners, which emphasizes externalizing behavior problems, the CBCL version also includes scores for internalizing behaviors of children. Since not all parents gave permission for school contact, and because not all contacted teachers responded, sample size for teacher data was reduced.

Although not all families were represented by Conners ratings, all of them did provide academic information in the course of interviews about the children and as a part of their completion of the CBCL. Also, when schools did report information it was commonly represented in a variety of forms: letter grades, numbers, percentiles, grade level based on test scores, and the like. To systematize diverse information, we devised two 5-point scales, one for Academic Performance and one for School Behavior. The scales ranged from serious problems (rated 1: grade failure; expulsion) to superior functioning (rated 5: exceptional grades or strong performance in gifted classes; good behavior at school, responsive and appropriate). Mid-range scores reflected specified problems such as suspension or placement in special classes for academic or discipline problems. An interrater reliability analysis was conducted on a subset of 25 children. Pairs of independent raters reviewed the records and assigned scale ratings, achieving 100% agreement within one scale point. Pearson correlations were .82 ($p < .001$) for the Academic Performance rating and .77 ($p < .001$) for the School Behavior rating.

Children's Cognitions

The Piers–Harris Children's Self-Concept Scale (Piers & Harris, 1969) was administered to obtain relatively stable self-attitudes in children. The scale contains 80 true–false items covering personal behaviors and traits, school performance, physical appearance, and popularity; it yields an overall score of positive self-concept. The scale, which is widely used in research and school applications through grade 12, has been shown to have good levels of internal consistency and test–retest reliability, as well as convergent and construct validity (Piers, 1977; Piers & Harris, 1969).

An experimental task for self-schema assessment was based on the levels of processing incidental memory task, adapted by Hammen and Zupan (1984) for children from procedures employed with adults (e.g., Derry & Kuiper, 1981; Hammen, Miklowitz, & Dyck, 1986). The task is based on the hypothesis that an information-processing schema about the self is stored in memory and guides the selective encoding and retrieval of information about the self, so that self-descriptive adjectives that are consistent with the schema are recalled better than schema-irrelevant words. The procedure consists of reading to the child 44 self-descriptive adjectives, half positive and half negative in content, under one of two encoding instructions: self-referent ("Is this like you?") or structural ("Is this a long word?"). Children check yes or no on a response sheet after each question. At the end of the presentations they are unexpectedly asked to remember as many words as possible. The proportion of words marked as self-referent that are recalled is then computed for positive adjectives and negative adjectives and is hypothesized to represent the strength of attitudes about the self.

The Children's Attribution Style Questionnaire (CASQ; Seligman et al., 1984) presents items regarding hypothetical events and two possible causes of each event that vary on attributional dimensions of internality, stability, and globality. The child selects the causal explanation that indicates what she or he would think if the event actually occurred. A score of 1 is assigned to each response representing an internal, global, or stable cause for each of the negative event items of the scale. Each such response is viewed as an indicator of a depressive attribution style. Only the negative event items were administered, and the composite scale was scored. Seligman et al. report modest levels of internal consistency reliability, and relatively stable scores over a 6-month period. Evidence for the construct validity of the scale is reviewed in Hammen (1990-b).

Owing to theoretical and procedural developments in research on adult depression, we devised a new procedure for assessing children's self-schemas that was introduced after the study was already under way. Thus for some of the children (and a similar procedure was given to their mothers), the procedure was completed during the follow-ups, although for most of the sample it was administered at the initial evaluation. Based on procedures developed for college students (Hammen, Marks, Mayol, & deMayo, 1985), it also assumes that information retrieved from memory can be used to infer the presence of an organizing principle, or schema, that facilitates the retrieval of memories. Children were asked to recall and give specific examples of each of four kinds of events that had occurred within the past week: times they felt good about themselves, times they felt bad about themselves, times that felt they didn't do as well as they thought they should or criticized themselves for something they did or failed to do, and times they felt alone or as if they needed to have someone there or felt that people didn't care about them. These four cues were counterbalanced and presented orally to the child by the interviewer following examples to make sure the child understood the task. In order to end on a positive note, a final question was asked but not scored: give examples of times you felt like you really enjoyed yourself or did things that made you feel really happy.

Judges rated the content of each recalled example according to whether its content and intention were primarily interpersonal (involving behaviors or feelings about other people or social situations) or achievement (involving behaviors or feelings about performance with respect to standards, or in terms of levels of skills, self-regulation, or healthy functioning). In a reliability analysis, independent judges' ratings of the classification of 274 recalled examples yielded 91% agreement overall.

Following procedures used by Hammen, Marks, Mayol, and deMayo (1985), totals of interpersonal or achievement memories were tallied across the four recall tasks, and children were then classified, according to the simple preponderance of examples, as "interpersonally vulnerable" or "achievement vulnerable."

Children completed the Parent Perception Inventory (PPI; Hazzard, Christensen, & Margolin, 1983), an assessment of their perceptions of 18 important maternal behaviors. Nine of the behaviors were positive (e.g., giving comfort, time together, allowing independence), and nine were negative (criticism, threats, commands). The instrument has been found to have adequate levels of internal consistency reliability and of convergent and discriminant validity (Hazzard et al., 1983). An overall score was computed that reflects the balance of positive behaviors over negative.

Assessment of Mother–Child Interactions

Two tasks were selected to represent different types of situations in which mother–child interactions might be observed. One task was intended to be an achievement task that would elicit cognitions and behaviors of possible relevance to depression vulnerability (e.g., a self-control model, implicating dysfunctional standard-setting, self- and other evaluation, and expectations). Children were blindfolded and seated in front of a stack of wooden blocks of various shapes and colors. Their task was to stack the blocks in a particular order, by feel alone, by following their mother's instructions to build the same model as the one in a photo she was given. Children were told that most kids can stack eight blocks (although in reality this is extremely difficult to do).

Prior to the task children and their mothers were separately given a questionnaire concerning their expectations, aspirations, standards of success, and similar items; after the task they were given a different questionnaire to probe their evaluations of their performance.

There were two difficulties with this task. One was that the task itself greatly constrained the interaction behaviors, so that there was little variability across groups. The other is that some of the dyads took the task to be an achievement challenge, as intended, but others viewed it as a game to have fun with and therefore approached the task with different aims. For these two reasons, the verbal interaction data from the task were not considered further, although Chapter 4 presents some of the interaction questionnaire responses of the children.

Conflict Discussion Task

The mother and child participated in an unstructured interaction task in which they were asked to identify several topics on which they commonly disagreed. One of these was selected by the experimenter for discussion. Typically the topics involved routine household issues, such as chores, bedtime, and allowance. The pair was asked to discuss this topic for 5 minutes with the goal of working toward a resolution. The experimenter then left the room, explaining that videotaping of the discussion would allow us to view it later.

This is a very realistic and involving task. Indeed, six children refused to do the task, anticipating that it would unpleasant to discuss an area of disagreement with their mothers (three in the unipolar, two in the medical, and one in the normal group). Because the conflict discussion often elicited negative feelings in the pairs, following the discussion, the experimenter asked the two to identify some topic they agreed had been pleasant or fun recently, and discuss it. The latter, which was not videotaped, was intended to neutralize any negative experiences elicited in the conflict discussion.

In cases of two children from the same family participating in the study, the mother had separate interactions with each.

Scoring

Each utterance made by the mother and the child was scored separately. The first, third, and fifth minutes were used as the basis of most of the analyses that will be reported. The discussion was transcribed, and each utterance was coded into one of 21 mutually exclusive content categories adapted from the Peer Interaction Rating System (Whalen, Henker, Collins, McAuliffe, & Vaux, 1979), modified somewhat to apply to the current task. In addition, a few categories relevant to depression were added (e.g., self-critical comments).

To establish reliability of the scoring, raters blind to maternal diagnostic status coded 26 transcripts independently. Percentage agreements across categories ranged between .80 and 1.00. Subsequently, categories used too infrequently to permit meaningful analyses (less than 10% of the families) were omitted. Other categories with highly correlated or theoretically similar content were combined (e.g., positive task and positive personal feedback). The result was six superordinate categories that were scored for mothers and children separately:

Task involvement:
1. task productive comments
2. off-task comments

Affective quality of feedback:
3. confirmatory/positive comments
4. disconfirmatory comments
5. negative, critical comments

Self-commentary:
6. self-critical remarks

For these six categories, kappa coefficients of agreement between independent judges ranged from .85 to .95 (all p values $< .001$).

Task involvement comments included directions, suggestions, information, or opinions that were focused on the task at hand. What were termed off-task comments referred to nonfunctional comments related to the task or talk that was unrelated to the task. Affective feedback included disconfirmatory statements (corrections, feedback intended to redirect performance) and negative feedback. The latter included negative evaluative comments on the child's (or mother's) performance or on the individual's personal characteristics such as style or competence, accompanied by signs of irritation, frustration, sarcasm, or anger. Positive feedback included positive evaluations of the child's (mother's) task performance or personal style or competence, as well as statements intended to reinforce the child's behavior. Self-critical remarks referred to critical comments about one's own task performance, feelings, behaviors, or competencies.

For the analyses to be reported, scores in the various categories were computed as proportions of total utterances. This method controls for differing degrees of talkativeness of the individuals that might distort the picture of their interaction behaviors.

Follow-Up Procedures

Every 6 months the families were contacted and scheduled for follow-up interviews. Where possible, families were retained for up to 3 years. Of the original 96 children, 90 were retained for 1 year and 79 for 2 years; 70 completed all 3 years. The breakdowns of the sample sizes by year and by maternal group are presented with the diagnostic outcomes in Table 3.5. The primary reasons for discontinuing were refusal or loss due to moving out of the area. Several families joined the study fairly recently and could not be followed for the full 3 years.

The follow-up interviews were conducted by telephone, with separate appointments made with the child(ren) and the mother. As noted earlier, practical considerations necessitated telephone interviews during the follow-ups. Other studies have reported adequate diagnostic reliability for interviews conducted by phone (Paulson, Crowe, Noyes, & Pfohl, 1988; Wells, Burnam, Leake, & Robins, 1988). In our data collection, information obtained from mothers and children, and from other mental health specialists if available, was combined to arrive at final diagnoses. After the interviews were completed, the mother was mailed the CBCL to fill out for each child, and also completed the BDI. Children were either read the CDI over the phone or completed it and returned it, depending on their ages.

Assessment of Maternal Symptoms

Interviews following the SADS format were used to obtain symptom information about maternal functioning since the last contact. Details were obtained sufficient to make diagnoses and to date the onset and duration as precisely as possible. Also, as noted, the women completed and returned the BDI.

Assessment of Maternal Stressors

Methods of assessing stressful life event occurrence were modeled after Brown and Harris (1978), who attempted to evaluate the impact of each event by assessment of the context in which it occurred. Problems with simply checking items off a life event questionnaire include difficulties with memory, which might affect selective recall, and failure to obtain accurate dating of event occurrence, as well as an inability to evaluate the "objective" impact of the event in terms of its meaning to the individual. Therefore, interviews about one's circumstances can elicit details of date of events as well as information about what was going on in the person's life at the same time. Thus the interview covers standard probes about areas such as social/marital, finances, work, and home life. When an occurrence was noted within the 6 months since the last interview, information was systematically obtained about its expectedness, the person's resources for dealing with it, and the outcomes. Women were also asked to describe and rate the subjective impact of the event. A narrative report of the information was prepared, deleting mention of how the woman felt about the event.

Subsequently, a rating team read each report and assigned objective threat ratings, defined as the way a typical person would be likely to experience the impact of the event under similar conditions. The ratings ranged from no threat to severe threat on a 5-point scale. Team members were specifically not given any information about the woman's own reactions or her symptom status. These ratings can be completed with high levels of interrater reliability. We have used the methods extensively in this and other projects (e.g., Hammen, Ellicott, Gitlin, & Jamison, 1989; Hammen, Marks, Mayol, & deMayo, 1985).

Assessment of Children's Symptoms

Both the mother and child were interviewed, using the K-SADS, about the child's symptoms since the last follow-up. Details from the two sources were used to arrive at diagnoses and dates of changes in symptoms. Additionally, as noted, CDI scores were obtained from the child.

Mothers were also asked to complete the CBCL for each child, providing measures of symptoms across various areas, as well as overall behavior problems and social competence, as previously described.

Assessment of Children's Stressors

When questionnaires are used, problems with assessment of children's stressors are even more pronounced than with adults, because of the highly different meaning of events at different developmental stages. Therefore, we developed a procedure for interviewing children, based on the contextual threat approach of Brown and Harris (1978). The goal for children, as for adults, is to elicit sufficient detailed information about the timing and surrounding circumstances to be able to rate the impact of the event on the child.

Children were queried about whether they had experienced changes "or anything that has caused you some trouble or made you upset" in 12 areas: family life, friends, pets, school, health, neighborhood activities, moves, accidents, financial issues, problems with the law, problems with authorities, and major disappointments. Any event the child mentioned was accurately dated and, as with the mothers, detailed information was obtained about conditions surrounding the event, prior expectations, previous experience, consequences, and emotional and instrumental support. Events involving other family members were included only if they could be expected to affect the child directly through some objective consequence and not simply because of the other's distress. Both episodic and ongoing stressors were evaluated.

Mothers were also interviewed about events affecting the child. Judgments about event occurrence and objective threat were made in the same way as for the mothers. In an initial reliability study, two independent rating teams evaluated all events reported for the first 58 children in the study. Across 271 events, agreement within one point on the objective threat scale was 99%, with a Pearson r of .80 ($p < .001$).

Summary and Overview of Chapters to Follow

Based on the methods sketched in this chapter, each of the following chapters focuses on particular types of outcomes or conceptual areas. Chapter 3 presents the basic outcomes of the project: what are the diagnostic and psychosocial functioning outcomes of children at risk, and how do they look over time? Next comes a set of chapters each addressing a conceptual area thought to mediate children's risk for negative outcomes. In Chapter 4 the depression-vulnerability cognitions of the children—their role in predicting future outcomes, and their correlates—are presented. Chapter 5 explores the role of stress in the family: chronic stressful conditions affecting the mother, maternal stress, and children's stress; here stress is viewed as a determinant of behavior and outcomes as well as a consequence of behavior and personal characteristics and symptoms of the mother or child. Then the role of parent–child interactions and the quality of the relationship between the two are discussed in Chapter 6. What are the characteristics of the interactions of mothers with affective disorders and their children, and what are the correlates and implications of the observed relationship quality? We not only consider the impact of the mother and her characteristics on the child, but we also attempt to analyze reciprocal effects of the two on each other.

Chapter 7 considers the role of characteristics of maternal illness and family circumstances. Here the mother's background is explored, including her own family of origin and their psychopathology, as are the characteristics of her husband, the child's biological father. In Chapter 8 the issue of "resilience" is raised, along with its counterpart, "risk." What are the characteristics of the children who, despite various risk factors, appear to have favorable outcomes? Another approach to this issue is to consider pairs of siblings in which one fares well while the other has difficulties, and attempt to characterize differences between them that might account for different outcomes. Finally, in Chapter 9 the overall findings of the study are summarized, and integrated models are presented and tested that attempt to include some of the many and nonorthogonal factors that have been discussed. Limitations of the present study are acknowledged, and researchers are urged to address various gaps.

3 Diagnoses and Dysfunction in Children at Risk

In Chapter 1 the major studies of offspring of parents with affective disorders were discussed and their general findings were noted. Across the various projects a generally dismal picture emerged: children of mothers and fathers with depression or manic depression were significantly more likely to have diagnoses and impairment than were children of normal parents. In this chapter the findings are reviewed in greater detail, with primary interest in the studies that employed direct interview methods and DSM III criteria. Such studies permit us to compare rates of disorder across studies, by different parental diagnoses.

Following the review of recent offspring studies, the first set of results of the study is presented. These data represent the very first question addressed by the study—whether, under improved conditions of measurement and design, the children of women with affective disorders would display elevated rates of pathology, and whether their rates would be higher than those of offspring of chronically medically ill women. Additionally we asked what the diagnostic outcomes would be over a longitudinal follow-up and posed questions concerning unipolar versus bipolar outcomes and whether impairments in academic and social adjustment would also be observed.

Direct Interview Studies of Children's Lifetime Diagnoses

Children of Unipolar Parents

Tables 3.1 and 3.2 summarize rates of diagnoses in recent studies of children of unipolar and bipolar parents that have employed direct interview assessments. As Table 3.1 indicates, the overall rates of any diagnoses of unipolar offspring as reported by Keller et al. (1986) are 65%, and Weissman, Gammon, et al. (1987) report 73%.These figures, which are discussed later, are highly comparable to the 77% rate in the current study, and they indicate alarmingly high rates of disorder. Klein and colleagues (1988) found somewhat lower rates of all disorders in their adolescent offspring, compared with the other studies. However, they did report that their sample displayed more cases of dysthymia than any other condition (17%), and this figure is comparable to the 14% in the present study. The studies in Table 3.1 indicate moderately high rates of major depression; our figure of 41% is the highest of all such studies, although very similar to that of Weissman et al. (1987) at 38%.

The direct interview studies, like the current one, generally indicate elevated rates of conduct disorders, anxiety disorders, and substance use disorders in the offspring of unipolar parents. Overall, therefore, there is considerable consistency in recent studies in the patterns of disorders, suggesting high rates of depression, but also elevations in all other kinds of disorder. With the exception of the Klein et al. (1988) investigation, even the percentages across studies are relatively similar where it is possible to make direct comparisons.

Children of Bipolar Parents

The figures in Table 3.2 are not as directly comparable across studies as are the unipolar studies, because the results tended to be reported in somewhat different forms. The current study indicates that bipolar offspring have relatively high rates of any disorder, with particular elevations in behavior disorders, with similar but lower rates for affective and anxiety disorders. Gershon et al. (1985) and Klein et al. (1985) present results that appear to show a similar pattern with comparable rates, while the other studies do not present data in a form suitable for comparison. All of the studies are alike in suggesting very low rates or no diagnosable hypomania in the young offspring, although they hint that subsyndromal forms of bipolar disorders begin to make their appearance in adolescence.

Nondiagnosis Studies

Since the previous studies of offspring of parents with psychiatric disorders generally did not report outcomes in terms of diagnoses, some of the recent studies cannot be compared to them. However, the previous reports all indicated elevated levels of disturbance, for example, 58% "disturbed functioning" (Weissman et al., 1972); 53% of nonremitted parents had children with disturbances (Billings & Moos, 1985a); two-thirds of ill mothers saw their children as having clinical levels of internalizing symptoms (Lee & Gotlib, 1989a); 44% of toddlers had "substantive" problems (Pound et al., 1985); 33% of boys and 21% of girls had "persistent" problems (Rutter & Quinton, 1984). In their review of studies of depression in parents and children's outcomes, Forehand, McCombs, and Brody (1987) included not only offspring comparisons, but also studies of mood

TABLE 3.1. Lifetime diagnoses of children of unipolar depressed parents—Direct interview studies.

Study	Percent receiving diagnosis						
	Any diagnosis	Major depression	Dysthymia	Oppositional or conduct disorder	Alcohol/drug use/dependency	Anxiety	More than one diagnosis
Keller et al., 1986; Beardslee et al., 1987							
Patient	65	24	8	30	13	19	46
Normal	nr	nr	nr	nr	nr	nr	nr
Weissman, Gammon, et al., 1987							
Patient	73	38	nr	22	17	37	2.4[a]
Normal	65	24	nr	17	7	27	1.7
Klein et al., 1988							
Patient	51	9	17	13	11	15	26[b]
Medical	21	0	0	6	6	3	nr
Normal	24	0	0	0	8	5	nr
Orvaschel et al., 1988							
Patient	41	15	15	nr	nr	20	23
Normal	15	4[c]	nr	nr	nr	9	nr

Note: nr = not reported.
[a] Mean number of diagnoses. [b] Estimated: combination of affective and nonaffective disorder. [c] Represents all affective disorder (including dysthymia).

TABLE 3.2. Lifetime diagnoses of children of bipolar parents—Direct interview studies.

Study	Any	Major depression	Dysthymia	Hypomania	Oppositional or conduct disorder	Alcohol/drug use/dependency	Anxiety
	Percent receiving diagnosis						
Cytryn et al., 1982							
Patient	nr	23	46[a]	nr	nr	nr	23
Normal	nr	8	15	nr	nr	nr	8
Decina et al., 1983							
Patient	52	26[b]	nr	nr	nr	nr	nr
Normal	6	nr	nr	nr	nr	nr	nr
Gershon et al., 1985							
Patient	72	10	28[c]	3	17	28[d]	24[e]
Normal	51	14	24	0	7	24	14
Nurnberger et al., 1988[f]							
One ill parent	74	13	nr	3	nr	8 alcohol 5 drugs	nr
Two ill parents	67	0	nr	13	nr	33 alcohol 27 drugs	nr
Normal	31	0	nr	0	nr	3 alcohol 0 drugs	nr
Klein et. al., 1985							
Bipolar	43	3	8	"bipolar" 27	11	8 alcohol 11 drugs	5
Other psychiatric	18	5	0	"bipolar" 0	9	9 alcohol 9 drugs	5

Note: nr = not reported.
[a] Percent of families with diagnosed child. [b] Includes major and minor depression. [c] Atypical depression, includes dysthymia and cyclothymia. [d] Other, includes alcohol. [e] Separation anxiety. [f] Figures are for development of disorder during 2-year prospective follow-up.

symptoms in children referred for conduct problems as well as nonproblem children. They found that 55% of all of the studies indicated an association between parental depression and negative outcomes in the children. The strongest associations with poor adjustment occurred in the offspring studies, higher than in the clinic-referred child samples.

If anything, the more recent, direct interview studies indicate even higher levels of dysfunction in children if past diagnoses are used as criteria. Taken together, it appears that between half and three-quarters of school-age offspring of parents with psychiatric disturbance have significant disruptions in functioning, variously measured.

Since both nonstructured interview techniques and interviews regarding past histories may be subject to a certain degree of unreliability, it is particularly instructive to look at diagnostic information for current and recent functioning. It is also important to obtain information about the children at times when the parent is not acutely ill or hospitalized, so that the typical, rather than acute, consequences of parental illness are evaluated. urthermore, the stability of diagnoses over a longitudinal course is important information that has generally been lacking in studies to date.

Children's Diagnostic Outcomes in the Present Study

Developments in the systematic diagnostic assessment of children have made it possible to use rates of diagnoses as a reliable way to compare groups and to compare results across different studies. Most of the studies that have directly interviewed children and their parents have employed the Kiddie-SADS (Chambers et al., 1985; Orvaschel et al., 1982), a system initially based on Research Diagostic Criteria but modified to enable DSM III diagnoses to be made from the information obtained.

Interview information on children in the present study is derived from both the child and the mother, except for rare instances when the child refused an interview or could not be scheduled for a regular 6-month interview. We found that the mother and child provided similar information in the great majority of instances, and they were forthcoming, open, interested, and cooperative in giving information about a variety of potentially sensitive matters. On occasions when we learned that a child was in treatment for psychological problems we obtained permission to contact the therapist and asked for diagnostic information. All of the interviewers were clinically trained psychologists who had received additional instruction and supervised training in children's diagnoses with the K-SADS. For the most part when it was possible to do so, the same interviewer contacted the family on repeated evaluations over time, building a relationship with them that facilitated exploration of personal information. Although it was not possible to have interviewers blind to maternal diagnostic status after the initial contacts with families, the use of systematic interviews with the K-SADS, from both mother and child, inclusion of information from other professionals where warranted, and reviews of diagnostic information by the research team increase our confidence that the information obtained is valid and complete.

In the sections to follow, the information is presented for past, current, and follow-up diagnoses. The first section permits a comparison with other studies of offspring of parents with affective disorder where information is available in terms of DSM III diagnoses obtained directly from the child (and parent). Information about children's current diagnoses at the time of entry into the study gives us a glimpse of children's functioning when the mother is not in an acute episode of affective disorder or exacerbation of medical illness. Finally, although increasing numbers of investigations provide information on past and current functioning, the present study is unique in providing follow-up information for up to 3 years, based on our direct, regular 6-month interviews.

Past and Current Diagnostic Outcomes

Past History of Diagnosable Disorder

Table 3.3 summarizes children's diagnostic status for past history of diagnosable disorders. This table includes all 96 children in the study and is an updated version of information on a slightly smaller sample that was first reported in Hammen, Gordon, et al. (1987). Looking first at the category "any disorder" (excluding minor depression), the unipolar group children and the bipolar offspring have very high rates overall (77% and 67% respectively), whereas the medical group reported moderate rates (44%) and the normal group relatively low rates (24%). The differences between the groups were statistically significant, as indicated in the table.

Affective Disorders

As Table 3.3 indicates, there were no past diagnosable episodes of mania or hypomania, although possible cases of hypomania, not indicated in the table, were noted in a few instances. On the other hand, depression has clearly made its appearance in these youngsters at an early age, with major depressive episodes reported in 41% of the unipolar group children. This rate is much higher than in any other group, and the overall distribution was statistically significantly different, although it should be noted that there were cases of major depression in all of the groups, including the normal controls. Dysthymic disorder was also diagnosable in several children with unipolar depressed mothers. The overall rate of affective disorder was significantly different in the groups but clearly greatest in children with unipolar mothers, while the bipolar group offspring and the other groups were fairly similar with low rates.

TABLE 3.3. Past diagnoses of child by maternal group.

	Group								
	Unipolar (n = 22)		Bipolar (n = 18)		Medical (n = 18)		Normal (n = 38)		
Diagnosis	N	%	N	%	N	%	N	%	$\chi^2(3, N = 96)$
Any disorder[a]	17	77	12	67	8	44	9	24	19.16***
Affective disorders	10	46	3	17	3	17	3	8	12.74**
Major depression	9	41	3	17	2	11	3	8	11.19**
Dysthymia	3	14	0	0	1	6	0	0	7.46†
Mania/hypomania	0	0	0	0	0	0	0	0	0.00
Behavior disorders	4	18	6	33	1	6	3	8	7.85*
Attention deficit	2	9	1	6	1	6	2	5	.40
Conduct disorder	4	18	5	28	0	0	3	8	7.80*
Alcohol use	0	0	1	6	0	0	0	0	4.38
Drug use	1	5	0	0	0	0	1	3	1.48
Anxiety disorders	5	23	3	17	2	11	4	11	1.91
Separation anxiety	1	5	2	11	2	11	2	5	1.25
Overanxious disorder	1	5	0	0	1	6	1	3	1.11
Other	3	14	1	6	0	0	1	3	4.67

[a] Does not include episodes of minor depression.
* $p < .05$. ** $p < .01$. *** $p < .001$.

Behavior Disorders

Diagnosable conditions that are generally considered to be "externalizing" disorders appeared to be somewhat more rare in the sample than the emotional disorders but were significantly differently distributed across the groups. Children of bipolar mothers were especially likely to report such problems, particularly conduct disorders, whereas unipolar offspring were less likely to do so but more likely than the medical and normal group children to display such difficulties.

Anxiety Disorders

Disorders marked by separation anxiety, overanxious behaviors, severe phobias, or other kinds of anxiety reactions occurred in approximately 10–20% of the children. However, there were no differences in the groups in the frequency of occurrence of anxiety problems.

Conclusions

Overall, therefore, the past psychiatric history of the sample is one of depressive disorders, relatively concentrated in the unipolar group. Behavior disorders and anxiety reactions were less common but relatively evenly distributed across all the groups, except for conduct disorders, which were more common in the unipolar and bipolar samples.

Current Diagnoses of Children in Present Sample

Table 3.4 presents the rates of definite K-SADS–based current diagnoses of children in our study. The current status of the children represents their typical functioning, rather than response to acute distress in their mothers—in the sense that the mothers were recruited and scheduled to participate in the study no sooner than 3 months after discharge from the hospital or entry into treatment for acute episodes. The information on current and past diagnoses is also noteworthy because the interviewers of the children were blind to the mother's diagnosis at the point the evaluations were conducted.

As Table 3.4 indicates, overall rates of disorder (a figure that covers any definite diagnosis including minor depression) are fairly low with the exception of the unipolar group. A statistical comparison indicates that the rates are significantly different, owing apparently to the elevated rate of disorder in the unipolar group children.

Affective Disorders

Overall rates of depressive disorders were computed to include major depression and dysthymic disorder, but they excluded minor depression. None of the children displayed hypomania at the diagnostic evaluation.

TABLE 3.4. Rates of current diagnoses in children.

Diagnosis	Group								
	Unipolar ($n = 22$)		Bipolar ($n = 18$)		Medical ($n = 18$)		Normal ($n = 38$)		$\chi^2(3, N = 96)$
	N	%	N	%	N	%	N	%	
Any disorder	12	55	4	22	4	22	6	16	11.29**
Any affective disorders	6	27	0	0	1	6	1	3	13.77**
Major depression	1	5	0	0	0	0	1	3	1.48
Dysthymic disorder	5	23	0	0	1	6	1	3	10.47*
Any behavior disorders	3	14	1	6	2	11	2	5	1.64
Attention deficit	1	5	0	0	1	6	0	0	2.91
Conduct disorder	2	9	1	6	0	0	2	5	1.67
Alcohol use	1	5	0	0	0	0	0	0	3.40
Drug use	1	5	0	0	1	6	1	3	1.11
Any anxiety disorder	7	32	3	17	2	11	3	8	6.39†
Separation anxiety	4	18	2	11	1	6	3	8	2.15
Overanxious disorder	1	5	1	6	2	11	1	3	1.81
Other	2	9	0	0	0	0	1	3	3.78

Note: Children may receive more than one diagnosis.
* $p < .05$. ** $p < .01$. † $p < .10$.

The groups differed statistically, as Table 3.4 indicates, accounted for largely by the high rate of dysthymia in the children of unipolar mothers.

Behavior Disorders

There were no differences between groups on any of the separate categories of behavior disorder, and generally the rates of disorder were low. However, both the unipolar and medical groups had slightly elevated overall rates in comparison with the bipolar and normal groups.

Anxiety Disorders

As Table 3.4 suggests, anxiety disorders were more prevalent in the groups than were affective or behavior disorders. The pattern was especially true for the bipolar, medical, and normal groups. On the whole, the presence of anxiety-related disorders was only marginally statistically different in the groups, and the individual categories did not differ.

Conclusions

Overall, therefore, the picture of the children's functioning that emerges is that the unipolar offspring are especially impaired, while the bipolar, medical, and normal groups are very similar overall. The unipolar group youngsters are especially likely to display depression and anxiety, and a small subset of them have significant, ongoing behavior problems. The pattern continues the findings concerning past psychiatric histories, with the exception that bipolar offspring no longer display elevated rates of behavior disturbances. An obvious additional generalization that is easy to overlook is that *within* each group there are enormous differences between families in the incidence of disorder, and even within the same families there may be differences between siblings. A major emphasis of the research program is to explore such variation as a way to account for specific factors, besides maternal diagnosis, that may contribute to children's diagnostic status.

Longitudinal Follow-Up Diagnostic Status of Children in the Study

A unique feature of the present investigation is the systematic follow-up of children in the sample at regular 6-month intervals for up to 3 years. At the present time, only Billings and Moos (1985a) and Nurnberger et al. (1988) have reported follow-up data on their offspring samples, unipolar in the former study and bipolar in the latter.

Of the original 96 children studied directly, 70 completed the full 3 years, 79 completed 2, and 90 completed at least 1 year. The rates reflect various reasons for noninclusion at specific points, relatively evenly divided among refusal, moving out of the area, and recruited later into the study so that they haven't completed the full 3 years. The sample sizes resulting from attrition are reported in Table 3.5, where it is apparent that more of the bipolar families were lost than in other groups. Therefore, the Year 3 data are especially tentative, owing to small remaining samples of bipolar offspring.

The procedures for arriving at diagnoses, described fully in Chapter 2, included interviews of both the mother and child, and most of these were conducted by telephone because of the enormous practical problems associated with scheduling and arranging face-to-face contacts. Final diagnostic decisions were based on all available sources of information. Generally, mothers and children agreed fairly well in their reports of events and symptoms in the previous 6 months. However, when discrepancies did occur, we tended to favor the report of symptom occurrence. For instance, children were themselves more likely to report depression and antisocial or substance abuse behaviors than the parents did (or were aware of), especially for the older youngsters. Where possible we had the same interviewer follow the families over time, and the tradeoff between lack of "blindness" on the one hand and increased sensitivity and openness due to established rapport on the other clearly favored the latter in our judgment.

Table 3.5 presents the rates of DSM III definite diagnoses for each year of follow-up. The results for the Year 1 period indicate very few definite diagnoses in the normal group children, mild rates in the medical group, and more marked rates of disorder in the children of mothers with affective disorders. Overall, the comparison between groups on presence/absence of diagnoses during the first year indicates highly significant differences, as indicated at the bottom of Table 3.5.

It is particularly noteworthy that the children of unipolar mothers had more serious disorders, whereas the children of bipolar women tended to display relatively mild problems not listed in the table, such as minor depression. The four groups differed significantly in rates of major depressive disorder, χ^2,(3, n = 90) = 12.93, p = .0048, and dysthymic disorder, χ^2,(3, n = 90) = 14.17, p = .0027. In both cases, the children of unipolar depressed women had the highest rates. Overall, 10 of the unipolar group children (46%) had either major depression or dysthymic disorder (2 had both), compared with 7% of the bipolar, 17% of the medical, and none of the normal group children. It is also apparent that the unipolar children exceeded the other groups in percentages of conduct disorder (overall χ^2(3, n = 90) = 9.43, p = .02, and substance use disorders. For drug and alcohol use disorders the effect was only marginally significant, χ^2(3, n = 90) = 6.61, $p < .10$. On the whole, the groups did not differ on incidence of anxiety disorders, although none were reported in the normal group.

TABLE 3.5. Diagnosis of definite disorder during 3-year follow-up.

Group	n	Percent receiving diagnosis							
		Any[a]	Major depression	Dysthymia	Hypomania	Conduct disorder	Attention deficit	Substance use	Anxiety disorders
		Year 1[b]							
Unipolar	22	73	27	27	0	23	5	18	9
Bipolar	15	67	7	0	0	0	0	0	12
Medical	18	50	6	11	0	6	6	6	11
Normal	35	20	0	0	0	3	0	3	0
		Year 2[c]							
Unipolar	19	63	16	32	0	21	0	16	11
Bipolar	11	82	0	9	0	0	0	9	9
Medical	15	40	7	0	0	0	7	0	7
Normal	34	24	3	0	0	0	0	3	3
		Year 3[d]							
Unipolar	16	81	19	24	6	19	0	19	19
Bipolar	6	83	0	20	0	0	0	0	20
Medical	14	64	0	7	0	7	7	0	7
Normal	34	35	0	0	0	0	0	3	6

Note: Children may receive more than one diagnosis.
[a] Includes possible diagnoses and minor depression not shown in table. [b] Any versus no diagnosis, $\chi^2(3, N = 90) = 13.49, p < .001$. [c] Any versus no diagnosis, $\chi^2(3, N = 79) = 15.07, p < .002$. [d] Any versus no diagnosis, $\chi^2(3, N = 70) = 12.25, p < .001$.

Children of bipolar mothers were much more likely to report symptoms of anxiety disorders such as overanxious disorders and separation anxiety, or possible minor depression, than they were to display evidence of more severe disorders. They mostly received "possible" diagnoses, not shown in Table 3.5, and only one had a major depressive episode. In the Year 1 analyses, none were viewed as hypomanic or cyclothymic.

The proportions of diagnoses in Year 2 display similar overall patterns. The groups differed significantly in the presence/absence of diagnosable disorders. Unipolar group children showed moderate rates of disorders of all types, compared to the other groups. Forty-two percent of the unipolar offspring had some affective disorder, compared with only 9% of the bipolar group children. However, the groups did not differ significantly on proportions of children with major depression. Four children in the unipolar group received diagnoses of conduct disorder during Year 2, and this rate significantly exceeded those of the other groups, $\chi^2(3, n = 79) = 13.31, p < .004$. The unipolar group also had a higher rate of substance abuse, but the groups did not differ significantly. It should be noted that one unipolar child had a possible diagnosis of cyclothymia in Year 2.

For Year 2, children in the bipolar group mostly reported nondiagnosable levels of symptoms, not displayed in the table. It is noteworthy, however, that many displayed affective symptoms. Two children had possible diagnoses of hypomania, and one had possible cyclothymia; two reported possible minor depressions, and two displayed significant but nondiagnosable overanxious behavior.

Year 3 diagnoses continue similar patterns. It should be noted that several of the bipolar offspring are not included, owing largely to attrition

TABLE 3.6. Cumulative probability of major depressive episode—Survival curve estimates[a].

	Group			
Age interval at onset	Unipolar	Bipolar	Medical	Normal
0–4	0	0	0	0
5–9	.09	.06	.07	.05
10–14	.43	.20	.16	.12
15–19	.67	.33	.45	.12
Mean age	14.0 (*SE* = .6)	16.1 (*SE* = .6)	16.35 (*SE* = .9)	12.5 (*SE* = .3)

Note: From "Longitudinal Study of Diagnoses in Children of Women with Unipolar and Bipolar Affective Disorder" by C. Hammen, D. Burge, E. Burney, and C. Adrian (1990). *Archives of General Psychiatry*, **47**, 1112–1120. Copyright, 1990, the American Medical Association. Reprinted by permission.

[a] Kaplan–Meier method; comparison between survival curves, log rank test $\chi^2(3) = 11.64$, $p = .0087$.

(i.e., moving out of the area). For the most part, the children show slightly higher rates of disorder in Year 3 than in Year 2. Overall, the groups differ in presence/absence of diagnosable disorder, $\chi^2(3, n = 70) = 12.25, p = .0066$, with the affective disorders groups showing highest rates of diagnoses, the medical group moderate levels, and fewest in the normal group. Of 16 children of unipolar mothers, 7 had some form of affective disorder, mostly major depression or dysthymia. The groups overall differed marginally significantly on proportion of major depression, $\chi^2(3, n = 70) = 7.52, p = .057$. Similarly, the groups differed marginally on substance use disorders, with the unipolar offspring showing highest rates of drug and/or alcohol abuse, $\chi^2(3, n = 70) = 6.74, p = .08$. Interestingly, in one family one sibling continued possible cyclothymia (from Year 2), while the other sibling in that family had hypomanic episodes that led to treatment with lithium.

The bipolar group children remaining in the Year 3 follow-up showed a continuation of previous patterns: 3 of the 6 had minor depression and overanxious symptoms, and 1 continued possible hypomanic symptoms (along with possible alcohol abuse).

Age of Onset

Hammen, Burge, Burney, and Adrian (1990) used survival analyses to project the estimated curves for probability of having a major diagnosis by age. This information takes into account the age of onset of first major diagnosis (excluding minor depression and nondiagnosable symptoms), regardless of whether it occurred prior to the study or during the follow-up observation, and regardless of when a child might have dropped out of the study. This figure also excludes two of the medical families (with a total of 4 children) in which the mother had experienced major depressive illness, in order to more clearly depict the correlates of medical illness rather than depression. Figure 3.1 presents the survival curves, and statistical analyses indicated that the four maternal groups differed significantly. As the figure suggests, early childhood onset is relatively rare, but unipolar children showed increasing frequency of onset from about age 8 and all onsets occurred by age 14. In contrast, the other groups showed gradual increases in onset, with most occurring later. The unipolar group clearly fared the worst in terms of probability of disorder, while the normal group children were the least likely to be diagnosed.

Similar survival analyses were computed for the onset of major depressive disorder. Omitting the 4 children of depressed medically ill women, there were 22 cases of major depression over the course of the study, and 10 of these occurred to unipolar offspring. Table 3.6 presents the survival curve estimates, indicating the proportion of children likely to be diagnosed with major depressive episode at each age interval. These figures confirm the relative rarity of early childhood onset of major depression

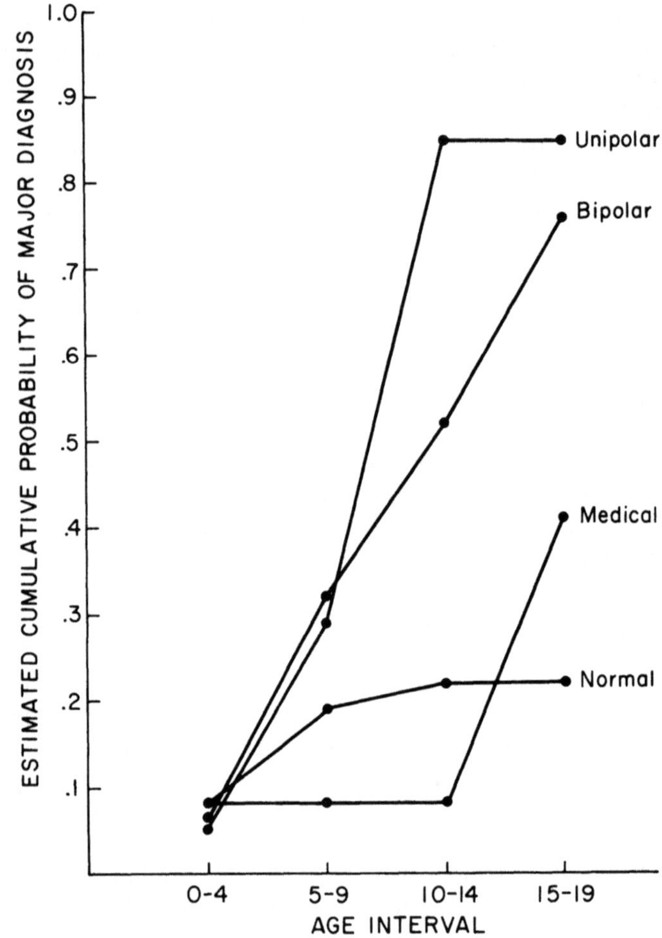

FIGURE 3.1. Survival curve estimates of major diagnosis by age interval, for children of unipolar, bipolar, medically ill, or normal mothers. From Hammen, Burge, Burney, and Adrian (1990). Longitudinal study of diagnoses in children of women with unipolar and bipolar affective disorders. *Archives of General Psychiatry*, **47**, 1112–1120. Copyright, 1990, the American Medical Association. Reprinted by permission.

as reported by others and indicate relatively earlier onset for the unipolar offspring than for the others, consistent with the patterns observed by Weissman, Gammon, et al. (1987).

Patterns Observed over Time

Hammen et al. (1990) evaluated the characteristics of children's diagnoses during the follow-up period. Such information, obtained every

6 months, yields the most complete and reliable data about children's functioning. Table 3.7 presents the nature of the diagnoses during the follow-ups for children who completed at least 1 year of observation, characterized as new disorders, relapse, or chronic disorder. The unipolar offspring displayed strikingly high rates of both chronic and new disorders, and 5 youngsters had recurrences of major depressive episode. Of the 12 new disorders in unipolar children, 6 were internalizing disorders (major depression or onsets of overanxious or dysthymic disorders) and 6 were externalizing disorders (conduct and substance abuse disorders). The other three groups had similar, relatively low rates of disorders during the follow-ups.

Overall, the pattern data generally indicate that there is considerable consistency in children's diagnoses across a 3-year span (or even longer, considering the lifetime psychiatric history data collected on all of the children). While the severity of the disorders may ebb and flow over time, it was rare for a child to suddenly develop symptoms of a disorder that had not made an appearance earlier in her or his life. Additionally, although some of the children seemed to improve with time, the majority of children who were diagnosable continued to display difficulties at least intermittently.

Additional Issues in Children's Diagnostic Outcomes

Treatment and Severe Negative Outcomes of Children in the Study

During the initial contacts with the families in the study, information was gathered concerning treatment the children had received. This information provides an additional way of confirming the existence of dysfunctional behaviors and maladaptive reactions in the children. Fully 25% of the sample had previously been in treatment with some mental health professional for psychological difficulties. The actual percentages of children differed significantly in the different maternal groups ($\chi^2[3, n = 96] = 11.58, p < .01$). As might be expected, the children of unipolar mothers had the highest proportion of treatment (46%), compared with 33% in the bipolar group, 28% in the medical group, and 8% of the normal children. At the time of the initial interview, only 4 children were currently in treatment, 2 from the unipolar group and 2, the medical group.

There are additional, more dramatic ways to portray the diagnostic outcomes of children exposed to maternal disorder. In the initial evaluations the mothers were queried not only about their children who were in the study (between the ages of 8 and 16), but also about other older or younger children. As reported by Hammen, Gordon, et al. (1987), Family History Research Diagnostic Criteria were applied to an additional 50

TABLE 3.7. Number of diagnoses of major disorders during the follow-up.

	Unipolar n = 22	Bipolar n = 15	Medical n = 14	Normal n = 35
Chronic disorder	13	1	2	2
Relapse/recurrence	5	1	1	0
New onset	12	3	4	4
None or minor	9	10	10	30
At least one disorder[a]	13 (59%)	5 (33%)	4 (29%)	5 (17%)

Note: Children may receive more than one diagnosis, but were not counted more than once for the same diagnosis over time. Chronic disorder refers to ongoing symptoms that may vary in severity but the child has no more than several weeks symptom-free. Relapse/recurrance refers to onset of major depressive episode. New onset refers to onset of diagnosable disorder that had not been observed before.

[a] Based on sample with at least one year of follow-up.

Note: From Hammen, Burge, Burney, and Adrian (1990). Longitudinal study of diagnoses in children of women with unipolar and bipolar affective disorders. *Archives of General Psychiatry*, **47**, 1112–1120. Copyright, 1990, the American Medical Association. Reprinted by permission.

siblings in the first 58 families seen in the study. These were children who were too young or too old for the age range, or they were additional children in the age range who were excluded when we limited inclusion to two per family; a few were excluded because they had serious medical problems or lived elsewhere with their fathers. In general, these children had rates of diagnosable disorder that were very comparable to those of children studied directly. Additionally, we obtained treatment information on the excluded offspring. In the total sample of offspring, combining included and excluded children, we learned that 10 children had been hospitalized at some point for psychiatric reasons. Eight of the hospitalizations occurred in the unipolar group (and one each in the bipolar and normal groups).

Even more tragically, suicide occurred in several of the families: two offspring had committed suicide prior to the study—one child of a unipolar mother and one child of medically ill mother. During the follow-up phase of the study, one teenager committed suicide following hospitalization, and the mother was in the unipolar group.

Additional evidence during the follow-ups regarding children's severe impairment came to light. Four children were hospitalized for psychiatric problems, and at least six youngsters were arrested for various crimes such as drug dealing and theft. At least several other children stole money from their parents but were not prosecuted, and there were numerous instances of serious academic and behavioral problems. The following vignettes represent a few, but by no means all, of the severe outcomes of children in the study. Unfortunately, some of the rich clinical detail has to be omitted so as to preserve confidentiality, but the essential elements of the stories are retained.

Adam was 12 at the time of entry into the study and had a history of depression and separation anxiety and school difficulties that had led him to be considered "educationally handicapped." During the follow-up period he was hospitalized 3 times. He was incorrigible at home and at school, would refuse to go to school or get into fights with teachers and other students. He would steal from his mother, and if angry, would demolish the furniture or kick holes in the wall, or even hit his mother. He used drugs and sold drugs. When depressed, he'd often be unable to get out of bed, and would be extremely sensitive, fly into rages if he felt offended, and worry that he couldn't go back to school because the other kids would make fun of him for having problems. Finally, at some point the mother got public services involved, and he was placed in a group home with therapeutic foster parents and attended a special school. He would come home on weekends. Although there was some improvement, over time he increasingly got into fights at the placement and ran away, escalating into expulsion from the facility. Since he was a ward of the court, the alternative was juvenile hall, and when he learned this he ran away and lived on the streets for a time. His mother was contacted when he was brought to the hospital in serious condition after being beaten up in circumstances that were never entirely clear. Temporarily at home, he continued angry and destructive acting out and increasingly got into drug use and thefts, blown drugs deals, and arrests. Eventually he ended up in juvenile hall.

Alice was 16 at the time of initial contact and apparently had a history of minor depressions, but nothing severe. However, soon after her mother's remarriage, she became depressed. As she became more withdrawn, sleepless, and made a minor suicide attempt by cutting her wrists, she was hospitalized. After a long period of hospitalization, and maintenance on antidepressants, she returned to school where she seemed to have friends, began dating, and got a job. At home, her relationship with her mother was very negative. She graduated from high school and was accepted in college, and then, before she left, we were informed that she had committed suicide.

Alan, who was 11, his 16-year-old sister, and their mother were all hospitalized within close proximity to each other. On recovery, he appeared to have poor social skills, very low self-esteem, viewed the world as a hostile place, and seemed to have little capacity for enjoyment. Although his relationship with his mother was very conflicted, he was quite fearful of separation. He was doing poorly in school in special classes. As the follow-ups progressed, his fearfulness and somewhat paranoid attitudes intensified, and he would often fly into rages and believed that the house would be broken into while he was there and he would be harmed. He was continued on medications, which seemed to help stabilize his moods, but even when he was functioning better he would go for long periods of time not speaking to certain members of his family. Eventually, he began to show increased perceptual acuity and other odd beliefs. He thought he could "hear" electricity running through wires, and thought that he had special powers. These behaviors were interpreted as hypomania by his doctors, and he was put on lithium.

Comorbidity in the Follow-Up Period

It was relatively common for children to display more than a single type of symptomatology. For instance, of the children who were found to have histories of diagnosable disorders in their past, 24% had more than one diagnosis. For children who were currently diagnosable at the time of the initial evaluation, 58% had more than one diagnosis.

For a more detailed analysis of comorbidity in the children, diagnoses from the longitudinal follow-ups were examined. In the Year 1 follow-up, counting only definite diagnoses (and excluding minor depression), only a few youngsters displayed affective disorders alone: 3 in the unipolar group, 1 in the bipolar group, 1 in the medical group, and none in the normal group. Even fewer showed only "externalizing disorders" such as conduct disorder or substance use disorders, and a few displayed only anxiety disorders. By contrast, the more typical pattern was for a mixture of affective and nonaffective disorders. There were 6 such children in the unipolar group in Year 1, displaying major depression and/or dysthymic disorder, along with conduct disorder and/or substance use disorder.

Viewing the sample available for all 3 years of the follow-up, children were classified as showing "internalizing" disorders only (affective and/or anxiety disorders) versus presence of "externalizing" disorders (conduct disorder, substance use, attention deficit, with or without concurrent emotional disorders). Taken as proportions of children who had diagnosable disorders, internalizing patterns appeared in 58% of the unipolar children, 80% of the bipolar, 25% of the medical illness group, and 70% of the normal children. The groups did not appear to differ in proportions of children with the various patterns of disorder.

Age and Gender Effects in the Present Sample

Sex of Child

In the initial evaluations of past and current diagnoses, no significant gender differences were observed, although boys were somewhat more frequently diagnosed than girls. For instance, 52% of boys and 44% of girls had received past diagnoses. For current problems, more boys (35%) than girls (20%) met diagnostic criteria for one or more disorders. Hammen et al., (1990) reported that the overall cumulative probability of disorder as characterized by survival analyses indicated a rate of .41 for boys compared with .39 for girls, suggesting that the overall lifetime rates were not different. In the age interval of 15 to 19, however, girls' rates (.69) exceeded those of boys (.41). In general, within the various maternal groups there were no significant differences in boys' and girls' rates of disorder, and the various disorders did not show significant gender differences. For example, among all the children who displayed a major depression at some point during the follow-ups, 5 were boys and 6 were girls.

Age Effects in Diagnoses

As expected, older children tended to display more evidence of disorders. For instance, when the children were divided into preadolescent (8 to 12 years) and adolescent (13 and older) groups, the older children were more likely to have a past diagnosis (55%) than were the younger ones (42%). Similar trends were apparent for current diagnoses, with older children diagnosed at the rate of 30%, compared to 25% of the younger ones.

In the follow-up period the older children (59%) were significantly more likely to be symptomatic in the Year 1 follow-up than were the younger children (37%), $\chi^2(1, n = 90) = 4.26, p = .04$. However, these differences were not significant in the Year 2 and Year 3 follow-ups. After 3 years of follow-up there were still 13 children below age 13, of whom 39% were symptomatic, compared with 60% of the older children still available for follow-up, but the effect was not statistically significant. As indicated previously in the discussion of age of onset, the school-age years 8 to 12 tended to be the most likely period of onset, accounting for about 60% of onsets, with 20% before age 8 and 20% during adolescence.

Comparisons Between Groups in Children's Outcomes

Comparisons with Medical Control Group

A particular question raised by the present study is whether children of women with affective disorders are uniquely at risk due to parental affective illness or whether risk is generally associated with any chronic illness. To test this question, the chronically medically ill group offers a comparison, since children are exposed to mothers with severe chronic symptoms and impairment of functioning, with periodic exacerbations sometimes requiring hospitalization. The children of diabetic mothers or severely arthritic mothers often find their parent restricted in activities, unable to perform certain tasks that may require vigor and energy. Sometimes the children of diabetic mothers have found them semiconscious; children of arthritic mothers realize that their parent suffers great pain and immobility. In both kinds of illness the children are often required to take on household tasks and responsibilities, and there may be overt or covert resistance to children's efforts to separate themselves and become more independent of the family.

Children in the medical illness group were compared with children of unipolar mothers on rates of past diagnosis. Statistical analyses failed to show significant differences in rates across broad categories, or specific ones. The sole exception was a marginally significant difference between the two groups on rates of major depression, $\chi^2,(1, n = 40) = 3.04, p < .10$.

With respect to follow-up diagnoses, as Table 3.5 indicates, rates of presence/absence of disorder were moderately high for the medical group children; there were no statistically significant differences in comparisons with the unipolar group each year. In Year 1, the unipolar group children were significantly more likely to have a diagnosis of affective disorder than were the medical group offspring, $\chi^2(1, n = 40) = 3.74, p = .05$. However, there were no differences in other diagnostic categories in Year 1 or in Years 2 and 3.

Since the bipolar offspring had even lower rates of disorder in general than did the unipolar children, we conclude that past diagnoses are relatively nonspecific to children with ill mothers. That is, although the rates of disorder are higher for the unipolar children than the medical group children, the differences were not significant statistically. In the follow-up, there is some suggestion that unipolar children are uniquely likely to experience depressive disorders, but the statistical effect attains significance only in one year. Taken together, the results suggest that psychiatric risk to children may be more a function of maternal disability than of affective disorder as such. Nevertheless, despite few statistical differences between the medical and unipolar groups, the latter appeared to be seriously affected compared to more moderate rates of disorder in the medical group children.

Unipolar Versus Bipolar Comparisons

Inspection of the tables indicates that the offspring of unipolar mothers generally had more diagnosable disorders than did children of bipolar mothers. However, as reported by Hammen and Anderson (1990), the groups did not differ statistically significantly in any category of past diagnoses. Current diagnoses, on the other hand, suggested that unipolar children had elevated rates, and the effect was marginally significant for presence of any diagnoses, $\chi^2(1, n = 40) = 3.07, p < .08$, Yates's corrected. Also, they had significantly higher rates of current affective disorder, $\chi^2(1, n = 40) = 3.83, p < .05$, primarily reflecting dysthymic disorder.

With respect to follow-up levels of disorder, as indicated in Table 3.5, the rates of overall presence of significant symptomatology are similar for the unipolar and bipolar offspring, and there were no significant differences between the two groups for any of the follow-up periods. This overall pattern largely reflects the presence of mild problems, such as minor depression and "possible" but not definite diagnoses in the bipolar group children. Looking at specific diagnoses, in Year 1 the unipolar group children displayed significantly more definite affective disorders (major depression or dysthymia) than did the bipolar offspring, $\chi^2(1, n = 37) = 6.42, p = .01$. Unipolar children also reported more conduct disorder ($p < .05$) and marginally more drug use disorder ($p = .08$) than bipolar children in Year 1. In Years 2 and 3, however, the groups did not differ significantly, although the unipolar children continued to have higher rates of specific diagnosis.

In general, it appeared that the bipolar offspring tended to have more mild and transitory symptoms compared to the unipolar children, and they were especially likely to report fewer major depressive or dysthymic disorders. Thus it is not so much rates of disorders as it is persistence and severity of disorders that tend to mark the differences between the groups. As we shall see later, in a discussion of psychosocial functioning socially and academically, this observation is borne out. The bipolar children fared significantly better in terms of functioning, seemingly less impaired by their disorders than were their unipolar counterparts.

Psychosocial Functioning

Although diagnoses can be construed as a summary, or an index, of a variety of symptoms reflecting impairment of functioning, a more direct method of examining children's psychosocial behaviors is desirable. Various cognitive measures were obtained and are reported in Chapter 4. For our current purposes, analyses of social competence and academic/school behaviors characterize children's adjustments in typical situations. Consider the following vignettes of children in the study, where the symptomatic behaviors are both a cause and a consequence of difficulties in school and in peer functioning.

Jeff had been diagnosed with attention deficit and hyperactivity disorder while still a toddler, and in early childhood had a history of stealing, vandalism, firesetting, and fighting, as well as truancy. At the time of the initial contact he was 14 and had recently begun regular classes at school (formerly he had been placed in learning disabilities classes). He was fairly cheerful and seemed to have a solid sense of self-esteem. Through the follow-up period of 3 years, we saw him have increasing difficulties with high school. He found high school difficult and failed many classes, with escalating amounts of truancy and drug use. At one point, with the insistence, if not threats, of his mother, he got into therapy and there seemed to be a period of improvement in grades and reduced drinking. However, such gains proved temporary, and by the 4th follow-up he was considerably behind in units needed to graduate. He was unable to make them up in summer school due to nonattendance. The school referred him to a juvenile diversion program, and eventually he seemed to give up. He became very depressed about not graduating with his class and that his mother would not let him get a driver's license.

Jill was 10 at the initial evaluation, a thin, worried-looking girl who had a history of major depression and nondepressed emotional disorder. Jill was an average student academically, but she worried a great deal about things going on at school and often felt that she was picked on by the other children or by the teachers. She would often complain of stomach aches or other maladies so that she could stay home from school. As time went on, she had periods of school refusal where she would stay home for several days at a time. Her grades seemed to suffer accordingly.

Through the use of objective indicators of psychosocial functioning, Social Competence subscores of the Child Behavior Check List, based on maternal report, were computed at the initial evaluation and at each 6-month follow-up. Such scores were averaged over available data for each year; they reflect children's social activities, participation in hobbies and pastimes, and to some extent academic performance. Additionally, of Academic Performance and School Behavior ratings were obtained yearly, based on information from all sources, including school follow-ups and records as well as mother and child reports. The 5-point scales used to combine information not otherwise comparable are described in Chapter 2.

Table 3.8 presents the means for the three scores by maternal group, across various assessment points, based on information reported in Anderson and Hammen (1990a). Although means are presented for all 3 years, the reduced sample size available for Year 3 impaired the reliability of statistical tests, and therefore the overall repeated measures analyses of variance are based only on the initial assessment and Years 1 and 2 assessments.

For CBCL Social Competence, the mean scores are presented as standardized *T* scores. There was a significant difference between groups on mean scores, $F(9, 162) = 2.07, p < .05$. Specific comparisons between groups indicated that the unipolar offspring were seen as having significantly lower levels of social competence than the children of bipolar, medically ill, and normal mothers (p values $< .01$); the latter groups did not differ from each other. The analyses also confirmed what the table

TABLE 3.8. Mean scores on psychosocial variables over the follow-up period by maternal group.

Variable	Initial	Year 1	Year 2	Year 3
CBCL Social Competence				
Unipolar	35	36	37	36
Bipolar	52	52	49	47
Medical	50	51	49	44
Normal	49	52	49	45
School Behavior				
Unipolar	2.6	3.1	3.0	3.5
Bipolar	4.3	4.3	4.2	3.6
Medical	4.0	4.1	4.1	4.0
Normal	4.1	4.4	4.2	4.2
Academic Performance				
Unipolar	2.9	3.1	2.7	2.9
Bipolar	3.7	4.2	3.9	3.6
Medical	3.8	3.7	3.8	3.5
Normal	4.1	4.3	4.3	3.7

Note: From "Psychosocial Outcomes of Children of Unipolar Depressed, Bipolar, Medically Ill and Normal Women: A Longitudinal Study" by C.A. Anderson and C. Hammen, (1990-a), manuscript under review.

indicates: scores were relatively stable over time and no temporal effects (interaction of time and group) were significant.

School behavior ratings refer to conduct at school and degree of participation in regular classes compared to difficulties in attendance or deportment that might lead to suspension or placement in special classes or schools. As Table 3.8 indicates, the unipolar children scored significantly lower—indicating more problems—compared to the other groups, $F(9, 225) = 4.19$, $p < .001$. As with Social Competence, they differed from all the other groups, and the other groups were similar to each other. The effects were quite stable and did not differ significantly across the various assessment points. Academic Performance scores reflect grades and level of performance. Not surprisingly, the groups differed significantly overall, $F(9, 225) = 2.77$, $p < .005$, with the unipolar children performing at a lower level than all other groups.

To express these findings in a more concrete way, consider that scores of 1 or 2 on the School Behavior Rating indicate repeated suspensions or truancy, or expulsion, dropout, or placement in special schools due to conduct difficulties. From the total of 96 youngsters, 7 had such outcomes at some point during the study and follow-up, and 5 of the 7 were in the unipolar group. On the Academic Performance Rating, a low score of 1 or 2 indicated serious problems such as failure in two or more subjects or threat of grade failure or actual failure or placement in learning disabilities class. Fully 22 of the 96 children evidenced such poor performance at some point during the follow-ups, and 10 of the 22 were in the unipolar group. Altogether, 45% of the unipolar sample had such academic difficulties at some point, compared to 17% of the bipolar, 22% of the medical, and 13% of the normal group children.

Summary and Directions for Further Research

The results of the study of children of unipolar, bipolar, medically ill, and normal women confirm our worst fears based on earlier research: children of women with affective disorders are more likely than not to experience major disorders at some point in their childhoods. The risk for diagnosable problems is equal for boys and girls overall, and the presence of multiple diagnoses was the rule rather than the exception.

The effect needs to be qualified in two important ways: the unipolar offspring appear to be considerably more impaired than the bipolar children, and the medically ill children have increased rates of problems that often distinguish them from normal parent families. The children of unipolar depressed mothers were more likely to display affective disorders in the past, current, and follow-up assessments, and they tended to have elevated rates on all disorders as well. Although the bipolar children displayed high rates of relatively mild, nondiagnosable symptoms, they tended to have later onsets and fewer chronic or recurrent major problems. Also, the bipolar children did not differ from normal children and offspring of medically ill mothers in terms of psychosocial functioning in social and academic settings. In contrast, the children of unipolar mothers were impaired both by diagnostic criteria and by relatively stable levels of low functioning socially and academically. While the bipolar children may not yet have passed into the age of risk for bipolar forms of the disorder—and indeed several appear to display mild mood disturbances of both depressive and hypomanic kinds—their relatively superior functioning interpersonally and at school provides a solid foundation. Many of the unipolar offspring, by comparison, appear to have embarked relatively early on a chronic course of impaired functioning that bodes ill for adult adjustment. Children must master a variety of coping and adaptational skills, as well as acquiring beliefs in their worth and competence. Impairment of functioning in these realms is likely to have lifelong consequences.

The medically ill group offspring generally tended to show more diagnoses than did the normal group children, owing to the relatively dysfunctional behaviors that several of them displayed. Such results suggest that families of medically ill parents are subjected to stressful conditions that impair children's adjustment. Thus it appears that difficulties the offspring experience are not unique to having a clinically depressed mother.

Although the present data paint a grim and disheartening picture overall, many children exposed to the risk of parental disorder fared well, and in Chapter 8 we explore the sources of risk and resilience. Also, the present results do not reveal to us the contributors—and hence the targets of future prevention—to children's risk. We contend that negative outcomes are not primarily genetic and thus not immutable. Moreover, we do not view the women with recurrent unipolar depression as incapable parents. However, the task of unraveling the multiple and overlapping factors that contribute to disorder is formidable. Nevertheless, it is a necessary step. Most past studies of children of parents with affective disorders have stopped at precisely this point, demonstrating children's risk for dysfunction but going little beyond such description to tackle the questions of mechanisms.

In the chapters to follow, we attempt to explore some of the likely sources of impediments to normal functioning and adjustment. In Chapter 4, children's cognitions are explored, especially those associated with possible vulnerability to depression. In Chapter 5 we tackle stress—chronic family strains and mother's and children's episodic stressful life events as well as the mutual stress on each other that episodes of symptoms may cause. In Chapter 6 the issue of family relationships is explored, with primary emphasis on mother-child interactions, their quality, and their implications. In Chapter 7 we explore additional characteristics of the mother and the family that might affect children's behaviors; it is here that we tackle the often-neglected topic of the role of the father. Chapter 8 discusses risk and resilience and includes a consideration of well and ill siblings in the same family; finally, Chapter 9 attempts to integrate some of the major themes and findings into a general model of risk for psychopathology. Also, the shortcomings of the present study and the gaps and loose ends are noted, in the hope that other investigators will find sufficient challenge and reward in pursuing such issues, so that future studies will add substance to the tentative findings of this investigation.

4
Vulnerability to Depression: The Role of Children's Cognitions

One of the initial aims of the present investigation was to explore cognitive vulnerability to depression in children. The highly active research on cognitive perspectives on adult depression, briefly outlined in Chapter 2, provided models and tools for understanding how thoughts, beliefs, and interpretations of the self and the world contribute to depression. It seemed likely that such cognitive processes and dysfunctional cognitive content have their origins in childhood in many individuals. By extension, therefore, we predicted that some of the risk to children of women with depressive disorders might stem from dysfunctional cognitions. Thus the research reported here afforded an opportunity to examine potential vulnerability cognitions in high risk children, and the longitudinal design provided methods for testing the relationship between dysfunctional cognition and subsequent depression.

In this chapter several aspects of depressive cognitions in children in our study are explored: the descriptive characteristics of cognitions in the children, their correlates—with implications for the origin of the cognitions—and their consequences in terms of prediction of future depression. A feature of the current project is a particular emphasis on cognitions associated with the self. The implications and future directions of research on vulnerability cognitions are discussed.

Before presenting the results of studies of depression-relevant cognitions in the current sample, however, it seems useful to place the study in the context of findings and issues emerging from other investigators' studies of depressive cognitions in children.

Research on Depression and Cognitions in Children

Since the 1970s when such studies began to appear, most of the investigations of children's depressive cognitions have been direct extensions from the adult models to children. There have been three general trends. First, studies examined whether the cognitions in children were the same as those seen in depressed adults, much as investigators were beginning to explore whether depressive symptoms in children were the same as those seen in adults. Second, studies examined whether adult models of depression could be extended to children. Third, and relatively new, has been the study of the childhood origins of vulnerability to depression. In the sections to follow, these themes are pursued briefly in the context of each of several major versions of adult cognitive models of depression. A much more detailed coverage of the research on children's depressive cognitions is reported in Hammen (1990-a).

Beck's Information-Processing Model

The history, evolution, and contemporary developments in Beck's theory of depression have been explored in more detail elsewhere (Hammen, 1985, 1988a, 1990-b). However, it is important to note several issues here, because their status bears importantly on the past and future developments in the study of children's cognitions.

The original model, which emphasized the characteristic negative ways of construing the self, world, and the future (e.g., Beck, 1967, 1976), yielded a great deal of confirming descriptive information. Such research demonstrated that when depressed, individuals do indeed think in highly negative ways that often represent bias and distortion in interpretation of information. It seemed plausible that such self-deprecating and pessimistic thinking might intensify, or even initially cause, depressive symptoms.

However, it was only in a second wave of investigations that the etiological implications of the model were subjected to test, using a variety of questionnaire and experimental procedures, with patient and nonpatient samples, using both longitudinal designs and cross-sectional manipulations. When the data began to emerge, the model encountered difficulties requiring elaboration and refinement. For example, it became clear that the concept of stable, underlying cognitive tendencies that could *cause* depression required alteration. The various methods for assessing the allegedly stable cognitive vulnerability suggested that the cognitions were *not* stable, and that when no longer depressed, individuals did not display negativistic thinking. Studies suggested instead that depressive distortions, dysfunctional attitudes, or negative self-schemas are mood-dependent concomitants of depressive symptoms (e.g., Dobson & Shaw, 1987; Gotlib & Cane, 1987; Hamilton & Abramson, 1983; Hammen, Marks, deMayo, & Mayol, 1985; Hollon, Kendall, & Lumry, 1986; Lewinsohn, Steinmetz, Larson, & Franklin, 1981; Miller & Norman, 1986). Recently, Barnett and Gotlib (1988) concluded that there is little evidence of enduring global cognitive biases that cause depression. However, it remains possible that dysfunctional views of the self and the world might intensify ongoing depressive reactions, or that they are latent until primed by relevant negative experiences.

In response to the empirical shortcomings of the model as an etiological approach to depression, Beck and colleagues have refined their notions of dysfunctional thinking. There is now a differentiation between surface cognitions, which might reflect immediate distortions of circumstances and are best seen as concomitants of depression, and deeper processes such as beliefs and assumptions, which represent vulnerability. In the latter instance, negative self-schemas and dysfunctional attitudes are viewed as underlying vulnerabilities that if triggered, will activate depressive cognitive sets leading to the other symptoms of the dysphoric state. One recent, exciting extension of Beck's model (e.g., Beck, 1982), which is actually consistent with certain psychodynamic models of subtypes of depression, suggests an interaction of underlying vulnerability and the specific kind of circumstance that would trigger depression. Individuals might be "sociotropic," or "autonomous" in terms of the values, beliefs, and personal meaning attached to events relating to interpersonal relationships or achievement/autonomy. If negative events occur that impinge on the underlying domain of self-definition in such a way that the person interprets himself or herself as defective, deprived, or depleted, then depression will occur. If negative events occur that do not tap into the vulnerable area of self-relevance, then symptoms would be mild and transitory if they occurred at all. Support for this interaction of cognitive vulnerability and stress has been consistent (see Hammen, in press-c). Unfortunately, however, the mechanisms of the self-schema process have not been clarified, and their operation, development, and organization remain unexplored.

Recently Segal (1988) reviewed and analyzed the gaps in understanding the properties of depressive schemas. Pursuit of schema characteristics seems to be a fruitful direction because the schema process appears to capture the selective attention to negative information that is likely to intensify dysphoria. This information-processing model also accounts for the relative resistance of negative schemas to change through the incorporation of positive information. The link between mood and accessibility of information, the availability of somewhat primitive logic in depression (e.g., "all or nothing" thinking), the acquisition of self-schemas and their stability and complexity—these are among the questions that Beck's information-processing approach raises that have implications for developmental psychopathology.

Investigators of depression models not only note the conceptual gaps in Beck's approach but also urge alteration of the model to distinguish among potential subtypes of depression as well as differentiation of applications of the model to processes of onset, maintenance, relapse, and recovery. Also, there is a call for integration of cognitive approaches with actual environmental events, including the interpersonal context, and resources (e.g., Abramson, Alloy, & Metalsky, 1988; Barnett & Gotlib, 1988; Hammen, 1988a). As we shall see, there is even greater need to attend to these suggestions in the field of children's cognitions, since the achievements of that field lag behind those of adult depression research.

Studies of Cognitive Distortion in Children

The earliest extensions of Beck's work to children examined depressed youngsters' cognitions. Several studies, using versions of adult questionnaires adapted for children, did indeed find confirmation that relatively depressed youngsters display more depressive distortions or negativistic choices (Campbell-Goymer & Allgood, 1984; Leitenberg, Yost, & Carroll-Wilson, 1986; Roback-Moyal, 1981). Only one such study investigated depressed children in psychiatric treatment rather than high scorers on depression inventories in normal populations (Haley, Fine, Marriage, Moretti, & Freeman, 1985).

Cognitions specific to hopelessness are also directly related to Beck's model, and relatively extensive research has been conducted in child samples. Most such studies included clinical samples, and virtually all found the predicted association between depressive symptomatology and hopeless thinking (Asarnow, Carlson, & Guthrie, 1987; Benfield, Palmer, Pfefferbaum, & Stowe, 1988; Kazdin, French, Unis, Esveldt-Dawson, & Sherick, 1983; Kazdin, Rodgers, & Colbus, 1986; McCauley, Mitchell, Burke, & Moss, 1988).

Self-Concept Studies

Although Beck's original "cognitive triad" relevant to depression included cognitions about the world and the future in addition to the self, it is probably accurate to say that there is increasing emphasis on the self as the central ingredient of cognitive vulnerability to depression. As we shall see, this applies to other cognitive models besides Beck's, but the section on children's self-views is included here for convenience.

Self-esteem is a cognitive construct of critical importance in depression, referring to an evaluation of the worth of the self. Low self-esteem is not only a significant symptom of the depression syndrome, but it has also been hypothesized to be a cause of depression to the extent that self-blame and feelings of personal powerlessness contribute to the sadness and low arousal characteristic of depression (e.g., Rehm & Naus, 1990). Becker (1979) articulated a contemporary theory of depression based on self-esteem, although the psychoanalytic school had earlier emphasized the depletion of self-worth in depression (e.g., Bibring, 1953). Current models of depression are once again displaying an emphasis on self-processes, evolving from earlier versions of cognitive approaches, and with considerable convergence of perspectives—for example, Beck's self-schema model, the revised hopelessness theory of Abramson et al. (1988), Rehm's memory model with emphasis on self-schema processes (Rehm & Naus, 1990), and the vulnerable self-schema–life event model (e.g.,

Hammen et al., 1989). Such models are fairly well differentiated from each other in the particular form that self-conceptions take and their relation to event and individual content of vulnerable self-regard. However, the different models share a rejection of a global, trait model of self-esteem.

Descriptive studies of children's self-concept have commonly found associations between self-regard and depressed mood (e.g., Asarnow & Bates, 1988; Asarnow et al., 1987; Kaslow, Rehm, & Siegel, 1984; Kazdin et al., 1986; Koenig, 1988; McCauley et al., 1988; McGee, Anderson, Williams, & Silva, 1986; Saylor, Finch, Baskin, Furey, & Kelly, 1984). In an effort to go beyond the trait notions of self-esteem, however, researchers of adult depression have attempted to define and measure the self-schema process. This is an information-processing construct that postulates that self-views are represented in memory as a set of beliefs and propositions. Such schemas then shape the selection, interpretation, and retrieval of information so as to "fit" the preexisting template. A negative self-schema, for instance, guides the biased interpretation of information in a fashion that "confirms" beliefs in one's inadequacy and inefficacy. Initially tested by Kuiper (Derry & Kuiper, 1981; Kuiper & Derry, 1982), performance on an incidental memory task with adults supported the depressive self-schema hypothesis by demonstrating that relatively depressed individuals recalled more self-descriptive adjectives than structurally encoded words and more negative self-descriptive words than did nondepressed individuals. This pattern suggested that the self-schema had facilitated encoding and recall of material even when subjects did not expect to have to recall the adjective stimuli. Some of our own earlier work with depression in adults extended this self-schema approach in various ways (e.g., Hammen, Marks, deMayo, & Mayol, 1985; Hammen, Miklowitz, & Dyck, 1986).

In an effort to explore a specifically stress–diathesis approach to depression integrating both cognitive and environmental factors, we recently undertook a series of studies with adults, testing Beck's (1982) theory of sociotropy/autonomy in which depression can be predicted from the matching of specific types of events and vulnerability of self-worth to specific domains (reviewed in Hammen, in press-c). For instance, individuals who define their worth in terms of their relationships with others and social connectedness would be especially likely to experience depression if negative events occurred in the interpersonal domain. Persons who were especially likely to define themselves in terms of autonomous achievement would be vulnerable to depression if losses or failures occurred in the achievement realms. This approach has proved to be successful in predicting adult depression (e.g., Hammen et al., 1989; Hammen, Marks, Mayol, & deMayo, 1985).

To date, however, there are no specific studies of children's self-schemas and depression. Ours appear to be the only applications of such methods to children, and the results of studies with our high risk sample are reported in a later section.

Depressive Attributional Style

Like Beck's model, the learned helplessness model of depression has undergone several important revisions over time (e.g., Abramson et al., 1978, 1988; Peterson & Seligman, 1984; Seligman, 1975; Seligman et al., 1979). Early varieties of the learned helplessness model emphasized perceptions of noncontingency (helplessness) as a cause of depression. In a related vein, locus of control orientation, a traitlike characteristic capturing individuals' beliefs in internal or external control, was hypothesized to be related to depression.

In the more recent version of the learned helplessness model, the attributional reformulation, vulnerability to depression is seen as arising from a style of explaining the causes of events that emphasizes internal, global, and stable causal attributions for negative outcomes (Abramson et al., 1978). When a negative event occurs, the depressive attributional style leads to the expectation of future uncontrollability of negative events, and such hopeless/helpless cognitions are seen as the precipitant of depressive symptoms. A version of this approach emphasizes depressive attribution style as a vulnerability factor for depression (e.g., Peterson & Seligman, 1984; Seligman et al., 1979).

Initial support for the cognitive aspects of the model came from descriptive studies linking the cognitions with depressive symptoms. For instance, in a meta-analysis of nearly 100 studies, mostly correlational in nature, Benassi, Sweeney, and Dufour (1988) found consistent evidence of an association between beliefs in external locus of control and depression. There is generally support for an association between depression symptoms and depressive explanatory style (e.g., reviews by Peterson & Seligman, 1984; Sweeney, Anderson, & Bailey, 1986). However, both the methods of research and the theory have been criticized on various grounds. Among the concerns raised were the extensive use of largely normal unselected samples, use of measures of attributions about hypothetical rather than actual personally stressful negative events, inconsistent findings, limitations in the scope of the model and the questionable assumption of cross-situational attributional styles (e.g., reviews by Coyne & Gotlib, 1983; Hammen, 1985, 1988a). As we shall see, most of these concerns continue to be relevant to studies of depressive explanatory style in children.

More recent research on the attributional model with adults has attempted to test the crucial etiological hypotheses and the more fully articulated stress–diathesis aspects of the theory. Despite improved design and methods of investigation, including prospective investigations and use of clinical samples, however, there seems to be at best weak evidence of attributional style as a cause of depression in adults (e.g., review by Barnett & Gotlib, 1988). The problem of lack of stability of attribution style also undercuts the theory, in that remitted depressives do not appear to show the allegedly stable explanatory style. Meanwhile, Abramson et al.

(1988) have proposed revisions in the model, including specifying that it may be applicable only to a subset of depressed individuals and that it needs to consider personally significant events and their context and consequences. In short, much like Beck's model, the cognitive approach represented by the attributional model has become narrower in scope and more modest in the role assigned specifically to cognition, while the overall environmental context receives more emphasis.

Studies of Children's Attributional Style and Depression

Some of the earliest learned helplessness–related applications to children involved assessments of locus of control. Investigators found that relatively more depressed children in normal samples displayed more external locus of control construed as helplessness (Lefkowitz & Tesiny, 1980; Roback-Moyal, 1977; Tesiny & Lefkowitz, 1982). Leon, Kendall, and Garber (1980) assessed causal attributions in children and found that relatively more depressed children attributed positive events more to external causes and negative events to internal causes. When the Children's Attribution Style Questionnaire was developed (Seligman et al., 1984), a number of studies demonstrated the predicted association of the negative explanatory style and depressive symptoms (Blumberg & Izard, 1985; Kaslow et al., 1984; Seligman et al., 1984). In clinical samples, similar associations were also observed (Kaslow, Rehm, Pollack, & Siegel, 1988; Saylor, Finch et al., 1984). Interestingly, a study by Benfield et al. (1988) raised the question of whether the negative explanatory style is specific to depression and concluded that it is related to general psychopathology rather than to depression as such. Others, however, have reported that it is specific to depression (Asarnow & Bates, 1988; Kaslow et al., 1988; McCauley et al., 1988). Also, Asarnow and Bates (1988) and McCauley et al. (1988) suggested that the attribution style in children was specific to depressed states and was not present or as notable in remitted depression. Relatively few studies attempted to investigate the family correlates of attribution style. Two studies compared parents' and children's explanatory styles, and while Seligman et al. (1984) reported significant similarity between parents and children, Kaslow et al. (1988) did not find the same pattern.

Only one study was located that tested the role of attribution style as a vulnerability for the onset of depression. In a sample of normal children studied every 3 months for a year, Nolen-Hoeksema, Girgus, and Seligman (1986) observed a significant predictive relationship between prior scores and subsequent depression as well as partial evidence of an interaction between attribution style and negative events to predict depression. Also, children's explanatory style was correlated with teacher ratings and achievement behavior.

The gaps in the research literature on children's negative attribution style include study of the role of such cognitions as a vulnerability factor for later depression in clinical samples, and whether the negative attributions are specific to depressive disorders or general psychopathology. Moreover, there is inconsistency in the findings relevant to acquisition of explanatory style, with mixed findings of similarity between children and their parents. All of these questions are tackled in the present project, and the results are discussed in a later section.

Self-Control Cognitions

Rehm (1977) developed a self-control model of depression, derived from Kanfer's (1970) more general model. It emphasizes self-management skills and is intended to be a broader and more integrative cognitive-behavioral approach to depression than those initially focused largely on cognition or on behavior. Rehm originally proposed that depression often arises from maladaptive cognitions related to self-control, specifically to processes of self-monitoring, self-evaluation, and self-reinforcement. Thus a person who has very high achievement standards, who evaluates her performance as inadequate, or who fails to reward herself for successful achievement would be at risk for depression.

Reviews of research on self-monitoring aspects of the self-control process indicate general support for the idea that depressed adults may selectively attend to negative features of their environments, possibly displaying different criteria for interpreting or recalling positive and negative events (Rehm, 1988). Rehm notes, however, that depressed adults' perceptions may be veridical, because they may indeed be exposed to more negative experiences. Expectancies, self-efficacy, and self-evaluation have been subjected to considerable research. Rehm's review concludes that the expectancies of depressed persons are accurate and equivalent to those of nondepressed persons, but the former appear to set higher standards and thus are more negative in their self-evaluations.

Rehm's most recent speculations about the self-control approach give a central role to negativity about oneself (Rehm & Naus, 1990). Integrating research from a variety of sources on human information processing and memory, Rehm and Naus propose a general model of depression in which information is organized in memory so that emotions associated with the events are also stored with it. Prior experiences with depression are thus associated with events and cognitions that are readily accessible in new depressed states (similar to the model of Teasdale, 1983). Rehm and Naus propose that new models of self-management in depression would need to take into account not only memory-based inference and interpretive processes but social and historical data as well. Such emphases on self-schema processes within a broad social and historical context are compatible with our own approach (Hammen, in press-c).

Children's Self-Control Cognitions

Relatively limited research is available that has tested Rehm's hypotheses, but what there is has been generally supportive. Kaslow et al. (1984) found that relatively depressed children have more negative self-evaluation, lower expectations for performance, more stringent criteria for defining success, and greater likelihood of recommending punishment over reward. In their later study of clinically depressed children, Kaslow et al. (1988) observed that the depressed children had significantly more dysfunctional self-control cognitions than did the normal and nondepressed clinic children.

Cole and Rehm (1986) reported results of an investigation of observed self-control cognitions and behaviors in families of children in treatment for depression or nondepressed disorders and in normal comparison families. The child performed an achievement game called Space Maze while the parents were free to offer feedback and guidance. As predicted, parents of depressed children rewarded their child less than did the parents of nonclinic children (although the effect was statistically significant only for mothers). However, the groups did not differ on expressions of negative affect toward the child. There was no evidence that depressed children rewarded themselves less or punished themselves more. Further, while mothers of depressed children did set high standards for success, so did mothers of nonclinic children; these patterns also occurred in the children themselves, with depressed and nonclinic children displaying high standard setting. The authors interpret the results as partial support for the etiological role of dysfunctional self-regulatory cognitions, acquired in mother–child interactions, in the origin of children's depression.

In our own sample somewhat similar methods and hypotheses were employed to test questions of standard setting and self-evaluation; the results are presented in a later section.

Summary and Gaps in Current Research on Children's Cognitions

The research available on children's depressive cognitions clearly supports the hypothesis that depressive symptoms are accompanied by negativistic ways of construing the self, including negative self-evaluation and self-blaming tendencies. Like adults, relatively dysphoric children appear to selectively focus on self-devaluing and pessimistic content.

Going beyond such descriptive results to speculate about vulnerability to future depression is perilous, however, since speculations are hampered by several methodological and conceptual gaps in the field. Methodologically, much of the children's cognition research lags behind adult depression research in the overreliance on normal samples, cross-sectional designs, and use of questionnaire measures of cognitions. Some of the more recent studies have examined cognitions in clinical samples of children, and yet even that methodological improvement is limited by the problem of comorbidity of symptoms in youngsters. Additional research that separates subgroups of children who differ both on diagnoses and on dysphoric symptoms is necessary to address the issue of the specificity of negative cognitions to depressive symptoms.

Probably the greatest limitation is the dearth of longitudinal designs. The adult research has clearly indicated that most of the measures of depressive cognitions are mood-dependent, suggesting that cognitions are concomitants of the depression syndrome. Thus longitudinal studies are sorely needed to determine whether cognitions play any predictive role in future depression. It would also be useful to study the stability of depressive cognitions and the personal, family, and environmental factors that may be associated with their development and expression. Research on depressive cognitions in children raises unique and intriguing issues about the origin of dysfunctional attitudes and the potential formation of vulnerability schemas. Several of these gaps are addressed in at least a preliminary way in the present research.

Results of the Study

Assessment of Vulnerability Cognitions

There were several methods of assessing potentially important cognitions in the children in our sample, summarized in Table 4.1. Most were derived from theories of adult depression and extended in application and assessment to children. The measures of children's self-concept, testing an aspect of Beck's theory, and attribution style, had been developed by the time the investigation began. Also, it was possible to develop several measures of the self-control constructs based on similar methods reported by Rehm and colleagues. However, measures of the schema construct that had been developed for adults had not yet been applied to children, and therefore preliminary questions about their suitability needed to be addressed.

Developing Measures of Children's Self-Schemas

In a preliminary study based on normal schoolchildren, Hammen and Zupan (1984) explored whether 8- to 12-year-old youngsters would show evidence of a "self" process that was available as an organizing principle to facilitate judgment about personal traits and to facilitate recall. Based on adult research in both cognitive and social psychology, an incidental recall experiment with depressed nonpatient and patient samples had demonstrated that information encoded as self-descriptive facilitated recall compared to information encoded according to structural or semantic

TABLE 4.1. Cognitions relevant to depression vulnerability assessed in current project.

Variable	Procedure/origin
Positive self-schema	Incidental recall task; proportion of positive traits rated as self-descriptive that were recalled of all positive traits administered (from Zupan & Hammen, 1984)
Negative self-schema	Incidental recall task; proportion of negative traits rated as self-descriptive that were recalled of all negative traits administered (from Zupan & Hammen, 1984)
Self-concept	Piers–Harris Children's Self-Concept Test; sum of 80 items (Piers & Harris, 1969)
Negative attributional style	Sum of internal, stable, and global responses to hypothetical negative event items; Children's Attributional Style Questionnaire (Seligman et al., 1984)
Interpersonal/achievement self-schema	Relative proportions of social or achievement content across four tasks of memory for recent events (adapted from Hammen, Marks, Mayol, & deMayo, 1985)
Self-control variables	Questionnaire prior to Achievement task; scales measuring desired and expected performance, standards for success

properties of the words, and that mood state affected the quality of the self-descriptive information recalled (e.g., Derry & Kuiper, 1981; Hammen, Miklowitz, & Dyck, 1986). When the procedure was applied to children, we also found that self-descriptive words were recalled better than words encoded as part of a structural or semantic task (Hammen & Zupan, 1984). This suggested that children as young as 8 can make differentiated judgments about their own characteristics and that such self-related judgments seem to be stored in memory in a way that is consistent with a schema organization. Moreover, there was some evidence that children's current depressed or nondepressed mood state interacted with the judgments, such that more positive moods were associated with recall of more positive self-descriptive traits compared with trait words encoded under structural conditions. Relatively depressed children, on the other hand, did not show better recall of positive self-descriptive adjectives, tending—although not quite statistically significantly—to recall more negative self-descriptive traits.

In the first analysis of the cognitive vulnerability hypothesis tested in the present project, Zupan, Hammen, and Jaenicke (1987) explored the self-schemas of the children using the incidental memory task, based on a subsample of the first 81 children. As predicted, children demonstrated the schema effect, in that self-referent encoding facilitated recall, compared to encoding based on structural, rather than meaning, properties of the trait adjectives. There was also a significant interaction of depression level and recall of self-descriptive adjectives. The more depressed youngsters recalled more of the negative self-referent words than structurally encoded words but did not show the effect for positive self-descriptive adjectives. The nondepressed children showed the opposite effect. The results suggested that depressed children have easy access to negative images of themselves but less access to positive constructions of themselves. These findings are consistent with the information-processing view of depression, which suggests that when depressed, individuals may find themselves locked into a vicious cycle of "depressive" thinking about themselves. Children appear to display the same process even at a young age.

An entirely different approach to assessment of vulnerable self-schemas was based on developments in the adult research on depression that occurred after the present study was under way, testing the interaction of specific areas of vulnerability and specific life events (e.g., Beck, 1982; Hammen et al., 1989; Hammen, Marks, Mayol, & deMayo, 1985). On the basis of methods that Markus originally developed for construing self-schemas (e.g., Markus, 1977), we reasoned that a highly salient value could be inferred as an organizing schema for recalling the content of recent events. The procedure as applied to the children in the study is described more fully in Chapter 2. After interviewing children about specific recent incidents reflecting each of four different themes, all of the memories were coded according to predominance of interpersonal or achievement content. As we had found earlier with college students (Hammen, Marks, Mayol, & deMayo, 1985), most of the youngsters could be classified by a predominant theme. Of the 64 children who provided data for the analyses, 33 had more salient interpersonal content (19 girls and 14 boys), and 31 had more salient achievement content (16 girls and 15 boys). Nine additional children could not be classified because they either could not give examples or gave equal numbers of the two kinds of incidents (Hammen & Goodman-Brown, 1990). Thus the results of the classification suggested that salient values and personally relevant themes can be elicited from children, potentially indicating content areas of vulnerability. Tests of the relationship of the "vulnerable" area to life event occurrence and subsequent depression are reported in a later section on consequences of cognitions.

Overall Comparisons Between Depressed and Nondepressed Children

One of the initial goals of the current project was to characterize the cognitions of relatively depressed and nondepressed children. Then, if the predicted negative cognitions occurred in children as they do in depressed adults, our next aim was to proceed with the exploration of the potential origins and consequences of such cognitions.

Table 4.2 summarizes the children's cognitions, based on groups formed from Children's Depression Inventory scores at the initial family research session. Children scoring 9 or higher ($n = 20$) on the CDI were compared with those scoring below 9. (Table 4.4 presents similar comparisons, based additionally on diagnostic evaluations of depression as well as self-reported CDI; such results are discussed in the section on specificity.)

As seen in Table 4.2, self-schema scores on the incidental memory test of trait adjectives indicated that relatively dysphoric youngsters recalled higher proportions of negative adjectives they had rated as self-descriptive, compared to the nondysphoric children—although the between-group difference was nonsignificant. However, the within-subject comparisons indicated that the relatively depressed children recalled higher proportions of negative than positive self-relevant traits. The nondepressed children did not differ in recall rates for the two kinds of content.

As anticipated, the relatively dysphoric children were significantly more negative in their Piers–Harris self-concept scores. They were also more likely to display negative attribution style on the negative items of the Children's Attribution Style Questionnaire than were nondepressed youngsters. The scales for assessing the self-regulation cognitions prior to the block-stacking achievement task indicated no group differences. To a slight extent, the relatively depressed children expected to perform less well and had slightly higher standards for success than the nondepressed children, but the effects were nonsignificant. There were no differences in depressed and nondepressed children's evaluations of their performances.

TABLE 4.2. Assessment of depressed and nondepressed children on various cognitive variables.

	Group		
Variable	Depressed (CDI > 9)	Nondepressed (CDI < 9)	*t* scores
Incidental momory task			
Percent negative recalled	.45[a]	.32	$t(90) = 1.27$, ns[b]
Percent positive recalled	.27	.33	$t(90) = 1.20$, ns
Piers–Harris self-concept	50.8	68.2	$t(92) = 8.05\ p < .0001$
Children's Attribution Style Questionnaire	9.1	6.1	$t(91) = 4.41, p < .0001$
Self-control congitions			
Aspiration	5.8	5.7	$t(93) = < 1$, ns
Expectation	4.4	4.7	$t(93) = < 1$, ns
Standard for success	7.9	7.7	$t(93) = < 1$, ns
Self-evaluation	3.7	3.6	$t(93) = < 1$. ns

Note: CDI = Children's Depression Inventory.
[a] Within-subject comparisons: depressed group, $t(16) = 1.79$, $p < .05$, one-tailed; nondepressed group, $t(74) < 1$, ns. [b] Between-group comparisons.

Overall, therefore, relatively dysphoric children tended to display more negative cognitions measured in the various ways. The effects were more apparent for the measures of negative cognitions about the self (self-concept, self-schema, and self-blaming tendencies) than they were for self-regulatory cognitions.

Comparisons Between Children in Maternal Groups

A further major question posed in the initial goals of the present investigation was whether children of women with affective disorders would display evidence of vulnerability cognitions. That is, we reasoned that one mechanism for explaining the risk to children for depression is the acquisition of negative cognitions. Thus we predicted that there would be differences in the groups on the indicators of negative cognitions.

Jaenicke et al. (1987) compared children in the four maternal groups. The mean scores and comparisons are reported in Table 4.3. It is apparent that children in the unipolar and bipolar groups have significantly more negative views of themselves than children of medically ill and normal women. The negative self-schema score based on the incidental recall task did not differentiate between the groups, probably because recall of negative traits was relatively infrequent and therefore not a sensitive task for comparison. However, the recall task did indicate that relative absence

TABLE 4.3. Mean scores on cognitive vulnerability by group[a].

Variable	Group				Significant comparisons[b]	
	Unipolar	Bipolar	Medical	Normal		
Piers–Harris self-concept	58.37	60.17	65.00	67.06	1 vs. 3	1 vs. 4
	(10.88)	(14.50)	(9.97)	(10.32)	—	2 vs. 4
Children's Attribution Style Questionnaire negative total	7.58	8.67	6.12	6.33	1 vs. 3	1 vs. 4
	(1.95)	(4.74)	(2.06)	(2.75)	2 vs. 3	—
Negativity self-schema	.09	.09	.06	.07	—	—
	(.10)	(.08)	(.09)	(.12)	—	—
Positivity self-schema	.20	.20	.33	.30	1 vs. 3	1 vs. 4
	(.14)	(.15)	(.20)	(.18)	2 vs. 3	2 vs. 4

Note: Adapted from "Cognitive Vulnerability in Children at Risk for Depression" by C. Jaenicke, C. Hammen, B. Zupan, D. Hiroto, D. Gordon, C. Adrian, and D. Burge, 1987, *Journal of Abnormal Child Psychology*, *15*, 559–572. Copyright 1987 by Plenum Publishing Corporation. Adapted by permission.

[a] Standard deviations are in parentheses. [b] Planned comparisons were conducted between the unipolar group and each of the two nonpsychiatric groups and between the bipolar and nonpsychiatric groups; *ps* < .05, one-tailed.

of a positive self-schema was more characteristic of the unipolar and bipolar group children than of the others. Children in the unipolar and bipolar groups were significantly lower in self-concept and had more negative attribution styles. The effects were especially pronounced for the unipolar group children, who differed from both the normal and medical groups on three of the four measures. Thus there is evidence for more negative cognitions about the self in the offspring of women with affective disorders, and most notably in children of unipolar depressed mothers.

Specificity of Negative Cognitions

The issue of whether negative cognitions are specific to depression in children, or more generally to psychopathology, is a complex one to investigate. As reviewed earlier, studies had compared children with depressive diagnoses to those with other diagnoses, and some found that negative cognitions were elevated only in the depressed groups, whereas others did not find this to be true. However, a child might have a nondepressive diagnosis but also experience significant dysphoric symptoms, and it is very common for children to have concurrent diagnoses of affective and nonaffective disorders. A clear test of the specificity question, therefore, would require samples of children who do not show comorbidity and who also experience (or do not experience) subjective dysphoric symptoms. Thus both diagnostic and current subjective assessments are required. No study to date has reported such a separation of groups to test the specificity question.

In the present sample, we were hampered by a high incidence of comorbidity and, like most such studies, by the fact that subjective depression as measured by the Children's Depression Inventory does not agree entirely with interview-based diagnoses. However, based on presence or absence of current depression diagnoses, or nondepressed diagnoses, along with CDI scores, the following three groups were compared:

1. Children who currently were diagnosed as dysphoric or experiencing a major depressive episode or minor depressive episode, *and* whose CDI score was 9 or higher ($n = 8$).
2. Children who were diagnosed with a nonaffective diagnosis at either a definite or probable level (e.g., conduct disorder, substance use disorder, anxiety disorder) *and* who did not currently have a diagnosable affective disorder as described above, *and* whose CDI score was less than 9 ($n = 9$).
3. Children who had no probable or definite diagnosis of any kind, and whose CDI score was less than 9 ($n = 59$). Children with mixed internalizing and externalizing diagnoses were omitted from the analyses.

Planned comparisons between each of the symptomatic groups and the nonsymptomatic group, and between the depressed and nondepressed

TABLE 4.4. Assessment of depressed, nondepressed, and asymptomatic children on cognitive variables.

Variable	Group: Diagnosed depressed, CDI > 9 (n = 8)	Diagnosed nondepressed, CDI < 9 (n = 9)	No diagnosis, CDI < 9 (n = 59)
Incidental memory task			
Percent negative recalled	.48	.40	.30
Percent positive recalled	.24	.32	.34
Piers–Harris self-concept	50.4[a]	61.0[b]	69.6[c]
Children's Attribution Style Questionnaire	7.6[a]	6.1[a,c]	6.2[b,c]
Self-control cognitions			
Aspiration	6.0	5.4	5.7
Expectation	3.9	4.2	4.7
Standard for success	7.6	7.6	7.8
Self-evaluation	4.0	3.2	3.7

Note: Groups sharing the same superscript are not significantly different.

group, were conducted, and the mean scores for the cognition measures are reported in Table 4.4. The statistical comparisons are, of course, colored by the small sample sizes of the two symptomatic groups. There were no significant differences between the groups on the negative and positive self-schema recall scores, although the means suggest that the depressed children were most negative and least positive. The nondepressed symptomatic children resembled the normal children on the positive self-schema and were midway between the groups on negative self-schema scores.

A similar pattern occurred for the Piers–Harris self-concept scores, indicating that the depressed children were significantly more negative than both the nondepressed and the nonsymptomatic groups, and the nondepressed children were also more negative than the nonsymptomatic children (p values $< .001$). Depressed children were markedly more self-blaming on the attribution style measure than both comparison groups, but the effect attained statistical significance only for the difference between the depressed and normal children. For the self-control cognitions, none of the effects attained significance at the .05 level, although it is noteworthy that the depressed children had higher aspirations and yet lower expectations of success than both the other groups.

Overall, the results suggest that the most depressed children did indeed display the most negative cognitions, and generally more so than the nondepressed but symptomatic children. The latter, however, on several measures displayed some degree of negative views of themselves. Thus it would appear that negative cognitions that reflect self-evaluation are most pronounced in depression, but they are not unique to depression. Children experiencing nonaffective kinds of symptoms tend to view themselves more negatively than do normal children, but not as markedly as do depressed youngsters. There is a suggestion that cognitions reflecting other aspects of the self besides global self-evaluation are more specific to depression. Such measures include the attribution style, positivity of self-schema, and achievement aspiration.

Correlates of Children's Cognitions

How did the children's cognitions arise? What are the origins of depressive views of the self? Questions such as these are central to the understanding of vulnerability to depression from a cognitive perspective. Unfortunately, no definitive answers can be provided in the present study, since we are able only to take a cross-sectional look and did not have the capability of studying the temporal and developmental processes involved in the acquisition of views of the self. It is likely, for instance, that the essential processes begin shortly after birth. Although truly causal processes of the development of cognitions about the self cannot be clarified in the present work, we can at least begin explorations of likely possibilities.

Quality of Mother–Child Relationship

Perhaps one of the most likely possibilities is that views of the self are shaped by the mother–child relationship. There is considerable convergence in emphasis, although not in content or process, among psychodynamic, cognitive social learning, and developmental theorists on the importance of appropriate attachment, separation/individuation, and interaction quality in the formation of views of the worth and competence of the self. Both direct and indirect experiences with the mother can teach the child "you are bad/undesirable/incompetent." A basic question that can be posed within the limitations of the present cross-sectional design concerns the association between current representations of the self and quality of the mother–child relationship.

There are two measures of relationship quality. One is the child's subjective appraisal of the nature of the parent's behavior toward him or her, based on the Parent Perception Inventory (Hazzard et al., 1983). The other consists of direct observation, using scores for maternal criticism from the Conflict Discussion task and the Achievement task. The results of preliminary analyses were reported by Jaenicke et al. (1987). As predicted, there were significant relationships between children's perceptions of overall positivity of the mother's behavior toward them and their self-views. For example, self-concept correlated very highly with positive PPI scores ($r = .72, p < .001$), inversely with negative attribution style ($r =$

$-.38$, $p < .01$), inversely with negative self-schema ($r = -.21$, $p < .07$).

Even more convincing was the finding that the observed higher proportion of maternal criticism in the interaction tasks was associated with more negative self-concept ($r = -.28$, $p < .01$), more negative attribution style ($r = -.34$, $p < .01$), and low positivity of self-schema ($r = -.34$, $p < .01$), and marginally associated with negative self-schema ($r = .23$, $p < .10$). Overall, therefore, it seems that both the child's perceptions of the quality of interaction and the actually observed quality of interaction in terms of maternal criticism were associated with having negative cognitions about the self.

The Environmental Context of Self-Cognitions

A second area of focus concerned the context of children's lives. It was expected that self-views are greatly shaped by the kinds of actual experiences to which the child is exposed, with the likelihood that highly stressful circumstances and unrewarding environments have a negative influence on the child's views of the worth and competence of the self. This topic is an enormously complex one, and well beyond the scope of the current discussion. Again, however, diverse theoretical positions would agree that beliefs in one's worth and competence arise not only in reflections from the mother and significant others but also in mastery or adversity experiences.

Several environmental variables, therefore, were analyzed for their associations with children's cognitions about the self to provide a gross index of the underpinnings of such views. For instance, maternal history of depression was considered an adverse condition likely to affect in various ways the child's views of the self. Lifetime depressive experiences were rated on an overall 7-point scale, capturing relatively mild and transient depressions in the nonpsychiatric women as well as clinical episodes in the women with affective disorders. Overall, Jaenicke et al. (1987) found more severe depressions in the mother were significantly associated with more negative attribution style ($r = .32$, $p < .01$), inversely related to positive self-schema scores ($r = -.30$, $p < .05$), and marginally inversely related to self-concept ($r = -.20$, $p < .10$).

Exposure to ongoing stressful conditions was also hypothesized to be related to children's self-cognitions, in the sense of reducing the likelihood of mastery experiences and creating adverse and demoralizing experiences. Maternal stressful conditions may not only expose the child to negative conditions in the family but might also reduce the availability of the mother as a caretaker. As expected, higher levels of chronic maternal stress (see Chapter 2 for assessment details) were significantly associated with self-concept ($r = .35$, $p < .01$), and less positive self-schemas ($r = .40$, $p < .01$); however, stress was not associated with attribution style or with negative self-schema scores.

As a further examination of the correlates of self-perceptions, we predicted that actual school-related experiences would be associated with self-concept. Children's successes in academic matters, as well as their ability to conduct themselves according to appropriate norms of behavior, are likely to be important determinants of self-perceptions. As expected, there was a strong and significant correlation between the self-concept score and a scaled score of academic performance ($r = .49$, $p < .001$). Similarly, a rating of school behavior (ranging from normal classroom placement and excellent conduct to placement in special classes for behavior problems and expulsion) was also strongly correlated with self-concept ($r = .51, p < .001$). The cognitions assessed by the attribution style questionnaire were also examined; negative attribution tendencies were modestly correlated with school behavior ratings ($r = .27, p < .01$), but academic performance was unrelated to negative attribution style ($r = .13$, $p > .05$). Although the direction of causality cannot be determined, we expect that self-cognitions are both shaped by the rewardingness or adversity of school-related experiences and in turn contribute, in a reciprocal fashion, to behaviors that perpetuate the self-concept.

An additional question of interest was the differences between children who were classified as achievement-vulnerable or interpersonal-vulnerable and those who were "mixed." Using the methods of classification based on memory for recent personally significant events, the groups were compared on the cognitive measures and several demographic and mother–child interaction measures. The children in the groups did not differ in age, and the interpersonal and achievement children were similar in cognitions (positive self-schema, attribution style, and self-concept). However, in comparison with the small subgroup of youngsters who had "mixed" schemas and could not be classified, an interesting pattern emerged. The mixed schema vulnerability children had the lowest self-concept scores (F [2, 79] $= 3.96, p < .05$) and tended to report the most negative interactions with their mothers. When the mother–child interaction data on the Conflict Discussion task were coded to form overall indices of negative and positive quality of interaction, mixed vulnerability children received fewer positive comments and more negative comments from their mothers. A summary score for the balance of negative and positive comments was statistically significant across the groups, $F(2, 51) = 3.50, p < .05$. Also, it appeared that the mixed group children were actually more symptomatic, as viewed by their mothers (significantly lower CBCL Social Competence) and teachers (a nonsignificant trend toward more behavior problems on the Conners Teacher Rating Scale). The mixed vulnerability children were significantly lower functioning on the summary Academic Performance Rating. Although the results cannot clarify the direction of causality, it is intriguing to note that children who are vulnerable in both the achievement and interpersonal domains are apparently struggling in both domains, showing difficulties in their relationships with their mothers and in school functioning.

Similarity of Mother-Child Views of the Self

A third hypothesis regarding the acquisition of vulnerable cognitions is that children are learning from modeling. For instance, a depressed mother might exhibit self-deprecating cognitions or views of the world that the child observes and then applies to himself or herself. We did not administer cognitive measures to the mothers in the study and therefore do not have direct ways of comparing mothers' and children's cognitions. However, Jaenicke et al. (1987) reviewed the observation data for the mother–child interactions to see if mothers and children showed similar tendencies to make self-blaming remarks. The correlations between the two were nonsignificant. On the other hand, there was a strong association between children's self-critical commments in the Conflict task and maternal criticism ($r = .51$, $p < .0001$). Jaenicke et al. also found that maternal criticism in the observation task was significantly associated with children's self-blaming style on the attribution style measure ($r = .42$, $p < .001$). Rather than acquisition through observational learning, a more direct explanation is that maternal criticism causes children's self-critical remarks. Obviously, this causal explanation requires confirmation in a non–cross-sectional design.

The most direct opportunity to observe similarity of mother and child cognitions was the block-stacking achievement task. Children and their mothers were given questionnaires before and after the block-stacking task, assessing their aspirations, expectations, and standards for success. There were no significant correlations between mothers' and childrens' cognitions on these measures. Nor were there similar cognitions for mothers and children in the separate subgroups of depressed and nondepressed children, or across maternal groups. Thus the present study offers little evidence that children acquire their mothers' standards for self-regulatory cognitions.

Consequences of Negative Cognitions in Children

Hypotheses of the cognitive vulnerability approach to depression were tested in several ways in the present study. The longitudinal design offers an opportunity for a true test of whether cognitions at one point in time are associated with onset of depression at a later point. Few of the studies of cognitions in depressed children to date have tested the etiological aspects of the cognitive vulnerability models.

All of the analyses were conducted in the context of a stress-diathesis version of the cognitive model. That is, it was assumed that whatever cognitions might be relevant to depression require activation by a stressful condition. For those who are not vulnerable, stressors might give rise to mild or transitory symptoms, but for those who are vulnerable, the occurrence of a negative event gives rise to dysfunctional interpretations of the meaning and consequences of the event, and it is these negative thoughts that are considered to be the cause of depression.

Attribution Style

The first such study tested the hypothesized role of negative attribution style. As noted earlier, the reformulated attribution model of depression had been extended to children, with the prediction that the tendency to make internal, global, and stable causal attributions for negative outcomes would serve as a vulnerability factor for depression. Hammen, Adrian, and Hiroto (1988) undertook the analyses for a special issue on attributions and depression for the *British Journal of Clinical Psychology*. Stressful life events and symptoms were assessed during the first 6-month follow-up, using procedures described in Chapter 2. Nearly one-third of the children in the sample had diagnosable symptoms during that period, consisting either of new onsets or continuing conditions—either depressive or nondepressive disorders. Children's outcomes were assessed using two methods: the Children's Depression Inventory score at the follow-up, and diagnostic status as scaled on a 4-point scale. The latter scale was used to separately rate depressive disorders and nondepressive disorders (substance use, conduct disorders, anxiety disorders). A stressful life event score was computed for each child based on the objective threat totals from the life stress interviews. All events in the 6-month period were counted, unless they occurred after the onset of symptoms (in which case

Table 4.5. Hierarchical multiple regressions to predict diagnostic status in 6-month follow-up–Piers-Harris Self-Concept scores.

Predictor variable	R^2 change	Standardized regression coefficient	t[a]	p
Prediction of diagnosable depression				
Initial diagnosis	.25	.50	5.02	.0001
Piers-Harris self-concept	.04	−.22	2.12	.04
Stress threat	.06	.26	2.59	.01
Threat × self-concept	.01	.79	1.16	ns
Multiple $R = .60$, $F(4, 72) = 10.35$, $p < .0001$				
Children's Depression Inventory	.06	.24	2.16	.03
Piers-Harris self-concept	.07	−.48	2.52	.01
Stress threat	.12	.35	3.36	.011
Threat × self-concept	.02	1.01	1.37	ns
Multiple $R = .52$, $F(4, 72) = 6.60$, $p < .0001$				
Prediction of nonaffective diagnosis				
Initial (nonaffective) diagnosis	.33	.57	6.06	.0001
Piers-Harris self-concept	.00	−.04	.40	ns
Stress threat	.03	.20	1.97	.05
Threat × self-concept	.08	−2.10	3.33	.001
Multiple $R = .67$, $F(4, 72) = 14.64$, $p < .0001$				

Note: From "Self-Cognitions, Stressful Events, and the Prediction of Depression in Children of Depressed Mothers" by C. Hammen, 1988, *Journal of Abnormal Child Psychology, 16*, 347–360. Copyright 1988 by Plenum Publishing Corporation. Reprinted by permission.
[a] t-test for increment in R^2 after control for previously entered variables.

only those events rated as "independent" were included so as to exclude those possibly due to the child's symptoms). The hypothesis of cognitive vulnerability was tested with hierarchical multiple regressions, entering initial symptom rating first, followed by negative attribution style score, then total life event score, and then the interaction of attribution style and event score. Contrary to prediction, neither attribution style alone nor its interaction with stress made a significant incremental contribution to the prediction of depression (although both initial symptoms and stress total were significant predictors of the overall multiple R of .56). The same analyses, using CDI scores instead of diagnostic ratings, yielded similar results. On the other hand, unexpectedly, the prediction of *non-depressive* disorders did include the interaction of stress and attribution style as a significant contribution (incremental R^2 = .06, overall R^2 = .40). Inspection of the interaction suggested that negative attribution style increased the child's likelihood of having a nondepressive diagnosis only when coupled with high stress.

Overall, the results do not support the typical predictions of the attributional model of depression. Yet the negative explanatory style may have some relevance as a vulnerability marker for other kinds of children's outcomes. Since children often have multiple diagnoses, often mixtures of both internalizing and externalizing disorders, further studies in carefully composed diagnostic groups need to be undertaken to explore this finding.

Negative Self-Cognitions

The analyses reported by Hammen, Adrian, and Hiroto (1988) clearly indicate that children's stress is predictive of changes in symptomatology but suggest that attribution style is not predictive of vulnerability to depression as such. In a further test of prediction of depression, Hammen (1988b) performed similar analyses of follow-up symptoms and stress, using different markers of cognitive vulnerability, the self-concept score based on the Piers–Harris measure, and the positive self-schema score based on the incidental memory task. Results of the self-concept score as a vulnerability marker are reported in Table 4.5.

As indicated, stress and self-concept scores both make significant incremental contributions to the prediction of changes in children's depression over time (controlling for initial symptoms). The interaction term does not add significantly, suggesting the additive effect of the two variables. Moreover, although self-concept did not directly predict nondepressive diagnoses, the interaction of self-concept and stress did. As with the attribution style score noted previously, the effect of negative cognitions is relatively unimportant for nondepressed outcomes, except when negative cognitions encounter high levels of stress. Both studies suggest that depressive outcomes are associated with stress, but nondepressive outcomes are associated only with the high stress–high vulnerable cognition combination. In addition, subsequent depression is associated with lower initial self-concept.

Hammen (1988b) also found that the positive self-schema score was not a reliable vulnerability marker for subsequent depression. It is possible that the psychometric properties of the measure reduce its sensitivity. An even more likely possibility is that it is a marker of the depressed state, having limited predictive power. Studies of the incidental memory task of self-schema for adults, as well as investigations of attribution style in adults, have strongly suggested that these measures capture current depression rather than underlying vulnerability (e.g., Hamilton & Abramson, 1983; Hammen, Miklowitz, & Dyck, 1986; Hammen, Marks, deMayo, & Mayol, 1986).

The success of a self-concept measure as an indicator of cognitive vulnerability to depression requires that it also not be merely a measure of depression. Certainly low self-esteem is one of the symptoms of depression, so the two constructs overlap in that way. It is also true that several of the items of the Piers–Harris self-concept test appear to be mood symptoms. Factor analyses provided by the authors indicate an anxiety cluster and a happiness–satisfaction cluster, while the remaining items appear to be more specific to children's behaviors and attributes. Therefore, the analyses were recomputed, omitting the items in the two clusters from the total self-concept score. Results were virtually the same as with the original total self-concept score (see Hammen, 1988b). Therefore, it appears that a relatively enduring (not merely mood-specific) self-concept captures cognitions about the self that represent vulnerability to develop depression. The present analysis looked only at a 6-month period, and since it was based on a sample of children at risk (who mostly experienced some stressors), it remains to be seen whether similar results would occur in other populations and over longer periods. It is also noteworthy that by far the greatest predictor of symptoms was prior level of symptoms. Self-concept made a significant incremental contribution, but in clinical terms the implications are clear: past depression is an enormous vulnerability factor for later symptoms. Cognitions may be a part of this predictive package, but a host of additional possibilities, such as genetic susceptibility, acquired biological vulnerability, and other psychosocial factors, are also likely to be important risk predictors. As noted earlier, the adult depression field has begun to grapple more fully with the inadequacies of overly broad and inclusive cognitive models (e.g., Barnett & Gotlib, 1988; Hammen, in press-c, 1990-a).

Vulnerability to Specific Stressful Events

In addition to the shortcomings of cognitive models that stem from mood-dependent measures and overly broad inclusion, a further difficulty is apparent. Despite being called stress–diathesis approaches, most of the cognitive models had offered little conceptualization of the role of stressful events in triggering depressive reactions. By the same token, most of the life stress researchers had generally paid only obligatory attention to perceptions and appraisal processes in the stressful event–depression relationship (see Hammen, 1988a). Several years ago an effort was made by Beck (1982) to integrate life stress and psychodynamic formulations with a cognitive perspective, in predicting that two kinds of vulnerability to depression can be separated—one associated with depletion of the self stemming from interpersonal loss, conflict, or inadequacy, and the other resulting from failure or blockage in the autonomy or achievement domain. Hammen and Goodman-Brown (1990) extended the formulation to include the children in the current project. Using methods described earlier for characterizing each participants' most salient/vulnerable areas, we next identified those children who had or had not experienced a significant change in depressive symptoms during the first follow-up. Thirteen youngsters did become more depressed, as indicated by clinical interviews, and 51 of the other available children did not. Stressful life events that occurred prior to the symptom onset or change were noted (and for the youngsters who did not become depressed all their events in the 6-month period were included). The events were characterized according to their predominant content, as interpersonal or achievement events. The predominant event content in the period of observation was noted, and its "match" with the child's schema subtype, based on earlier classification, was determined. That is, a child who had given predominantly interpersonal examples to the schema task described earlier was considered "interpersonally vulnerable," and if he or she also experienced a predominance of interpersonal events, compared to achievement events, during the follow-up observation period, a "match" was said to occur.

A chi-square analysis of depressed–nondepressed by event matching–not matching indicated a significant effect. Children who became depressed were significantly more likely to have experienced more of the events that were congruent with their vulnerability type than noncongruent events, while youngsters who did not become depressed were equally likely to have had more congruent or noncongruent events. Unfortunately, the sample size of the children with depression onsets was too small to evaluate the effect separately for the two schema subtypes. However, it appeared that children who were most likely to become depressed were in the "interpersonal" schema group. Also, interpersonal events were much more likely to occur than were achievement events.

Such patterns require further study to determine whether it is simply more difficult to detect the "matching" effect for achievement because of the prominence of negative interpersonal events, or whether interpersonal events simply are more significant in their impact on children than they are for some adults. However, these preliminary findings suggest that children have begun to form views of themselves that invest particular importance and meaning in specific areas. It would prove to be very interesting to explore the origins, processes, and stability of these areas of potential vulnerability in children. These preliminary results also reinforce our efforts to more fully integrate the occurrence of stressful life events in formulations of depression, increasing our ability to predict the when and where of depressive reactions.

Summary and Directions for Further Research

Depressive cognitions in children parallel those reported for adult samples and indicate that the depressive experience is not only a mood disorder but also one defined by gloomy and self-deprecatory thinking. Results from the present study extended findings based on earlier, mostly cross-sectional analyses of normal children. We found that processes consistent with a self-schema organization can be observed even in young children, suggesting at least that to someone in a negative mood state, relatively self-deprecating cognitions come to mind and are available in memory. Moreover, negative cognitions about the self as represented in a global self-concept score were a risk factor, along with stressful life events, for subsequent increases or onsets of depression. Contrary to prediction, however, negative attribution style did not predict subsequent depression. There was some observation of specificity of negative cognitions for depressive symptoms, but this matter requires further study. It was also observed that negative cognitions were not universally associated with exposure to depressed mothers, as might be implied by a simple observational learning model of acquisition, but more specifically were related to relatively negative quality of mother–child interaction and to maternal depression history and chronic stress. Such results are consistent with views that emphasize both parent–child attachment quality and environmental conditions in the formation of vulnerability to depression.

From the point of view of an information-processing perspective on depressive cognitions, the appearance of self-devaluing and pessimistic thoughts in children may merely be the tip of pernicious psychological iceberg. Negative cognitions may signal an underlying self-representation that is highly attuned to congruent negative information and resistant to input that does not confirm self-devaluing thoughts. If we find that self-schemas form early and perpetuate themselves, especially if reinforced by difficult life circumstances, we would expect them to exert considerable impact on subsequent development. Negative views of the self and of the future may serve to diminish a child's effort, persistence, and coping capabilities in the face of challenges. Moreover, our present research on children's cognitions in the context of high risk family environments suggests that negative views of the self probably indicate difficult life situations including dysfunctional parent–child relationships and ongoing stressful conditions. Such surrounding circumstances contribute to the likelihood of self-perpetuating dysfunction in the child. Thus research with children cannot afford to overlook the context and consequences of cognitions, because of the high potential for a vicious cycle of maladaptation.

Exploration of cognitive hypotheses of vulnerability to depression in child populations lags behind studies with adult samples in both conceptualization and methodology. Not only is there catching up to do, but, ironically, studies of children offer unique but untapped opportunities not available in studies of depressed adults. Three areas that seem especially fruitful for further exploration in juvenile samples concern content, operation, and acquisition of cognitive vulnerability for depression.

Content of Cognitive Vulnerability

One issue is the specificity of the cognition–depression link. The specificity issue goes to the heart of the question of why some children develop depression and others develop different disorders. Under what conditions do children develop depressive reactions, in contrast with externalizing disorders, or even other internalizing disorders such as anxiety states? Research from the current project, as well as a review of existing studies, suggests that self-deprecatory cognitions are most pronounced in depressed children but are not unique to such youngsters, occurring also in children with externalizing disorders. There may be particular kinds of self-relevant cognitions associated with depression, or self-critical and self-devaluing beliefs might be particularly prominent. The present research suggests that not global views but particular domains of self-evaluation might be especially vulnerable. Obviously the specificity question is related to a more general etiological question of whether cognitions play a role in the onset of depression compared to other disorders, and under what conditions might cognitions lead to depression if other risk factors are also present? Moreover, further studies of self-representation in children might contribute to the understanding of disorders besides depression.

Operation and Mechanisms of Vulnerability Schemas

Related to the specificity question is the matter of the process and mechanisms of cognitive vulnerability. The current research reports findings compatible with the stress–diathesis approach, indicating that the combination of stressors and vulnerable cognitions is relevant to depression. The results heighten our interest in the relationship between stressors and vulnerability but shed little light on the actual activation of vulnerability and processing of information leading to depressive reactions. Considerable further work is needed to clarify such mechanisms (see also Segal, 1988).

Such studies should also address the issue of the continuity of mild and major depressive experiences as well as that between childhood and adult experiences of depression. One of the most robust findings in adult depression is that the best predictor of future depression is past depression, and the implications of this pattern for the study of children are enormous. Several perspectives are currently available to guide future research. In one model, Teasdale (1983; Teasdale & Dent, 1987) suggested that depressive cognitions are acquired through learning, and that life circumstances shape the extent to which dysphoric states are accompanied by self-deprecation and other depressive cognitions. For instance, a critical parent, or the absence of a comforting adult who provides encouragement, may contribute to the availability and impact of negative cognitions during a dysphoric state. Associated in memory with depressed mood, such negative cognitions may be activated along with the mood, and may serve to intensify or prolong dysphoric states. For such children, even mild or typical failure, loss, or disappointment experiences might increase the availability of negative cognitions, thereby affecting the severity of symptoms.

Another model, represented by Cicchetti and Schneider-Rosen (1986), emphasizes the effect of depressive experiences as interfering with normal development. As each stage of development provides competencies that are integrated into later structures, conditions that interfere with adaptation at one level may have considerable impact for subsequent development. The authors provide a complex and rich array of speculations about the implications of depression for later development, integrating biological, cognitive, and environmental variables. An even more biological model, such as that of Gold, Goodwin, and Chrousos (1988) emphasizes the role of early traumatic experiences on alterations of the brain, such that childhood depressive reactions may alter later biologically based stress reactivity. Cognitive processes are seen as mediating the impact of stressors on the sensitized maladaptive biological system.

All of these models propose a way of viewing depression as an experience that alters the likelihood of future depression. Although additional research is needed to verify the hypothesis of continuity between childhood and adult depression, it is highly likely that cognitions mediate the effects of early depressive experience on subsequent vulnerability. Studies of the organization and differentiation of mood–cognition linkages, and the processes by which stored cognitive representations are activated, are sorely needed to understand both normal and dysfunctional development.

Acquisition of Cognitive Vulnerability to Depression

The acquisition of vulnerability cognitions raises important questions for both normal and dysfunctional development. How and when are schemas regarding the self formed? What role might dysfunctional self-views play in children's development? The present work suggests in part that children seem to process information in a way consistent with the operation of a self-schema from a young age (as young as 8, as studied in our samples). However, it is not clear how stable such mechanisms are, or exactly how malleable or selective they might be. Cognitive vulnerability processes depend on the structure and content of memory organization (e.g., Dent & Teasdale, 1988; Rehm & Naus, in press; Teasdale, 1983; Teasdale & Dent, 1987).

It would be of interest to consider the developmental progression of differentiation of self-evaluative processes (e.g., Leahy, 1985b) with particular reference to depressive content (see also Digdon & Gotlib, 1985). To what extent do both normal and high risk children acquire positive as well as negative self-views, how can the diversity and flexibility of such self-images in terms of particular domains be assessed, and what are their correlates? Moreover, the inference processes that children use with respect to the self change over the different age periods. For instance, Leahy (1985b; Leahy & Shirk, 1985) proposed a structural-deveopmental theory linking conceptions of the self to cognitive development (see also Cicchetti & Schneider-Rosen, 1986). Early self-schemas are hypothesized to form at the preoperational level, and negative self-views may therefore be characterized by an all-or-nothing quality and an inability to refocus on disconfirming positive information that would modify the content of the self-schema. Additional cognitive skills acquired over time may accentuate the child's self-critical thinking. Leahy's (1985a) model includes Beck's self-schema notions of depression, integrated with cognitive-developmental theory. Further research within the framework of such an integrated approach not only would help to characterize the acquisition and operation of self-schemas and dysfunctional inferences in children but would also contribute to the understanding of adult depressive thinking.

Issues of the acquisition of vulnerability processes also include research on the context in which such processes develop. Our study emphasized the role of parent–child interactions and quality of communication in self-schema formation and suggested that the interaction quality itself is affected by background factors that include characteristics of the parents as well as the current environment as it impinges on the family. Such context also includes the child's own stressors, as well as academic and social functioning. Children are likely to acquire further information, whether distorted or veridical, about their competence and worth through observation of their functioning in a variety of circumstances that are important to them.

5
Family Stress

It is of course a truism that when bad things happen to people, people feel bad. But the obviousness and simplicity of this statement belie interesting and puzzling complexities. There is disagreement about what "stress" means, and in many ways it is simply a shorthand term to describe a variety of conditions that tax people's coping capabilities—even though each separate type of circumstance may elicit its own complex responses. In the families we studied, there were horrific events—violent abuse, death, suicide, molestation—as well as countless personal and domestic adversities that are the normative, if unwelcome, aspects of living. And yet some people become very depressed while others do not, even when very troubling events occur. Some people appear to become depressed from events that others may find relatively trivial. Events themselves do not necessarily happen by fate; sometimes it appears that individuals may instigate or contribute to the occurrence of negative events. Not only must we consider significant episodic events that happen with a definite beginning, but we must also investigate the role of ongoing chronic strains. Every individual and family experience recurring or continuing challenges in certain realms, such as financial security or quality of relationships.

From such observations, certain questions arise that have yet to be answered with certainty by research: Why do some people become depressed by stressors when others do not? Are there ways of understanding events that have unique significance to individuals, whose occurrence would cause particular vulnerability? Can we detect individuals who seem to play a role in the happening of negative events? Are there characteristics of families that seem to create additional exposure to stressful conditions? What about people who are already chronically burdened by continuing stressful conditions: Are such stressors also likely to contribute to depression, and how do chronic stressors and episodic events relate to each other? What about children's reactions to stress in their families? What about children's own stressful events and circumstances: Are there particular vulnerabilities? What are children's reactions?

The families in this study present an enormously challenging context to initiate exploration of these and related questions. For one thing, most of these families have built-in stressors in the form of chronic illness, either psychiatric disorders that recur or medical ailments that require ongoing care. Additional families, even without ongoing illness, faced ongoing severe marital, occupational, or financial problems. Many of the women in the study were divorced, raising families by themselves or with limited assistance. Altogether, the challenges faced by many of the women in the study are staggering, and our goal of attempting to determine the role of stress as a cause and a consequence of psychiatric impairment in mothers and children can only partly do justice to the magnitude of the problems faced by the families.

A second major challenge of the present population of families is simply that: They are families. The vast majority of research on stress and depression focuses on individuals. Although the stressful events they experience sometimes concern family members, the orientation is toward the person studied outside of the family context. The limitations of such a strategy are even more glaring in the case of children. The present study not only attempts to examine the effects of stressors on individuals but also considers that the reactions and symptoms of mothers and children may themselves prove to be stressors for the others in the family. Moreover, since the investigation is longitudinal, we attempted to capture some idea of changes and processes over time, including the potential "causal" relationship between characteristics of the person (including symptoms) and events.

Before turning to the analyses and results of our investigation, a brief review is presented of research on stress and depression, for adults and children. Then some of the gaps in the field are noted, including methodological limitations and conceptual shortcomings. Together, the findings and the limitations set the stage for the issues and methods pursued in the present investigation.

Stress and Depression

Stress and Depression in Adults

Reviews of research on the association between stress and depression have consistently found significant links between the variables, in community samples and in patients (e.g., reviews by Billings & Moos, 1982; Lloyd, 1980; Thoits, 1983). Refinements in methods and samples over the years have led to increasingly more focused conclusions: depression is especially linked to negative events, to major events with long-term threat consequences, to social exits (and to losses and other disruptions of interpersonal functioning), and to personally meaningful events (e.g., Barnett & Gotlib, 1988; Brown & Harris, 1978; Hammen, 1988a; Paykel,

1979). Moreover, we have begun to learn that different kinds of samples may show different stress–depression relationships. Thus, for example, much of the association of stress and symptoms may be contributed by those with prior depression or chronic symptoms, and the responses of the different samples may differ in magnitude and duration of depression and respond to stressors of differing magnitudes (e.g., Depue & Monroe, 1986; Goplerud & Depue, 1985; Hammen, Mayol, et al., 1986; Lewinsohn et al., 1988). In a related vein, there is increasing recognition of the need to differentiate between stress and its association with different aspects of depression: onset, maintenance, relapse, and recovery.

Some of the best-developed programs of research on stress–depression relationships involve large-scale studies of community residents, followed over time, with clinical evaluations of their status. The work of three investigators will be briefly noted as examples of emergent findings and recommendations. The English sociologist George Brown and his colleagues have provided the most intensive study of stress–depression relationships, based on extensive interviews of event occurrence in the context of the person's life. Initially, Brown and Harris (1978) found that onsets of clinically significant depression in women were typically preceded by events considered severe in impact. Subsequently, such results were replicated (e.g., Brown, Bifulco, & Harris, 1987), with the further refinements that risk for depression was increased when the event was a loss experience or was linked to an ongoing difficulty (somewhat analogous to a chronic strain). Moreover, Brown and colleagues found that negative self-evaluation, which they believe is associated with early childhood deprivation experiences and results from the presence of demoralizing chronic stressors, further increases the likelihood of depression associated with major life events (see also Brown, Bifulco, Harris, & Bridge, 1986). Although requiring replication in independent studies, the work of Brown is especially rich in hypotheses linking developmental experiences that underlie vulnerability with adult psychosocial experiences. His analyses also include speculations and preliminary data on individuals' tendencies to involve themselves in maladaptive environments (Bifulco, Brown, & Harris, 1987) suggestive of self-perpetuating patterns of distress–life events.

The research of Moos and colleagues has used a variety of questionnaire measures of stressors, chronic conditions, resources, and symptoms, supporting the link between depression (including relapse/recurrence) and stressors (e.g., Billings & Moos, 1984, 1985b). A recent longitudinal study is noteworthy for illustrating such associations, indicating that negative life events contribute to changes in symptoms, while self-confidence and other protective factors such as family support were negatively related to symptoms (Holahan & Moos, 1987). This study is additionally noteworthy because it examined the impact of parental life events and functioning on children's outcomes. Holahan and Moos found that 1-year follow-up changes in children's psychological adjustment were not related to parental life events but were significantly associated with maternal depression and negatively related to family support.

The work of Lewinsohn and colleagues, also using a community sample, included not only questionnaire assessments but diagnostic evaluation of depression. Among the many variables included in the longitudinal research, life stress appeared to be a predictor of the onset (or recurrence) of major or minor depression; twice as many individuals experiencing high levels of stress became depressed as those who experienced low levels (Lewinsohn, Hoberman, & Rosenbaum, 1988). Prior depression, being female, and elevated depression levels were additional predictors of onset of depression. Lewinsohn, Zeiss, and Duncan (1989) speculate that it is exposure to stressful life events, rather than simply enduring personal traits, that explains why some individuals become depressed, or have depression relapses, compared to others. Lewinsohn challenges researchers to pursue questions such as why women are especially likely to relapse compared to men, and what accounts for sustained susceptibility to relapse after a first episode (e.g., Lewinsohn et al., 1989).

A relatively new entry in the stress–depression arena is the study of stressors and episodes of bipolar affective disorder. A few retrospective cross sectional analyses suggested that, at least for initial episodes of the disorder, stress appeared to play some triggering role (e.g., Ambelas, 1979; Bidzinska, 1984; Kennedy et al., 1983). Recently, our research group reported results of one of the few longitudinal studies of bipolar patients, which found a significant association between relapse or recurrence and high levels of stressful life events (Ellicott et al., 1990). Such findings indicate a need for further examination of the role of stressors in both unipolar and bipolar patients, rather than relegating manic depression to the biological realm of allegedly "endogenous" episodes.

In addition to the methodological and empirical improvements in the field in recent years, there have been important gains in the conceptualization of the stress–depression relationship. More and more, investigators have converged in the view that cognitions about events—not simply events impinging on individuals—determine the responses to the circumstances. Events must be perceived as threats, losses, or as somehow meaningful, and the appraisal processes that lead to such interpretations may be determined both by the actual situation and by historical-psychological characteristics of the person (e.g., Beck, 1982; Brown & Harris, 1978; Hammen, 1988a; Lazarus & Folkman, 1983). Proposed mechanisms for characterizing and explaining cognitive vulnerability—and its role in stress-diathesis approaches to depression—were discussed in Chapter 2 and elsewhere (e.g., Alloy, 1988; Hammen, 1988a). Recently, in the context of our cognitive-environmental perspective on depression (Hammen, in press-c) we have hypothesized and tested a model of stress-reactivity that explicitly integrates stressful life event and cognition perspectives. Borrowing both from psychodynamic and cognitive formulations of distinctive depressions associated either with autonomous/self-critical or sociotropic/dependent themes (e.g., Arieti & Bemporad, 1980; Beck, 1982; Blatt, Quinlan, Chevron, Mcdonald, & Zuroff, 1982), we predicted that depression would occur only when the event content matched the vulnerability type. We speculated that domains of the self that represent the person's source of self-worth are also the region of vulnerability if that realm is threatened by loss or depletion. Hence a person may construe herself to be worthwhile and competent to the degree that she is successful and independent in her work, but job failure triggers cognitions about diminished self-worth, leading to depression. For the same person a divorce, on the other hand, may be an unsettling and unhappy event but only temporarily or mildly depressing to the individual to the extent that she does not construe her worth in terms of adequate and continuous intimate connections with someone. Support for the proposed life event–vulnerability congruence hypothesis has been reported in a longitudinal study of college students (Hammen, Marks, Mayol, & deMayo, 1985) and unipolar depressed outpatients (Hammen et al., 1989).

An additional line of research with promising conceptual contributions concerns the role of interpersonal functioning in depression. Although not, strictly speaking, in the tradition of life stress research, recent emphases on the interpersonal dysfunctions of depressed individuals warrant consideration in this context. The work of Coyne (e.g., Coyne, Kahn, & Gotlib, 1987; Coyne, Kessler, et al., 1987) is especially noteworthy for its emphasis on the responses of others to the depressed person. Depressed individuals appear to elicit reactions from others that, at least eventually, are negative and thereby may contribute to the further symptomatology of the depressed individual. Barnett and Gotlib (1988) recently reviewed research on interpersonal functioning of depressed persons and concluded that dependency and introversion, low social integration, and marital distress are found to be common in depressed persons. Such interpersonal deficiencies may in part be consequences of depression, but they may also characterize qualities of the person that disrupt relationships with others. Thus symptoms, attributes, and behaviors of the depressed or depression-vulnerable person might actually contribute to the occurrence of negative interpersonal stressors that in turn intensify depression. To the degree that individuals may attach interpretations of self-worth and efficacy to their functioning in interpersonal relationships, experiences of conflict, disruption, dissatisfaction, and loss are construed as personal depletions leading to depression. The interpersonal, life event, and cognitive approaches are thus clearly complementary and compatible.

A more complete discussion of the theories and findings of contemporary life event research is beyond the scope of this discussion. However, in a later section a brief review of conceptual gaps in the field sets the stage for some of the research that was conducted in the present study.

Stress and Depression in Children

Following the lead of researchers of adult illness and psychopathology, the study of associations between stressors and symptoms in children has expanded greatly in the past few years. A variety of investigations have reported significant associations between stressors and negative outcomes, including behavioral symptoms, somatic and physical ailments, and non-specific distress symptoms (reviewed in Adrian, 1988). Only a portion of the research, however, has investigated depression symptoms—and to date virtually no such research exists on diagnosed clinical depression in youngsters. The studies that exist, nevertheless, find significant associations between depression or internalizing symptoms and negative life events in cross sectional studies based on retrospective reporting; Pearson correlations typically range between .20 and .30 across studies of both children and adolescents (reviewed by Compas, 1987). On the other hand, results are less clear in the relatively few prospective studies, most of which are based on adolescents rather than younger children (see Compas, 1987). Some found no relationship when initial symptoms are controlled (e.g., Swearingen & Cohen, 1985; Wagner, Compas, & Howell, 1986), although three did find the expected association (e.g., Cohen, Burt, & Bjork, 1987; Compas, Howell, Phares, Williams, & Giunta, 1989; Compas, Wagner, Slavin, & Vanatta, 1986). Interestingly, several found that symptoms are better predictors of subsequent events, rather than the reverse (Compas et al., 1986; Swearingen & Cohen, 1985; Wagner et al., 1986).

In addition to research on the impact of heterogeneous accumulations of stressors, other lines of investigation have examined the consequences of specific stressful events. Large bodies of research exist, for example, on the effects of divorce or marital conflict on children, or starting school, chronic physical illness, and the like—not to mention studies of the effects of single-parenting, stepparenting, maternal employment, child abuse, teen-age parenting, and other reflections of domestic strain. Although beyond the scope of the current discussion, such studies remind us to attend to the varieties of mediating factors that create risk, but also resilience, in children exposed to such adverse outcomes (e.g., Compas, 1987; Felner, Gillespie, & Smith, 1985; Garmezy & Rutter, 1983).

Studies of Parental Stress and Symptoms Related to Child Outcomes

It is somewhat ironic that although research on children at risk because of parental psychopathology provides an opportunity to explore the effects of stressful conditions on children, relatively little of this research has explored these factors as such. One exception from the Weissman offspring study (Fendrich, Warner, & Weissman, 1990) found that certain family stressors, such as marital difficulties, are predictive of children's diagnoses.

However, despite the relatively little direct exploration of stress factors in families of parents with affective disorders, several studies have explored the effects of parental symptoms as a stressor having an impact on children or the joint effects of parental stressors and parental symptoms. The work of Rutter and colleagues (e.g., Rutter & Quinton, 1984) admirably illustrates the complexities of attempting to disentangle various adverse conditions that typically coexist in families with parental psychiatric disturbance. The work suggests, however, that the impact of exposure to psychiatric disorder was greatly intensified in the presence of marital discord and hostility, and where at least one parent showed personality disorder in the form of disturbance of interpersonal functioning. These results suggest that multiple stressful conditions accompanying parental psychiatric disturbance contribute to children's negative outcomes.

Billings and Moos (1983) demonstrated in their follow-up of depressed patients that the children of parents treated for depression were likely to experience adjustment problems, and that if the depressed parent also faced high levels of stressful life events, the rates of child disorder were significantly higher (see also Daniels, Moos, Billings, & Miller, 1987, for similar outcomes for children with rheumatic disease exposed to parents with depression and high life stress). Several other investigations of women experiencing highly adverse conditions such as marital disruption, immigration status, and poverty—while also raising young children—similarly indicate that both maternal depression and highly stressful life circumstances were predictive of disturbances in their young children (Fergusson, Horwood, Gretton, & Shannon, 1985; Longfellow & Belle, 1984; Pound et al., 1985; Williams & Carmichael, 1985).

Recently, well-developed methods for studying stress in children and adolescents have been employed by Compas, Howell, Phares, Williams, and Ledoux (1989). Their emphasis on the transactional nature of stress processes led them to study the reciprocal patterns of symptoms and stressors in families, between parents and children. Although their recent cross-sectional study included behavior problems (rather than depression symptoms) in a sample of 10- to 14-year-olds, the results are instructive for two reasons. One is that "daily hassles" appeared to mediate the relation between stressful life events and behavior problem symptoms, suggesting that such daily minor events are even more important predictors of symptoms than are major events. Second, parents' psychological symptoms in response to their own life events and daily hassles were associated with children's symptoms. At least for fathers, the association of their own symptoms and children's symptoms was significant, but the association did not obtain for mothers. Children's stressors were also associated with parents' symptoms (except for the association of girls' daily hassles with fathers' symptoms). Together, these results offer a promising glimpse of the mutual associations between stress and symptoms in family members, but they need to be expanded to encompass more clinically significant symptoms including depression as well as younger populations.

Limitations in Stress–Depression Research in Adults and Children

Methodological Shortcomings

Adult Studies

There have been important improvements in assessment of stress–symptom relationships in recent years. Originally investigators relied on lengthy periods of up to several years of retrospective reporting of events and tended to use questionnaires that were tainted with "events" that really might be symptoms. Additionally, such questionnaires included both positive and negative events, and some items were ambiguous enough that individuals might interpret them differently. Moreover, the severity of stress tended to be judged by assigning "objective" weights collected from "normative" samples, without consideration of the personal meaning that events might have to individuals. It is beyond the scope of the present chapter to document the developments in methodology, but suffice it to say that considerable sophistication now marks most stress–depression research. Most efforts focus not on change as such, but on negative events, assessed over a relatively brief (e.g., often 6 months) retrospective period, with questionnaires commonly edited to remove symptom items, and frequently including individual subjective ratings of the impact of the event. Improved efforts to measure symptoms include the use of standardized questionnaires and clinical evaluations in both community and patient samples. Moreover, individual investigators have emphasized assessments not only of episodic major stressors but also of "microstressors," sometimes called "daily hassles," and more enduring, chronic strains and difficulties.

Methodological refinements have paved the way for posing more complex questions, and as a result of such complex questions there are three methodological issues that need to be emphasized. First, because stressors have their effects on individuals as a function of their meaning to the person, simple questionnaire measures of event occurrence do not supply adequate information. "Illness of family member" may be a standard entry on a questionnaire, but its significance varies greatly if we know that a subject's mother had a heart attack, and they had always had a troubled relationship, and even in the hospital when the subject wanted to express her caring for her mother the latter was rejecting. Or the illness of a family member might refer to a brother-in-law's ulcer, which has little impact on the subject's own life. Clearly, interview methods that can probe the context of the event's occurrence and significance can identify more closely the relevant psychological impact of events. Perhaps previous questionnaire studies that reported correlations of .20 to .30 between events and symptoms were simply reporting that events in general do not have much impact, but that certain events may have great impact.

A second important methodological gap has been the relative neglect of methods for assessing chronic stressors, the ongoing conditions that affect individuals on a daily basis, imposing limitations, determining decisions, and likely eliciting emotional reactions that can affect functioning in major roles. A few investigators have attempted to measure such conditions (e.g., Brown & Harris, 1978; Pearlin et al., 1981), but each approach seemed to have limitations. Although episodic stressors are critical, their effects might be potentiated by baseline, chronic conditions. For families—especially children—the consequences of ongoing difficulties may be enormous: layers of worry, strain, demoralization that deflect the parent's attention, availability, energy, and warmth.

Third, longitudinal methods seem essential to go beyond some of the simple descriptive relationships between stressors and symptoms, to investigate the truly causal relationships. The next section explores conceptual issues to be addressed, some of which require longitudinal designs.

Studies of Child and Adolescent Stress

To a great extent the methods of studying children's stressors have lagged behind developments in adult research. Therefore, it is not surprising that one of the notable gaps is the overreliance on self-report questionnaire measures of stressful event occurrence. There are several problems with this approach. First, the items included on the instruments may have been selected by adults, rather than children, and may therefore not represent a meaningful sample of events that are significant to children. Compas (1987) notes that most of the questionnaires in current or recent use have indeed been developed from items selected by adults. Second, this difficulty is compounded by the relative neglect of the developmental level of the child in selection and evaluation of events. Clearly children at different ages attribute different significance to the same event (e.g., "got lost" or "ignored by the opposite sex"). What is the best way to determine the impact of events for children at different ages? Relying on normative standards for children of a certain age may fail to consider the child's developmental status and the unique context of the child's life that could influence the threat of the event. Asking the child herself about the subjective impact is a commonly used remedy, yet such reports run the risk of confounding dependent and independent variables. As Brown and Harris (1978) noted with respect to adult reporting, "effort after meaning" may lead individuals to ascribe significance to events simply because they believe that their distress must have been related to events. Moreover, children of different ages may face developmentally appropriate and expected life events as well as atypical events, but questionnaires may not adequately sample these domains equally for children of different ages. A third difficulty with the existing questionnaires is that they generally fail to present evidence of psychometric adequacy (Compas, 1987).

The psychometric problems may constitute unique challenges with children. Reliability of reporting, for example, may be impaired by the child's less developed memory, which might make it difficult to recall either the occurrence or the dates of events. Nor is the extent to which children may be biased toward omission of painful or embarrassing events known. Thus it would be highly desirable to include reports of event occurrence from independent sources who are in a position to know the child's circumstances; however, such methods are rarely employed.

An additional gap in the assessment of children's stress is the relative neglect of minor events and chronic events, compared to the intensive focus on major life events. Compas and colleagues (Compas, Howell, Phares, Williams, & Giunta, 1989; Compas, Howell, Phares, Williams, & Ledoux, 1989) noted that adult research on distress symptoms had found that minor hassles may be more related to symptoms than were major events, and they applied this approach to adolescents. They found that their measure of "daily events" (comparable to the adult hassles scales) was indeed associated with children's distress symptoms, and they suggested that such minor events may mediate the impact of major events.

Chronic, ongoing conditions have apparently not been evaluated in children, even though the impact of continuing, unresolved threats and strains has been shown to be related to adult depressive symptoms (e.g., Brown & Harris, 1978; Hammen, Davila, Brown, & Gitlin, 1991; Pearlin et al., 1981). Methods are lacking for assessing the impact of such continuing conditions, but this would seem to be a vital area to pursue, since the exposure to these conditions is likely to have a significant impact on the family environment that provides the support, socialization, and attachment foundations for the developing child.

Finally, a significant methodological gap remains in the design of many stress–symptom studies of children: overuse of cross-sectional measurement. It is widely acknowledged that prospective studies are needed in order to more clearly disentangle the event–symptom relationships that can be obscured by obtaining both kinds of data at the same time. Additionally, such longitudinal designs permit the evaluation of initial symptomatology, so that differences in symptom patterns between onset, change, and chronic states with respect to stressors can be evaluated. Also, prospective studies that employ relatively frequent assessments may help to reduce the inaccuracies of reporting due to memory that occur when lengthy retrospective reporting is called for. Finally, in view of the observation that the stress–distress link may be somewhat different for adolescents than for adults (with relatively stronger support for the effect of symptoms on subsequent events) (Compas, 1987), longitudinal studies permit the further evaluation of this process.

Methodological Contributions of the Present Study

In view of the shortcomings that were identified in the methods of investigating the impact of stressors when the present study began, the following procedures were included, and more detailed discussions of the methods are presented in Chapter 2.

Interview Assessment of Event Occurrence and Meaning

Both adult and child stressors were measured using procedures initially developed by Brown and Harris (1978) for adults. No previous use of these methods had been developed for children; indeed, there were no interview procedures for studying depressive outcomes to stressful events with children.

The interview method queries occurrence of events in a variety of domains, and when an event is identified, its timing and surrounding circumstances are assessed in detail. In this way, the "meaning" of the event in context can be evaluated in terms of its objective threat—defined as how it would be experienced by a typical person under identical conditions. The contextual assessment is especially useful for measuring the impact of children's events, because the developmental level of the child, which determines the meaning of the event, can be taken into account.

An independent rating team subsequently reads the narrative reports of each event occurrence; each report has been edited to exclude any reference to how the individual reacted to or felt about the event. The team rates each occurrence on a 5-point threat scale, ranging from mild to severe. Items are scored only if they have some objective negative consequences, remain unresolved for at least 24 hours, and for children, must have been more than an ordinary event for children of that age. The team also rates on a 5-point scale the likely extent to which the event's occurrence was independent of the person's behavior or characteristics. For example, death, illnesses happening to other people, and most personal illnesses are considered independent occurrences, but most interpersonal events involving others are considered to be "mixed" unless there is clear evidence to the contrary. Certain events that clearly reflect the person's own volition or characteristics, such as starting back to school or finding a new job, would be considered dependent events. Only events with a negative impact were included in the data. Finally, individuals rated each event according to a "subjective impact" scale ranging from 1 to 5.

Dual Assessment of Mother and Child About the Child's Events

In view of the possibility that children are incomplete or inaccurate reporters of events, we interviewed both separately about events that happened to the child. Events were included if either or both of them reported. Mothers did not always know of, or attach significance to, the same events a child might report, so that both sources of information were believed to yield a superior representation of the true experiences of the child than either alone.

Chronic Stress Assessment

An interview procedure was developed, covering seven areas of major role functioning, that permitted assessment of the level of ongoing difficulties in each realm for the mother. The circumstances had to have existed for at least the past 6 months. The scale yielded a total chronic strain score, or individual items could be used to characterize areas of functioning. Children's stressful life events were characterized as episodic or ongoing, so that separate measures of the two were obtained.

Longitudinal Design with Frequent Assessment

Life stress evaluations were conducted every 6 months. Although a shorter interval would have been preferable, such frequent evaluations would have been prohibitive. However, we are confident that over a 3-year period complete information was obtained, and the continuity provided by typically having the same interviewer likely improved rapport and accuracy.

Conceptual Gaps in Understanding the Stress–Depression Link

No student of stress processes will ever be without work, since stressful occurrences—significant and often unwanted changes—are part of normal life and provide an endless laboratory of experiences to draw upon. The question of whether one would *want* to be a life stress researcher is an entirely different matter. It is difficult to imagine an area of clinical psychological research more fraught with impossibly conflicting demands. Life stress research and conceptualization must be broad and integrative, yet it must be narrow and specific. We need to look at the big picture, but we need to see the microscopic. We must understand the individual's responses, and we must view the person in a larger context. We need precision about the interrelationships between elements of the person, reactions, and life context, but at the same time the flowing, changing, transactional (reciprocal) relationships must be considered, measured, and understood.

A major conceptual challenge for life stress research is simple: if all people responded the same way to stressful events and circumstances, we would have little problem, but since they do not, a major mission is to understand individual differences. There have been significant inroads into this question, involving not only differences in the types of events, but also in understanding differences in appraisal processes and other mediators such as coping resources, including social supports and coping capabilities. Even the same environmental events may be seen to have very different impact on individuals with different areas of self-vulnerability, coping resources, and supports. Thus we have greatly improved the predictability of the stress–depression association by learning more about the individual differences in mediating factors. However, to continue to develop the theoretical and practical goals of prediction of who becomes depressed and under what conditions, additional ingredients seem to be needed.

One of the first noteworthy conceptual gaps in the field is insufficient integration of models. While it is a necessary strategy at the beginning of a complex research paradigm to extol the virtues of a single variable, maturity of the field requires increasing complexity. It would seem safe to say that maturity has been reached, and simple models should be eschewed in favor of integrations of factors from various levels. For instance, simplistic cognitive or life event or biological or psychodynamic approaches to depression vulnerability should give way to integrative efforts (e.g., see Hammen, 1988a, and Lewinsohn, et al., 1988, for further statements). It would seem timely to include the historical/developmental origins of vulnerability experiences; as developmental psychopathologists and high risk researchers alike can remind us, the early environment provides the context for acquiring basic skills and resources of attachment, self-concept, problem-solving, and emotion regulation—among many—that would seem to contribute to vulnerability to dysfunction. Stressful life event occurrence, including exposure to adverse parenting experiences, may severely disrupt those processes necessary to the growing child.

In addition to the historical/developmental factors that ought to be included in integrative approaches, biological processes also present an area for integrative activities. Indeed, it is difficult to construe a complete model of the mechanisms of stress reactivity without knowing a great deal more about how the brain responds, both normally and dysfunctionally. Post, Rubinow, and Ballenger (1984) and Gold, Goodwin, and Chrousos (1988) are among those who have suggested that early childhood trauma may alter the brain and the neurobiology of stress responsiveness in such a way as to increase the likelihood that future stressful events, and perhaps especially those cognitively appraised as similar to initial traumas, will precipitate depression. Other models (e.g., Goplerud & Depue, 1985) suggest individual differences, possibly genetically or constitutionally mediated, in depressive responses to stressful circumstances (see also Palermo, 1989). Thus a complete model of the association between stressful events and depression needs to consider the biological substrate and its contribution to individual differences in the process.

A second gap is also one that has been raised by others but has been incompletely implemented: the need for more fully contextual and transactional models (e.g., see Brown & Harris, 1978; Compas, 1987; Coyne, Burchill, & Stiles, 1990; Lazarus & Folkman, 1984). The contextual component here refers to understanding the meaning of an event's occurrence by knowing the circumstances of the individual's life. However, the context also refers to the need for understanding that within families, the occurrence of an event to one member may have important effects on other members as well. This isssue has been largely neglected in high risk studies of affective disorders, in which the parental illness is rarely considered as a circumstance that itself affects others (an important exception, however, is the work of Rutter). Moreover, a child's negative events put demands on the parents, commonly including not only problem solving but also responding to disruptive regulation of emotion by the child. A highly charged negative event such as divorce, for instance, involves not only the parents' experiences but the impact of the experience on others in the family and the reverberations of those experiences and reactions on the parents. The transactional aspect of stress research attempts to capture this idea of mutual and changing influences and processes—both between individuals sharing the same ecology and within the person. In a transactional framework, a question that is as intriguing as the traditional events–cause–depression relationship is the impact of the person on events: To what extent and in what ways do people cause events that in turn may cause distress? Our tools for handling such complexities are poor, but the attempts to include contextual factors and transactions between individuals, over time, are welcomed.

Finally, increased precision is an additional need in the research on stressful life events. Important inroads are being made, but the point needs to be emphasized nonetheless. One aspect of the issue concerns precision in the scope of models, as applied to defining populations and stage or level of depression. Echoing themes raised by others as well, it is important to distinguish between symptoms and clinical states: Can we assume they differ on a continuum of severity? Some would argue not (e.g., Hammen, 1990-b; Lewinsohn et al., 1988), but this is an empirical question. It is further important to distinguish between samples of chronic and episodic depressions, between children and adults (and between children and adolescents), between unipolar and bipolar, and the like. Moreover, because of the enormous heterogeneity of unipolar depression, precision is needed in distinguishing between subtypes of depressed persons. Further, differences in the stress–symptom relationship should be predicted separately for the never-depressed, those at risk for relapse, and those with chronic conditions (e.g., Depue & Monroe, 1986). Thus grand theories at the level of complexity and integration are needed, but precision at the level of application and generality are also needed. Finally, precision of constructs is also necessary, and here advances are apparent in distinguishing between chronic, episodic, and microstressors or between mild, moderate, and severe depression.

In view of the enormously intricate conceptual and methodological issues raised by this brief review, the goals of the present research are, by necessity, modest. Only tiny portions of some of the vastly intriguing unresolved issues have been addressed. The following report represents, therefore, a preliminary approach to studying stress and its role in vulnerability to depression in both mothers and children in high risk families. Additional chapters will also consider aspects of the stress–symptom relationship: Chapter 6 explores the impact of stressors on mother–child interactions, and certainly quality of the relationship may be a stressful condition; Chapter 7 discusses aspects of the effects of parents' and childrens' symptoms as stressors affecting the timing of episodes; Chapter 8 considers coping and resilience factors that may mediate the impact of stress and risk conditions on children; Chapter 9 presents an integrative model of children's risk for disorder in which stressful conditions play a prominent role.

Results of the Study

Children's Outcomes Associated with Family Stress

Chronic Stress as a Covariate

All families experience certain kinds of continuing difficulties that color daily lives, especially for the parents, because the circumstances raise problems to be solved or their presence limits the members. For instance, many families experience chronic financial strains that affect a variety of daily decisions and choices. Other families may feel the ongoing effects of marital conflict between the parents, or there may be an ill family member whose health needs alter the lives of all members of the family in various ways. In the present study we recognized that families need to be characterized in the domains of chronic stressful conditions in order to compare them and to be able to assess the differences in outcomes that may be associated with such differences in the profile of strains encountered on a regular basis. Therefore, the chronic stress interview was developed, as described in Chapter 2, for the specific purpose of characterizing differences between families in terms of the chronic stressful conditions experienced by the mothers. The dimensions included marital/social functioning, finances, occupational functioning, relationships with children and with extended family members, and personal physical health and that of family members. These seven areas were evaluated separately on numerical scales indicating severity of ongoing difficulties, yielding chronic stress profiles as well as overall chronic stress totals.

Not only did we observe that families differed in their profiles of ongoing strains across the different domains of functioning, but also that the maternal groups differed from each other and varied widely within each group. For instance, the unipolar group tended to have the highest levels of overall stressful conditions; the normal group, the lowest. Yet within each of these groups there were families with relatively stable and strain-free functioning on most domains, along with others experiencing painfully high levels of chronic stress.

Examples of Family Differences in Chronic Stress

High Levels of Chronic Stress

Mrs. A. is widowed; some years ago her husband was killed in an accident. She remarried, divorced, and has intermittent relationships with men, and a wide circle of friends. However, she is isolated from her family and angry with them. Because of her condition, she was on public assistance and not working for some time, and she accumulated huge medical bills that are a struggle to pay. She started working for the first time in several years recently, and although she feels able to handle the job, there is a lot of pressure and she doesn't get along well with the boss. Her children have had difficulties; last year the oldest (21-year-old) son committed suicide while jailed for drug charges, and her daughter may have to be placed in foster care for unmanageability.

Mrs. B. has no psychiatric problems. She is divorced from an alcoholic man who comes and goes from her life (and is in and out of jail). She works full-time and supports the family of three children by herself. Because of job stresses she is looking for new work. She seems to have good relationships with her family members, but she has been burdened with the care of her elderly father, who had a stroke, and recently had him sent to a convalescent home.

Low Levels of Chronic Stress

Mrs. C. has an affective disorder with recurrent episodes, but is in good physical health and gets along with relatives and immediate family (except for tension with her mother-in-law). Her husband of many years is supportive of her, and they have a good relationship. They are comfortable financially. The husband owns a business, and there were difficulties such that they needed for her to return to work to supplement the family income. Although she had previously enjoyed being a homemaker, she likes the new job and feels accomplished and appreciated.

Mrs. D. has been married for many years, and the relationship is solid and fairly unconflicted. Financially the family has enough to get along, but they are feeling a little shaky because of a new mortgage. She works full-time and likes her job, serving as a supervisor, and feels that the work conditions are good. Her children squabble with each other, but family relationships are strong, and everyone in the family, including her parents, enjoys good health.

To characterize the children's diagnostic and psychosocial functioning by group, it seemed useful to control for the effects of such striking differences between and within groups on chronic maternal strain. Therefore, the chronic stress mean across all domains (excluding relationship with children) was a covariate in the analyses. Table 5.1 presents the adjusted means for each of the seven measures of children's functioning at the time of the initial evaluation in the study, controlling for chronic maternal stress. One child was randomly selected from each family for those families that had two youngsters in the study, in order to avoid nonindependent observations when maternal stress was the covariate. Of the eight child variables, seven yielded significantly worse functioning in the affective disorders versus normal group comparisons when no chronic stress covariate was employed. However, as Table 5.1 indicates, controlling for stress differences reduced the number of significant contrasts to four. Thus when the potentially confounding effects of strain were controlled, the children in the affective disorders groups fared significantly more negatively in diagnoses and school-related functioning than normal group children. Without such statistical controls, the group differences may give an exaggerated view of the impact of maternal affective disorder.

Chronic Stress as a Predictor of Children's Outcomes

The results of the Hammen, Gordon, et al. (1987) analyses suggested that differences in chronic stress levels may not just be a nuisance factor to control in order to get at the "true" differences that can be related to maternal diagnostic status. Indeed, we asked ourselves what maternal diagnostic status really means. It seems that diagnostic condition can be dismantled into several separate components. In the context of our present sample of women with longstanding and recurring psychiatric disorders, there seem to be at least three components, of which diagnostic status is an index: actual history of affective disorder, current depressive symptoms, and chronic stress. That is, for example, a woman in our study classified as

TABLE 5.1. Group means on children's outcomes adjusted for maternal chronic stress.

	Maternal group			
Variable	Unipolar	Bipolar	Medical	Normal
Diagnostic ratings				
Any disorder	1.9	1.3	1.1	0.9[a]
Affective disorder	1.9	0.9	0.9	0.8[a]
Psychological functioning				
Children's Depression Inventory	7.1	5.5	4.9	5.9
Child Behavior Check List—Social Competence	36.5	44.5	46.0	48.2
Child Behavior Check List—Behavior Problems	65.7	53.8	57.0	54.3
School and teacher ratings				
Academic Performance Rating	2.8	3.1	3.5	4.0[a]
School Behavior Rating	2.5	4.0	3.6	4.0[a]
Conners Teacher Rating	27.6	15.0	25.8	11.6

Note: From "Maternal Affective Disorders, Illness, and Stress: Risk for Children's Psychopathology" by C. Hammen, D. Gordon, D. Burge, C. Adrian, C. Jaenicke, and D. Hiroto, 1987, *American Journal of Psychiatry*, *144*, 736–741. Copyright 1987 by the American Psychiatric Association. Adapted by permission.

[a] Planned comparison $p < .05$: combined affective disorders group vs. normal.

unipolar depressed has a history of a certain number or course of episodes, she may or may not be currently depressed with some level of depressive symptoms, and she experiences some degree of chronic stressful conditions that may result from, and/or contribute to, her recurrent psychiatric disorder. We speculate that the various components of diagnostic status are typically confounded with diagnosis. In a medical model milieu, the emphasis on a possibly biological/genetic basis of children's risk for disorder is compatible with simply using maternal diagnostic status as a predictor. However, from an environmental/psychosocial perspective, diagnosis may be a marker of important variables that themselves have explanatory power. Thus we hypothesized that each of these components, measured separately, would contribute differentially to the prediction of children's outcomes.

Hammen, Adrian, et al. (1987) used hierarchical multiple regression analyses to predict each of several child outcomes, both from the initial evaluation and at the first 6-month follow-up. Each predictor variable—maternal history of affective disorders, maternal chronic stress, and current depressive symptoms—was entered last in equations. By entering each variable last, it is possible to determine its unique contribution to the outcome when the potentially overlapping effects of the others were statistically controlled. One variable, lifetime history of affective disorders, was scaled on a 7-point scale taking into account number of major depressive episodes and number of hospitalizations for psychiatric reasons. All of the women in the unipolar and bipolar groups scored 6 or 7 on the scale, and no other women scored that high, although many of the remaining women in the medical and normal groups had experienced some periods of depression that could be characterized between 2 and 5 on the scale (1 represented no history of any level of depression lasting more than a day). The current depression score, based on the Beck Depression Inventory, indicated considerable variability across and within groups. Some women in the unipolar and bipolar groups, for instance, were currently relatively symptom-free; some of the women in the other two groups showed elevations. The chronic stress measure was the mean across all domains (excluding relationships with children) covering conditions for at least the past 6 months.

Table 5.2 presents the increments in R^2 that were statistically significant when each variable was entered last. All of the overall regression equations were statistically significant, indicating that the three maternal variables together can predict children's outcomes moderately well. Lifetime disorder—the variable capturing psychiatric status of the mother—was a unique predictor of only one child outcome: history of any diagnosable disorder. On the other hand, current depression was the most frequent unique predictor of outcome, both for current and follow-up functioning in the children. Chronic stress, as expected, was also a unique predictor of several outcomes, especially of diagnoses and behavior problems.

TABLE 5.2. Hierachical multiple regression analyses to predict children's outcomes.

Variable	Incremental R^2 when entered last[a] Lifetime disorder	BDI	Chronic strain	Overall R^2
Initial outcomes				
Current (any) diagnoses		.04*		.17
Current affective diagnoses		.05*		.16
Lifetime (any) diagnoses	.07		.08	.41
Lifetime affective diagnoses		.04*	.09	.44
CBCL Behavior Problems		.13	.08	.38
CBCL Social Competence		.16		.32
CDI		.07		.19
Conners Teacher Rating		.20		.28
Follow-up outcomes				
Any diagnosis		.05	.05*	.35
Affective diagnosis		.07	.03*	.32
CBCL Behavior Problems		.07*	.08*	.25
CBCL Social Competence		.11		.27
CDI			.09	.23

Note: BDI = Beck Depression Inventory; CBCL = Child Behavior Check List; CDI = Children's Depression Inventory. All Overall regression equations are statistically significant. From "Children of Depressed Mothers: Maternal Strain and Symptom Predictors of Dysfunction" by C. Hammen, C. Adrian, D. Gordon, D. Burge, C. Jaenicke, and D. Hiroto, 1987, *Journal of Abnormal Psychology*, *96*, 190–198. Copyright 1987 by the American Psychological Association. Reprinted by permission.
[a] Only statistically significant increments once other variables were controlled for are noted. (*$p < .10$)

In addition to drawing the conclusion that the relationship between maternal psychiatric condition and children's risk is more complex than typically represented, two other implications emerge. One is that chronic stress is a factor that seems to be separable and to be an important, independent predictor of negative outcomes for children. Chronic stress is also likely to be a consequence of chronic psychiatric conditions—although it may be a contributor as well. Thus when we encounter recurrent psychiatric disorder, we are also likely to encounter lives that have been disrupted in social, occupational, and financial functioning. A pernicious cycle of strain and symptoms is likely to develop, creating the conditions for a reciprocal interaction of difficulty and reaction to difficulty. We shall have more to say later about this process.

The second implication of the dismantling strategy reported in Hammen, Adrian, et al. (1987) is that the two strongest predictors of negative child outcomes are nonspecific. That is, the conditions of current depressive mood and chronic stressful conditions are not unique to individuals with diagnosed affective disorder. Such conditions may occur in the lives of women who are demoralized and stressed for a variety of reasons, in the present study including chronic medical illness and severe family stressful conditions. Thus, aside from the genetic contribution to affective illness in children, which cannot be denied as a possibility, it is likely that the major sources of risk to children of women with affective disorder are the same risks faced in other families under conditions of depressive symptoms and high degrees of chronic strain.

Chronic Medical Conditions and the Impact on Children

The study was designed to evaluate the impact of maternal affective disorders, with a control for the effects of chronic illness as such. The medically ill women served as a comparison for such chronic stressors as having an ill mother who experiences both chronic symptoms and limitations and episodic exacerbations of her condition that might even require hospitalization.

Examples of Medically Ill Women and Their Lives

Mrs. E. has severe arthritis, with disintegrating bone and joints in parts of her body. She has been divorced for several years, but the ex-husband comes around to help with the yardwork and the children. She feels tied to him, and is upset when he dates others; she herself doesn't date and is somewhat isolated because of her illness. Money is tight; she and the family exist mostly on disability and some support from the ex-husband. She has difficulty performing many of the household chores because of her disability, but her daughter helps a lot, including helping her with getting dressed. She is close to the children, but depends on them in ways that cause conflict when they push for independence.

Mrs. F. has juvenile onset diabetes that is poorly controlled by insulin treatments, and she has many medical complications. Many of her family members (e.g., father, sister, child, husband) also experience various medical ailments. Her marital relationship is solid, and although they are fairly financially comfortable, the family business is unstable, leading to lots of worry. She works full time, and finds it rewarding, but also stressful at times due to heavy work loads.

Comparisons between the medical group and the affective disorders group generally did not indicate significant differences. Hammen, Gordon, et al. (1987; Hammen, Burge, Adrian, & Burney, 1990) found that such families had moderate rates of disorder in the children (overall rate of diagnosis 50%) that were lower than those of children in the affective disorders but higher than children in the normal group. In the analyses reported earlier that controlled for chronic maternal stress, there were no significant differences remaining between the medical group offspring and the affective disorders offspring—not only in lifetime diagnoses but also in current psychosocial functioning. As reported in Chapter 3 in terms of children's outcomes during the 3-year follow-up, the same patterns generally continued. The medical group children reported fewer significant disorders than did the unipolar group offspring but continued to be somewhat more symptomatic than the normal group children (see also Anderson & Hammen, 1990a).

Overall, the best conclusion seems to be that maternal impairment, whether due to affective disorders or medical illness, is associated with increased risk to children for negative outcomes. As with affective disorders, however, we would argue that the adverse consequences are mediated by the chronic strain and depressive demoralization experienced by the mothers.

Impact of Children's Own Stressors

In Chapter 4 tests of the hypothesized cognitive vulnerability to depression, given stressful life events, were reported. Children's stressors in the first 6 months following initial evaluation were used to predict outcomes, along with depressive attribution style and other self-schema, self-concept measures. Hammen (1988b) and Hammen, Adrian, and Hiroto (1988) reported that stressful life events emerged as significant predictors of changes in depression, contributing as a main effect, and not in interaction with cognitive variables.

Examples of Children's Stressful Events over Follow-Up Period

During the 3-year follow-up period G. was 16–18 years old. During that period, she was a victim of a hit-and-run accident causing minor injuries, changed schools because of problems at the former school, and got arrested on suspicion of selling drugs. She was convicted, and went to juvenile hall for a time, but got into trouble soon afterward by using the mother's car without permission. About this time, her grandmother died, and her mother was experiencing a severe depressive episode. Later, G. was suspended at school for possession of fireworks, continued to have academic problems, and eventually dropped out of high school. She got a job, but got fired for shoplifting. The mother, a single parent, kicked her out of the home due to continuing conflict and problems, but she had no place to live except with friends. The mother filed for bankruptcy due to severe financial problems. G. continued to have difficulty holding a job, and she and her mother fought frequently. After dating the same guy for a year, the relationship ended.

H. was also 16–18 during the period of the follow-ups, but his stressors were somewhat less severe. The mother's psychiatric disorder resulted in intermittent symptoms and a hospitalization that caused severe financial problems leading to bankruptcy. They moved. The parents had marital difficulties. H. got a car, but ended up having to return it when the loan failed to go through. He graduated from high school and started at junior college. He had some difficulties with his girlfriend and they broke up, and he experienced intermittent conflicts with his parents.

I., by contrast, was 10–12 during the follow-up periods, and she experienced different kinds of events more typical of a younger child: her mother had numerous complications of her illness, and she was bothered by her mother's conflict with her mother-in-law. She had some difficulties with a group of friends, and quit playing with them. Medical problems led her to have various tests that were unpleasant. Also, she had a bike accident and broke her foot. Her best friend's father died, and her own aunt died. At school she did fairly well but had problems in math.

J., aged 9–11 during the follow-ups, had numerous events that were out of the ordinary. In addition to his mother's illness and recurrent hospitalizations for various treatments, he had a series of accidents: he got a concussion from falling off his bike, in another accident broke a finger, and later on fell off a swing and tore ligaments in his knee. He also was found to have an arthritic condition. The dog had a seizure, his grandfather had open heart surgery, and his uncle died of cancer. There was also conflict between him and his parents, and he got into fights with his brother. His grandmother became ill, and after returning from the hospital, moved in with his family.

A recent dissertation by Cheri Adrian (1990) focused on the assessment of children's stressors and their impact on children's symptoms. She used the entire sample, over the entire longitudinal course of study, to identify various ways to test the hypothesized association between stress and symptoms. For each child, she identified the worst onset or exacerbation of symptoms and measured amount of stress in the 3 months prior; for children who did not develop significant symptoms a randomly chosen follow-up period was used. Correlations between various measures of stress (number of events, subjective ratings, objective ratings) and depressive symptom levels were statistically significant, ranging from .30 to .67 for the total sample. Similar levels of significant association were obtained for symptoms of any disorder.

Additionally, Adrian (1990) reported that amount of objective stress in the 3 months before onset/exacerbation was significantly higher than in the preceding 3 months, $t(37) = 4.17, p < .001$, or in the 3 months subsequent to symptom onset, $t(37) = 6.01, p < .0001$. Thus symptomatic children experienced their greatest stress level in the period 3 months prior to symptom onset.

Type of event was also an important consideration. Logistic regression analyses were used to characterize the best predictors of children's symptoms. Adrian (1990) found that for *any* symptoms, failure events and family conflict were especially predictive, and for depressive symptoms, family conflict emerged as the best predictor with loss/bereavement also contributing significantly. Zero-order correlations indicated that depressive symptoms were associated with loss ($r = .47$), family conflict ($r = .49$), and change/move/adjustment ($r = .26$), all significant relationships. Thus failure experiences, although very rare, appeared to be discriminating, and family conflict overall was a major predictor of symptoms.

Vulnerability to Stress

One question that has considerable implications for understanding children at risk is whether children of depressed mothers are more susceptible to the impact of stress than are comparison group children. Adrian (1990) examined whether the groups differed in responses to high levels of personal stress and in responses to low levels of stress. High stress was defined as a score on the objective threat totals of 8, which was the empirical cutoff between children showing relatively few or no symptoms and those who showed major responses to stress. Under high stress conditions, the majority of children in all groups showed symptom increases (85% of the combined unipolar–bipolar children, 86% of the medically ill, and 100% of the normal group children).

Under low stress conditions, however, the picture was different. Children of unipolar and bipolar women showed a high probability of symptoms even under low stress conditions (75%), compared with medical (42%) and normal (33%) group children. Altering the cutoff for defining high and low stress made the differences even more pronounced. When the sample median of 6 objective threat points was used, 77% of the children of depressed mothers showed symptom increases at this level, compared with 0% of the medically ill group and 17% of the children of normal mothers.

Thus it appears that higher stress levels are needed to provoke symptom increases in children of normal mothers and medically ill mothers, whereas children of women with affective disorders respond symptomatically even at relatively low levels of stress. The children at risk due to maternal mood disorder therefore appear to be vulnerable because they have lower thresholds for responding to stressful life events. This provocative finding needs to be replicated and explored further, since its mechanisms of operation are not clarified by the present analyses.

Potential Mechanisms of Stress Effects on Children and Families

The initial descriptions of children's diagnostic and psychological functioning indicated that family stress represented by chronic medical and psychiatric illness, as well as ongoing chronic stress unique to each family, is associated with adverse consequences. Now we turn to the question of how this process works its pernicious effects on children. Rutter and Quinton (1984) suggested several different mechanisms by which parental psychopathology may exert its effects on children: genetic transmission, the direct impact of parental disorder (e.g., children as victims of parental violence or neglect), the indirect effects of parental disorder (e.g., interference with parental functioning), and correlates of parental disorder (e.g., marital discord or social adversity). In the present chapter, we do not attempt to choose between such alternatives but rather consider the influence of several possible factors: stress exposure and the role of specific vulnerability of the children to types of stressors. We also briefly discuss parental symptomatology as a stressor. The impact of stress on maternal interaction and availability is briefly noted here and be pursued more fully in the next chapter.

Stress Exposure

One possible mechanism of children's risk for disorder in families with parental affective illness is that such families experience *more* stressful events and circumstances. Partly a cause of maternal depression, and possibly partly a consequence of maternal impairment, functioning, and characteristics, stress may simply accumulate in such families and present an unusual challenge to coping capabilities. Thus one of the first questions to explore is whether such families in fact differ in exposure to stress: chronic, ongoing difficulties, episodic stressors, and children's own stressful events.

Chronic Stress

As indicated in our previous analyses of children's outcomes, chronic stress differed between groups, and there was also considerable variability within groups. Table 5.3 presents the group means by specific role area and a total chronic stress score. Lower scores indicate lower levels of adequate functioning, and the highest score, 5, was given only for unusual and exceptional positive conditions. Statistical planned comparisons of the total chronic stress score tested the hypothesis that there would be more stress exposure in the unipolar and bipolar groups, especially the former, compared to the medical and normal groups, and that the medical group would display more than the normal group. All of these predictions were confirmed ($p < .05$), except that the bipolar and medical groups did not differ. Clearly, the unipolar group experienced the most chronic stress, and the effects were most pronounced in the realms of marital/social relationships, occupation, finances, and ongoing difficulties with children. Generally, differences between groups on health issues were not as pronounced, although of course the chronically medically ill women had more health impairment than the others. Nevertheless, it might be noted

Table 5.3. Mean chronic stress scores by maternal group.[a]

Variable	Maternal group			
	Unipolar	Bipolar	Medical	Normal
Marital/social	2.7	3.0	3.5	3.6
Job	2.7	3.1	3.5	3.7
Finances	2.9	3.2	3.5	3.6
Relations with extended family	3.4	3.7	3.9	3.8
Relations with children	2.5	3.1	3.3	3.6
Health, self	3.6	3.6	2.9	4.0
Health, others	3.4	3.9	3.7	3.7
Total chronic stress[b]	17.8	19.9	20.4	22.1

[a] Higher scores represent *less* stress. [b] Excludes relations with extended family due to extensive missing data.

that the women with affective disorders had more health problems than women in the normal group, and the unipolar women's family members experienced more chronic illness than any other group. Thus, overall, the stress exposure hypothesis suggests significant, ongoing exposure to chronic strain in most areas for the ill women, and especially significantly for the unipolar women.

Episodic Stressors

Exposure to episodic stress was assessed by comparing the occurrence of stressful events during the first year of follow-up evaluations (reported in Hammen, in press-a). Table 5.4 presents the group means according to different ways of measuring stressors. Total event impact scores indicated that the unipolar and medical group women experienced the highest rates of stress, with significantly higher scores for unipolar than normal women ($p < .05$). However, the groups differed markedly when they were compared, following Brown and Harris (1978), on number of events of major impact—those rated by the independent rating team as moderate or severe impact. Here, the unipolar women were significantly higher than all other groups (p values $< .01$), who did not differ from each other. The unipolar group women had an astounding 2.9 events of serious impact happen to them in the first year of follow-ups, compared with .96 to 1.4 for the other groups.

Especially noteworthy were differences in types of events. While the groups did not differ on events rated by judges as "independent" of their behaviors, the "dependent" events (those caused at least in part by the women), were significantly higher for unipolar women compared to the normal women and marginally higher than the levels reported by the bipolar and medical groups. Dependent events could be further subdivided into those that were primarily interpersonal. Here again, as expected, the

TABLE 5.4. Mean maternal episodic stress exposure in year 1 by group.

	Type of event category			
Group	Total all events	Independent	Dependent	Interpersonal
Unipolar	12.7	3.6	8.8	6.3
n = 14	(12.5)	(3.2)	(9.6)	(7.0)
Bipolar	9.1	3.6	5.5	3.2
n = 11	(6.0)	(2.7)	(4.8)	(3.2)
Medically Ill	11.6	6.6	5.1	3.0
n = 13	(6.5)	(6.1)	(5.5)	(4.3)
Normal	7.6	4.4	3.3	2.0
n = 22	(7.6)	(5.9)	(3.7)	(2.8)

Note: Adapted from Hammen, C. (in press-a). The generation of stress in the course of unipolar depression. *Journal of Abnormal Psychology*.
Standard deviations are in parentheses.

unipolar women had the highest levels of interpersonal stress, differing significantly from the other groups. Many such events involved conflict. It thus appears that the unipolar women are especially likely to contribute to the occurrence of their stressors—a stress generation effect that may perpetuate the stress–depression cycle in a reciprocal way.

Overall, therefore, stress exposure does indeed appear to be higher in the unipolar families. The unipolar and medically ill women both appear to have many events occur, but the unipolar women are especially likely to experience highly threatening events and events that are not independent of themselves. These findings suggest the potential for a vicious cycle of symptoms and events, contributing to the risk for all family members of ongoing symptoms and challenges to adjustment.

Examples of Women's Stressors

Mrs. K. presents a good example of frequent, severe events, some that are independent and some not, in which the activities of various family members have an impact on the others. In a 12-month period, her child's psychiatric problems worsened, and her husband left for one week and returned drunk. Fed up, she moved out and eventually sent the child to live with him due to considerable conflict. She filed for divorce, and the process, which involved dividing the property and resolving custody, was finalized. She got a new boyfriend and she got pregnant but had a miscarriage. She also had a car accident with painful whiplash, contracted pneumonia at one point, and had a second accident. Her grandfather died, and she found out she had failed to be promoted at work.

In contrast, although a number of negative events happened to Mrs. K.'s family in a 12-month period, many of them were independent of her. Her father was hospitalized for emphysema, and her mother-in-law died. Two additional relatives died; while she wasn't close to them, they were important figures to her children. She started back to school, and had important exams to take, and also as part of her training, had to work under highly upsetting conditions.

Children's Stressors

One of the hypotheses tested in the longitudinal phase of the study was whether children in high risk families experience more stressors than do their counterparts in non-ill families. Children's events include those that happen to family members as well as in various domains of their own living; thus increased risk for stressors might result from the problems of others including the mother, or from circumstances that affect the mothers as well as the other members of the family.

Viewing the entire 3-year period of observation, based on data from Adrian's dissertation, Adrian and Hammen (1990) reported four scores per child: objective threat total, average 6-month objective threat, the threat total for the 6-month highest stress period, and that for the lowest 6-month period. All of the scores, therefore, were based on the ratings assigned by independent judges of "objective" stress. The sample included 53 children (1 per family) for whom complete data were available. Table 5.5 presents the mean scores by group: combined unipolar–bipolar, medically ill, and normal.

All four measures of objective stress support the hypothesis of significant differences between groups. In all cases, the children at risk due to maternal affective disorders had significantly more stress than did the normal children (p values $<.001$). The children of medically ill women also differed significantly from the children of normal women (p values $< .05$), but the affective disorders and medical high risk groups did not differ from each other.

The 3-year objective threat totals were further subdivided by episodic and chronic/ongoing stressors. The chronic stress total for the affective disorders group (M = 17.2, *SD* = 10.2) and the medically ill group (M = 15.2, *SD* = 10.3) both differed significantly from the normal group (M = 3.9, *SD* = 4.9) but did not differ from each other. The episodic event mean of the affective disorders group (M = 37.5, *SD* = 15.9) differed significantly from the normal group (M = 23.0, *SD* = 10.9), but neither group differed from the medically ill group (M = 29.8, *SD* = 11.1). Note that for the affective disorders and medical groups, chronic stress represented about one-third of their total objective threat scores, but for the normal group children the chronic stress proportion was much lower (about one-sixth).

When the stress totals were subdivided by dependent/independent ratings, the groups were not different on occurrence of entirely independent events. However, they were significantly different on dependent events. The affective disorders group children (M = 34.7) had the highest levels, differing significantly from both the medical group children (M = 21.3) and the normal children (M = 8.8), and the latter two groups also differed significantly from each other. The vignettes of children's stressors that were presented earlier provide some flavor of the ways in which certain

TABLE 5.5. Mean child stress exposure over 3 years.

	Children's group		
Objective threat rating	Affective disorders	Medically ill	Normal
Total, 3 years	54.4	44.2	26.9
	(21.3)	(18.7)	(13.0)
Average, 6-month period	9.2	7.5	4.6
	(3.7)	(2.9)	(2.2)
High stress, 6 months	13.3	12.8	9.1
	(5.2)	(5.1)	(3.6)
Low stress, 6 months	4.9	5.2	1.6
	(3.1)	(2.4)	(2.9)

Note: From "Children of Depressed Mothers: Stress Exposure and Responses to Stressful Life Events" by C. Adrian and C. Hammen, 1990, unpublished.
Standard deviations are in parentheses.

children's own behaviors and characteristics contribute to the misfortunes that befall them.

The children's events were categorized by content to determine whether exposure to stressful events and circumstances affected some areas more than others. Six content types were examined: loss-bereavement, family conflict, peer conflict, change-move-adjustment, achievement failure, and other negative events (e.g., illnesses, accidents). An overall multivariate analysis of variance indicated significant group differences ($F[12, 88] = 2.82$, $p < .01$). Univariate tests, however, showed that the differences were significant for family conflict stress, peer conflict, and "other." The family conflict and peer conflict variables indicated significantly higher scores for the children of women with affective disorders compared with normal family offspring, while the "other" category was significantly higher in the medically ill children than the normal group children.

Overall, the children's stressors over the 3-year period of observation were remarkably similar to those observed for the mothers. Children at risk due to maternal illness, both medical and psychiatric, did indeed experience more stressful events than did normal group children. Generally speaking the effects were more pronounced for the affective disorders group than the medically ill group, but the effects were not always statistically significant. It was noted that children's exposure to stress included both episodic and chronic stressors, and the high risk groups were higher on both types. Additionally, interpersonal conflict—both family and peer—appeared to be an area of increased exposure. We might speculate that to a large extent, children's own characteristics and behaviors contribute to the occurrence of such events; indeed, the children of women with affective disorders had significantly higher levels of events considered "dependent" or at least partly dependent on their behaviors. Therefore, we conclude that stress exposure is one by-product of living in a family with an ill mother and thus a potential contributor to the children's dysfunctions. Moreover, to the degree that much of the stress took the form of interpersonal conflict, we may be observing an emergent pattern of reciprocal stress–symptom causation that heralds a pernicious course of development and adjustment for the youngsters.

Specific Vulnerability: Congruence Between Events and Self-Schema

As noted in Chapter 4, an integration of cognitive and life stress approaches to depression vulnerability led to the prediction that individuals whose beliefs and feelings of self-regard and efficacy were attached to particular domains of functioning would be especially vulnerable to develop depression if negative events occurred in that specific domain (but less so in other domains). Hammen and Goodman-Brown (1990) extended the hypotheses to children. We found that the youngsters in the present sample could typically be characterized as having salient themes related either to interpersonal events or to achievement events. Of the children who completed the procedures, 33 were classified as interpersonally vulnerable (19 girls and 14 boys) and 31 as achievement vulnerable (16 girls and 15 boys). An additional 9 children could not be classified, and 3 children were omitted from the analyses based on lack of events during the follow-up.

Children's stressful events and symptoms in the 6 months following schema assessment were compiled, and all events that occurred were independently judged as primarily interpersonal or achievement in content. Two groups of children were formed, 13 who became more depressed and 51 who had no depressive symptoms. (Of the 13 symptomatic youngsters, 7 had onsets of major or minor depression and 6 were exacerbations of ongoing dysthymic symptoms.) Stressful life events that occurred prior to symptom change for the depressed group, and for the entire 6-month period for the nondepressed group, were compiled and categorized by content. A chi-square analysis of depressed/not depressed by congruent/noncongruent events was computed. (The congruent events category meant that the child experienced more events of the same type as her schema type than of the nonschema type.) The overall chi-square was statistically significant, $\chi^2(1) = 3.02$, $p < .05$, one-tailed. Thus there appeared to be an association between depression symptom change and the congruence of events and schema type. Because of the small sample sizes, it was not possible to determine the effect separately for interpersonal and achievement schemas. However, it was apparent that most of the children who became depressed were in the interpersonal vulnerability group. Whether this pattern is unique to the sample, or unique to children of this developmental stage, remains to be explored. Additionally, since interpersonal events are more common than achievement events, and events of all kinds were more frequent in the children who became depressed, the data can be said to provide only suggestive support for the congruency hypothesis itself. Nevertheless, it does appear that for certain children who appear to base their views of themselves on interpersonal experiences, depression was associated with a preponderance of difficulties in the social domain.

Maternal Symptoms as Stressors

We hypothesized that the occurrence of significant symptoms in the mother might serve as a stressor for the child and hence be associated with onset of symptoms in the child. The expression of depressive or other distress reactions in the parent could be threatening to the child and could signal the withdrawal of support and availability of the parent. Thus, as a "threat" and "loss" event, we might predict that exacerbations of maternal symptoms would be associated with onset or increase of symptoms in the child.

TABLE 5.6. Hierarchical regression analysis to predict children's depression at 6-month follow-up.

Variable	R^2 change	Significance of R^2 change
Initial depression	.21	$t = 4.0,\ p < .0001$
Event stress total	.03	$t = 1.76, p = .08$
Maternal symptom stress	.10	$t = 3.73, p < .001$
Events maternal symptoms	.04	$t = 2.22, p < .05$
Overall $F(4, 79) = 11.75, p < .0001$, overall $R = .61$, $R^2 = .37$		

Note: From "The Relationship Between Mother and Child Episodes in a Longitudinal Study of Risk for Depression" by C. Hammen, D. Burge, and C. Adrian, (in press). *Journal of Consulting and Clinical Psychology*.

Moreover, when the child experiences stressful life events, the impact of maternal symptoms may be intensified because the child needs assistance from the mother, whose symptoms may interfere with her ability to respond. Thus there might be a direct effect of maternal symptoms, as well as an interactive effect of maternal symptoms and child events, in predicting the child's depression (see also Longfellow & Belle, 1985, who tested a "buffering" effect of maternal mood and maternal stressors on children's outcomes).

Table 5.6 presents the results of a hierarchical multiple regression analysis (Hammen, Burge, & Adrian, in press). Initial symptoms were controlled by entering level of depression first, then the child's objective threat stress total (prior to depression onset) and objective threat rating associated with maternal symptomatology, and finally the interaction of the two latter terms. All the data were based on the first 6-month follow-up period. As the table indicates, each of the variables was a significant incremental predictor, although the main effect of children's stress was only marginally significant. Of particular interest, the maternal symptom stress rating was highly significant as a predictor of children's depression, and the interaction term added to the prediction beyond that. Figure 5.1 presents the form of the interaction. As expected, children showed relatively magnified depressive reactions under the combination of high personal stress and maternal symptom stress.

The impact of maternal and child symptoms, construed as stressors, on each other is discussed further in Chapter 7. Also, the possible effect of maternal symptoms and stressful life experiences on the quality of the interaction between the mother and the child is considered. Chapter 6 examines this hypothesis in detail.

Summary and Directions for Further Research

A simple goal of the present investigation was to explore the role of stress as a predictor of children's risk for dysfunction. Maternal illness,

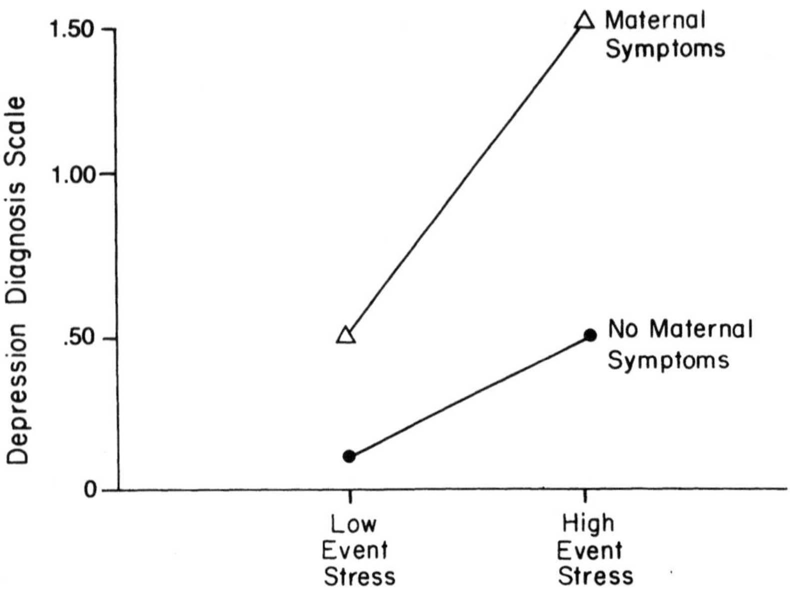

FIGURE 5.1. Children's mean depression diagnosis rating as a function of level of stressful events and Presence of maternal symptoms. From "The Relationship Between Mother and Child Episodes in a Longitudinal Study of Risk for Depression" by C. Hammen, D. Burge, and C. Adrian, in press. *Journal of Consulting and Clinical Psychology*.

both psychiatric and medical, may constitute stressful environments that challenge the family's adaptive capacities. In this chapter we saw that illness as a stress condition affects children's outcomes, and the effect is more pronounced for the affective disorders groups (especially unipolar depression) than for medically ill groups. Moreover, chronic stressors, which often accompany illness status both as cause and consequence, also contributed to children's outcomes. And even beyond that, children's own stressful life events contributed to their negative outcomes—and such analyses extend the methodological achievements of past research.

Additional findings emerged that provide considerable food for thought. Both mothers and children in families with affective disorders as well as chronic medical illnesses experience more stressful life events, objectively defined, than do normal family members. Increased exposure to stress certainly sets the stage for continuing distress. Moreover, it appeared that some of the women, especially those with recurrent unipolar disorder, contributed to the causation of stressful events. They were especially likely to be involved in interpersonal difficulties. Similar patterns were also observed in their children. Additionally, it was possible to identify in advance the children who had a particular vulnerability to interpersonal events, and those who experienced a preponderance of such events indeed appeared to become more depressed. Finally, the interdependency of the mothers and children in an interpersonal network of mutual impact was hinted at in the finding that children who were exposed to maternal symptoms as a stressor—and particularly when they had their own high levels of stress—became more depressed.

The results considered in the present analyses reinforce investigators' observations that the multiple, overlapping, adverse conditions which seem to trouble distressed families defy easy explication (e.g., Rutter & Quinton, 1984). Stressful life events occurring in high risk families, in the final analysis, pose more questions than answers. On the one hand, they represent disruptive circumstances, and we have some general notions that they function to create difficulties that challenge the coping capabilities of the individuals (e.g., Lazarus & Folkman, 1984). On the other hand, life events are also a *marker* of processes that we can only speculate about: They may get in the way of maternal "buffering" or attachment with children and therefore have their effects by impairing important mothering activities. Or they may indicate certain maternal characteristics that actually reflect interpersonal impairment contributing to event occurrence, and to possible parental impairment as well. Such complexities require us to revise the view of stressors as external events that merely "happen" to people.

6
Parent–Child Relationships and Depression

Over the decades depression has been variously characterized by the dominant etiological theory of the times as an intrapsychic disorder in response to loss, as a biological disorder of defective genes or neurotransmitters, as a cognitive disorder of dysfunctional thinking about the self and the environment. Recently, at least among certain psychologists, the emphasis has shifted again: depression is an interpersonal disorder. Depression undoubtedly involves some of all of these and other processes, for it is wise to consider that there are "different depressions," involving different origins.

The interpersonal emphasis is an especially important one, for it reminds us that people exist in the social world and cannot properly be understood, or treated, in isolation. There are three components to the interpersonal emphasis: interpersonal causes, interpersonal symptoms, and interpersonal consequences of depression. Theories of the social *origins* of depression cut across various philosophical viewpoints, including intrapsychic responses to interpersonal loss, reactions to interpersonal events, particular vulnerability to events involving attachment and social contact, or dysfunctional interpersonal skills that create or maintain inadequate interpersonal rewards (see in particular the work of Arieti & Bemporad, 1980; Brown & Harris, 1978; Bowlby, 1980; Lewinsohn, 1974; Paykel, 1979).

The *symptoms* of depression that are relevant to the interpersonal realm include loss of pleasure, which usually entails diminished enjoyment of formerly engaging relationships, often accompanied by social withdrawal, irritability that may be directed toward others, increased dependency on others as a result of feeling helpless and inadequate, increased sensitivity to perceived rejection or distancing by others. The individual's reduced energy and motivation commonly result in difficulty in sustaining effort or participation in activities, including interpersonal contacts. It becomes easy to give up, or to avoid effortful interactions. The cognitive characteristics of depressive thinking doubtless lead to evaluations of the self and others in pejorative terms. While longing for solace to ease the depressive feelings, the individual may nonetheless believe that others are incapable or insensitive—indeed, the individual is unlikely to feel comforted even if caring others provide support and encouragement.

Given these common symptoms of depression, it is hardly surprising that the *consequences* of depression involve impairment of social role functioning. Over time, the moderately or severely or persistently depressed person may be avoided by others who find the interactions aversive or who experience futility, feeling that nothing they can do is helpful to the depressed person. Depressed individuals are not fun to be around, and in addition may simply be unable to perform their typical role obligations—as responsive parent, loving spouse, or even instrumental adult. The work of Coyne and colleagues (e.g., Coyne, Kahn, & Gotlib, 1987) has characterized the dysfunctional transactions of depressed persons in their social context and provided data on the aversive consequences of interacting with depressed others (see also Billings & Moos, 1983; and Billings, Cronkite, & Moos, 1983, on consequences of depression on the family and on the positive role of supportive family relationships; Barnett & Gotlib, 1988, review and discuss the extensive data on interpersonal causes and consequences of depression; see also Gotlib & Colby, 1987).

Clearly, a general review of the data on interpersonal aspects of depression is beyond the scope of the current discussion. This general commentary sets the stage, however, for a fuller discussion of research specifically on *family relationships* and depression. Several strands of research from adult and developmental psychopathology are discussed briefly. In their suggestion of a link between depressive outcomes and disturbed family relationships, these early studies suggested the need for direct evaluations of family processes in our high risk sample. At the point that the current study began, there were virtually no such direct observations in families of children at risk. Subsequently, developmental psychopathologists and others have contributed theories and direct observation studies on the descriptive characteristics and possible processes involved in depressed parent–child interactions. Relevant work in such areas is discussed. Finally, data from this project are presented to answer a variety of questions about the nature and consequences of parent–child interactions in the high risk families.

Depression Associated with Negative Parent–Child Relationships

Some of the earlier indirect studies included methods such as retrospective questionnaire-based reports and interviews about behavior or attitudes.

Depressed Adults' Reports of Childhood Experiences

Burbach and Borduin (1986) reviewed 14 studies of retrospective reports by depressed patients of their parents' child-rearing practices. Although limited by the methodological weaknesses of the retrospective procedures, nonstandardized questionnaires, and lack of diagnostic evaluations of the adult patients, the reports contained uniform themes of negative qualities of parent–child interaction (see also Holmes & Robins, 1987; McCranie & Bass, 1984; Perris et al., 1986). There was some inconsistency across studies in the reported dimensions of parental care, owing largely to use of noncomparable instruments. Nevertheless, the most common themes included reports of low care (low involvement, withdrawal of affection) and use of negative or punitive strategies. None of the early studies presented information on whether the parents were depressed or suffered from other psychopathology.

A major limitation of restrospective accounts is that depressed persons may exaggerate negative experiences recalled from the past. To test this potential source of bias, Parker (1981) compared perceived child-rearing behaviors reported by subjects and their mothers. He found a significant degree of correspondence between mothers' own reports and those of subjects. A similar goal led Oliver, Handal, Finn, and Herdy (1987) to compare parental child-rearing practices reported by pairs of siblings. They found that while relatively depressed individuals did indeed recall more negative behaviors in their parents, their reports corresponded with those of their nondepressed siblings. Parker also reported test–retest reliability in samples of clinically depressed patients in their reports of negative child-rearing experiences and found that such reports were fairly stable and did not change much even when patients' depression level changed. On the other hand, Lewinsohn and Rosenbaum (1987) studied the recollections of community residents about their parents' child-rearing practices and found that nondepressed and remitted depressed individuals' perceptions did not differ. They concluded that reports of negative child-rearing practices may be biased by the depressed state; however, since their analyses did not include direct evidence of a shift in perceptions when mood changed, their speculation requires further testing. Overall, the preponderance of retrospective data consistently indicate some types of negative child-rearing experiences, but it seems important to pursue the matter with direct observation studies that would represent a more valid sampling of actual parental practices.

A final note concerning retrospective reports of depression associated with negative child-rearing experiences emerges from the vast array of studies on childhood loss. Although the experience of the loss of attachment figures in childhood has been theorized to be an important antecedent of depression (Bowlby, 1988), the research on the topic has yielded a mixed picture with considerable inconsistency of results with respect to adult depression. Recently, however, the quality of care received by the child following the loss has been implicated as the critical factor. Two recent studies suggest that lack of adequate parental care following the loss predicted adult psychopathology (typically depression); those who received good and supportive care in stable family situations were less likely to display evidence of disorder (e.g., Bifulco et al., 1987; Breier et al., 1988).

Ratings of Depressed Children's Relationships with Parents

A few studies attempted to characterize the quality of parent–child relationships in the families of children who were currently depressed. Several such studies involved clinical samples, although three such investigations lacked a comparison group (see review by Burbach & Borduin, 1986). None of the instruments used for making ratings was psychometrically evaluated. Thus such studies may serve mainly as suggestive sources of information for further analysis. Nonetheless, the findings were consistent; generally more negative, less affectionate, and even cruel or abusive relationships were reported by clinical raters (e.g., Kaslow et al., 1984; Poznanski, Krahenbuhl, & Zrull, 1976; Puig-Antich et al., 1985a,b).

Family Relationships and the Prediction of Relapse

Recently, considerable research mostly in the field of schizophrenia has suggested that negative parent–child relationships portend relapse in schizophrenic offspring returned to their families after hospitalization. Extensions of this research on the role of the so-called expressed emotion (EE) variable of parental criticism and/or overprotection have now been applied to affective disorders. Hooley, Orley, and Teasdale (1986) found that 59% of patients with high EE spouses relapsed during the follow-up observation. Adult bipolar patients returning to their families have been found to have higher relapse rates if they come from high EE families (Miklowitz, Goldstein, Nuechterlein, Snyder, & Mintz, 1988). One of the shortcomings of the expressed emotion construct is that it is overly general, however, and recently two studies have suggested that it is criticism about the patient that is the strongest predictor of relapse (e.g., Hooley & Teasdale, 1989; Spiegel & Wissler, 1986).

Overall, therefore, there is suggestive evidence that depression, both in adults and in children, may be related to dysfunctional relationships with the parents. The methods of the studies do not permit the conclusion that depression is caused by such relationships, since the data may be subject to depressive distortion, parents' (or spouses') behaviors may be a consequence of the child's or patient's behaviors, or both may be due to other, unassessed causes. Thus additional methods are needed to observe the relationships to directly characterize the qualities and to establish the causal connections between depression outcomes and parental/ interpersonal behaviors.

Impairment of Parental Functioning in Depressed Women

An additional link in the presumptive chain of associations between negative quality of parent–child relationships and depression comes from studies of children of depressed parents. Noting the growing body of research on the risk to children for psychopathology in such families, a few investigations have attempted to characterize the quality of the parent–child relationship, testing the possibility that depression impairs parental functioning and thus contributes to children's dysfunction. In the sections to follow this relatively sparse body of research is discussed briefly.

Depressed Parent Reports

The original research on dysfunctional maternal interactions with children was reported by Myrna Weissman and colleagues (e.g., Weissman et al., 1972; Weissman & Paykel, 1974), based on interviews with the clinically depressed women. Interviews of 40 depressed women and normal control women indicated that at all ages of children, women's depression was associated with greater friction and less positive involvement with their children. Even when the women had recovered from episodes of depression, they reported continuing interpersonal dysfunction in their relationships with their children and others. Unfortunately, little information about the children's functioning was provided, and no direct data were collected from the children about their conditions or their experience of their relationship with their mothers.

In addition to the depressed women's reports of dysfunctional parenting cited by Weissman and Paykel (1974), other investigators have indicated that depressed women feel ineffective or report more negative perceptions of their children (Davenport et al., 1984). A number of studies have shown that maternal depressed mood contributes to reports of more problems in children; relatively depressed women view their children's behaviors more negatively even when observations or independent reports failed to note objective differences between such children and the control group youngsters or suggested that relatively depressed mothers may exaggerate the extent of difficulties in their youngsters (e.g., Forehand, Wells, McMahon, Griest, & Rogers, 1982; Griest, Forehand, Wells, & McMahon, 1980; Griest, Wells, & Forehand, 1979; Webster-Stratton & Hammond, 1988).

Research by the Moos group on socioenvironmental predictors of the functioning of children of depressed adults is also relevant to a consideration of family relationships. Both the initial cross-sectional study (Billings & Moos, 1983) and the 1-year follow-up (Billings & Moos, 1985a) indicated that children's physical and psychological functioning was associated with parents' reports of family arguments. Overall, the remitted depressed families reported more positive attributes on the Family Environment Scale than did the nonremitted patient families; correspondingly, the children in the remitted depressed families functioned better than those in the nonremitted families.

Weintraub (1987) reported outcomes of school-age children of schizophrenia, unipolar, bipolar, and normal parents from the original Stony Brook High Risk study. He noted that "considerable deviance in family functioning, expressed in conflict, marital discord, and parenting skills, was characteristic of the families with an ill child, and this discord was related to child adjustment" (p. 439). However, little detail was presented, and no information was given on specific patterns within diagnostic groups. The general theme of the report emphasized nonspecificity of children's outcomes by parent diagnosis.

All of these studies provide suggestive but typically indirect information generally supporting the notion that depression in mothers or parents is associated with more critical and negative attitudes toward their children or family conflict. More compelling evidence, however, comes from direct observations of the patterns of interactions of depressed women and their children.

Observations of Depressed Women with Their Infants and Toddlers

Clinical observations and some of the earliest systematic observations based on high risk samples suggested that depressed women have great difficulties in their interactions with their babies. They appear overwhelmed, anxious, unresponsive, and uninvolved (e.g., Anthony, 1983; Cohler et al., 1977; Sameroff et al., 1982). Similar patterns have also been reported in observations of manic depressive women (or spouses of bipolar men) with their infants (Davenport et al., 1984).

Studies of women with elevated depression scores, rather than clinical diagnoses, also indicate evidence of caretaking difficulties with infants. Livingood, Daen, and Smith (1983), observing mildly depressed women with their newborns, and saw less unconditional positive regard toward their babies, compared with nondepressed women—although the groups did not differ on stimulation and contact. Field (1984) observed that relatively depressed women displayed reduced responding and less positive expressions toward their babies. Subsequent research has also indicated less responsiveness by the infants of depressed mothers (also Field, Healy, Goldstein, & Guthertz, 1990; Field et al., 1985, 1988). Bettes (1988) observed that relatively depressed mothers' speech directed toward the infant was delayed, compared to that of nondepressed mothers. Fleming, Ruble, Flett, and Shaul (1988) also observed that postpartum depressed mothers showed less reciprocal vocalization and affectionate contact with infants than did the nondepressed mothers.

In addition to these indications of unresponsiveness and relative withdrawal from their babies by depressed women, there is some indication of hostility. For instance, Lyons-Ruth, Zoll, Connell, and Grunebaum (1986) found that relatively depressed low income mothers displayed evidence of covert hostility and flattened affect with their year-old babies. Cohn, Matias, Tronick, Connell, and Lyons-Ruth (1986) also found angry and intrusive behaviors displayed by depressed mothers toward their babies. Cohn, Campbell, Matias, and Hopkins (1990) did not find that depressed mothers of infants were unresponsive, but rather they were more negative toward their infants (especially boys) and the infants, too, were more negative.

Maternal depressed behavior appears to affect the infants; studies of simulated depression indicated that infants react with protest responses (Cohn & Tronick, 1983). Field (1984) found that only babies of nondepressed mothers reacted, whereas those of naturally depressed women did not change. However, Field et al. (1990) observed that the infants of depressed mothers "matched" their mothers' state more often when she was negative and less when she was positive. Whiffen and Gotlib (1989) observed that infants of women with postpartum depression displayed lower cognitive development on the Bayley Scales of Infant Development, and they also displayed more negative emotional reactions during the testing periods.

Studies of depressed mothers and their toddlers also suggest dysfunctional interactions. For instance, unipolar and bipolar women were observed interacting with their 1- to 4-year-old children, and the children's attachment behavior was assessed in the Strange Situation (Radke-Yarrow et al., 1985). Compared with children of normal women, there were more insecurely attached children of diagnosed women, especially manic depressive mothers. There was a significant association between attachment and quality of affect expressed by the mother toward the child. Mothers of securely attached children expressed positive affect more often and negative affect less often than did the mothers of insecurely attached children. Observed at ages 2 to 3, the children and their unipolar and bipolar mothers spoke less, and the mothers tended to respond more slowly to their children's speech (Breznitz & Sherman, 1987). Also based on the same population, Kochanska, Kuczynski, Radke-Yarrow, and Welsh (1987) observed "control episodes," in which the mother attempted to influence the child's behavior during naturalistic interactions. They found that women with affective disorders were less successful in resolving such episodes compared with normal mothers. For instance, when control efforts by the mother were resisted, women with affective disorders were more likely to avoid confronting the child by dropping their demands; or, if they persisted, there was less likelihood of mutually negotiated compromise.

Goodman and Brumley (1990) observed 3-month- to 5-year-old children and their clinically depressed or schizophrenic or normal mothers in a sample of disadvantaged black women. Although not as impaired in parenting as the schizophrenic mothers, the depressed mothers displayed significantly less responsiveness, involvement, structure, or discipline compared to the normal mothers. The youngsters whose mothers displayed more positive affect, interest, and involvement with them had higher mental development IQ scores. Also, aspects of children's social behavior were associated with maternal responsiveness. Finally, in an English sample of depressed community women who were parents of 2- to 3-year-olds, Mills, Puckering, Pound, and Cox (1985) reported reduced proportions of reciprocated interactions between the depressed mothers and their children. The authors interpret the pattern as a failure by the mother to "recruit, sustain and expand the young child's attention and concentration"—a concept similar to many of the other studies' reports of lack of maternal responsiveness or speech contingency. Mills et al. also reported that the children with the greatest level of behavior problems had the mothers with the lowest proportions of reciprocated interactions.

Observations of Depressed Women with School-Age Children

Information available on the interactions of mothers of school-age and adolescent children is scant. Besides the current study, which is reported in a later section, only a few such studies were located. Webster-Stratton and Hammond (1988) observed mothers of 3- to 8-year-old clinic-referred children. The women were classified as depressed or nondepressed by a cutoff score of 10 or higher on the Beck Depression Inventory. Relatively dysphoric women made more critical statements toward their youngsters during the observation period but otherwise did not differ from nondepressed women on praise or other behaviors. Hops et al. (1987) collected systematic observation data in the homes of 52 families, of whom 27 of the mothers met RDC-SADS criteria for major or minor depression. The depressed women were further subdivided into those who were maritally distressed or nondistressed. The children were between the ages of 3 and 16. The distinctive features of this study are the extensiveness of the observations, covering ten 1-hour occasions, and the analyses of sequences of communications between family members. In addition to the observed dysphoric affect displayed by the depressed women in their interactions, a major finding was that mothers' sadness served to suppress the aggressive affect of other family members. Also, family members' aggressive affect appeared to suppress the mothers' dysphoric affect. The authors interpret this pattern to reflect mutually aversive interchanges that the family members find functional in the short run, but that are clearly maladaptive overall.

Panaccione and Wahler (1986) observed mothers interacting with their preschool children and found that maternal depression level (BDI score) was associated with how aversively the mother interacted with the child (disapproval, shouting, and other negative behaviors). The depression scores were also associated with maternal negative perceptions of the child's behaviors.

Cole and Rehm (1986) observed parents of 8- to 12-year-old clinic-referred depressed and nondepressed children and of normal controls interacting with their child in a structured task. This study is included here because at least half of the mothers of the depressed children (and a few mothers of the other children) met criteria for clinical depression. The brief observations were scored with methods intended to test Rehm's self-regulation model of depression. Of particular relevance here is the finding that mothers of depressed youngsters were significantly less likely to express positive feedback after their child's performance compared with nonclinic mothers. The groups did not differ, however, in expressions of negative affect and criticisms toward their children.

Noting the correlational nature of most of the observation data on effects of maternal mood on parenting behaviors, Jouriles, Murphy, and O'Leary (1989) attempted an experimental manipulation of mood. Observing mothers interacting with their 4- or 5-year-old boys following positive and negative mood induction, the investigators found significant differences in frequency of positive maternal communication (but not negative) in the two mood states. The mothers were more talkative overall in the positive mood induction condition than in the negative condition.

Conclusions and Gaps in Research on Family Interactions and Depression

The diverse studies of child-rearing deficiencies associated with depression, and depression associated with antecedent dysfunctional family relationships, all suggest disruption in the parent–child relationship as a cause and consequence of depression. Certainly, the consistency of reported difficulties encourages us to supplement the intense genetic focus in psychopathology research on affective disorders with further investigations of the family relationships. Nevertheless, the body of research briefly reviewed clearly raises far more questions than it answers.

Methodological Limitations

Research that would be most definitive is also that which is most lacking: direct observational analyses of parent–child relationships, analyses of associations between parent behavior and children's outcomes, using designs that permit inferences of causality including reciprocal influences of child–parent relationships and including clinically depressed parents. Naturalistic and longitudinal studies would be especially valuable, but cross-sectional and experimental methods that permit microanalyses of causal processes and address issues pertaining to mechanisms are also much needed.

Although methodological gaps in the existing studies are apparent (see also Burbach & Borduin, 1986; Downey & Coyne, 1990), it is clear that the field is rapidly expanding and moving in the direction of increased sophistication. Thus perhaps an even more pressing need is for the clarification of the conceptual gaps to be addressed to guide the use of improved methods.

Conceptual Limitations in Family Studies of the Antecedents of Depression

Several issues have not been adequately addressed, much less resolved, in recent research: explanatory mechanisms, direction of causality, and specificity to depression. These are noted only briefly here (but see also Burbach & Borduin, 1986; Downey & Coyne, 1990; Gelfand & Teti, 1990).

The consideration of explanatory mechanisms is enormously complex and must include two questions: What about depression affects maternal child-rearing practices? What about those practices affects the child, leading to dysfunction and to depression? As various clinicians have noted, depression refers not only to affect (sadness, irritability) but also to energy, motivation, cognition, interest. A depressed mother's tasks at different developmental stages of the child are different, and they may be differentially affected by her various symptoms. There are numerous avenues for exploration; two that have been in the forefront are attitudes of hostility, rejection, and criticism on the one hand and reduced energy, involvement, responsiveness, and contingency on the other. Downey and Coyne (1990), for instance, reviewed the mother–child observation studies and noted the reduced effort apparently shown by relatively depressed women with their infants, possibly owing to their own low energy. Such women may be highly self-focused and therefore inattentive and withdrawn, or they may be defective in the timing of the responsiveness to their children (e.g., Goodman & Brumley, 1990; Mills et al., 1985). The woman's lack of energy and negativistic beliefs about her abilities and motivations may reduce her persistence, patience, and willingness to persevere or be assertive in conflict resolution (e.g., Bugenthal & Shennum, 1984; Kochanska et al., 1987). Hostility and irritability, on the other hand, may reflect not only negative attitudes about herself and her children but also reduced tolerance for imperfections or noncompliance in the child (e.g., Forehand et al., 1987). Mood-related cognitions may affect the awareness, interpretation, and recollections the mother has about the positive and negative features of the child's behavior (e.g., Jouriles & O'Leary, 1990).

We need to study how the behaviors the mother emits are dysfunctional as well as how her symptoms affect her behavior. Among the numerous candidates for further exploration are emotional arousal and regulation of emotions in the mother and child (Zahn-Waxler, Kochanska, Krupnick, & McKnew, 1990), insecure or dysfunctional attachment (e.g., Radke-Yarrow et al., 1985), and internalization of self-esteem by the child. And of course the child's acquisition of appropriate problem-solving skills and social relationship capacities may not only be adversely affected but also may exert an ongoing pernicious effect on subsequent development (e.g., Beardslee, Schultz, & Selman, 1987; Pettit, Dodge, & Brown, 1988; Zahn-Waxler et al., 1990). Thus a great deal of the *how* and *when*—along with the *what*—needs to be subjected to systematic microanalysis.

The second major gap concerns the direction of causality. Most of the research designs of existing studies do not fully address the possibility that mothers are responding negatively to their deviant children or that both the maternal behavior and the child's behaviors represent reciprocal patterns of dysfunctional interaction (a major exception is Hops et al., 1987). Even studies that indicate deviant and noncompliant responding by the child do not clarify the origin of such behavior. Explorations of the beginnings of dysfunctional patterns are, of course, likely to require going back to the earliest days after birth, when the temperament of the child may elicit dysfunctional or "depressive" behaviors from the parents (e.g., Rutter & Quinton, 1984; Whiffen & Gottlib, 1989). Forehand et al. (1987) have suggested that for families of children with externalizing disorders, the direction of causality may be from child conduct disorders to parent depression; within families, different child characteristics may elicit or respond differentially to parent behaviors displayed while depressed. There is no lack of interest in the question of mutual influences of parent and child, yet research designs capable of exploring such patterns have been scarce.

Finally, the question of specificity remains to be tackled with the vigor it deserves. This issue has two aspects: specificity of depressive outcomes as a consequence of certain child-rearing practices and specificity of depression as a cause of certain child-rearing practices. The issue of whether depression in offspring is a specific consequence of particular behaviors (e.g., criticism, withdrawal) is entirely murky. Few studies have addressed the topic with methods permitting that kind of question to be raised. When appropriate comparison groups and sensitive outcome or process measures have been employed, studies suggest little evidence of specificity. For instance, the schizophrenia high risk studies have not identified qualitative differences in the parenting practices of patient parents associated with one disorder or another (e.g., Goodman & Brumley 1990; Weintraub, 1987). Virtually no high risk study has addressed the question of which childhood disorders are linked with particular kinds of parenting practices. Holmes and Robins (1987) reported that unfair, inconsistent, and harsh discipline was associated with both depression and alcoholism in adults. Overall, therefore, there is considerable room for exploring what parent–child relationship issues are related to depression outcomes or to other outcomes.

The other major issue of specificity is the question of whether the dysfunctional parenting alleged to result from depression is actually specific to depression. Downey and Coyne (1990; see also Chapter 5 of this volume) argue that stress, including marital distress or other ongoing stressful conditions, rather than depression as such, may contribute to dysfunctional interpersonal behaviors. It is critical to explore this issue, because an undue emphasis on depression—an intraindividual experience—to the neglect of stress—a contextual condition—could result in misleading conclusions on the nature of dysfunctional relationships and their treatment. Downey and Coyne review research on consequences of stressful conditions for parenting, concluding that there is evidence that parental dysfunctions arise in a variety of stressful conditions not specific to depression. Although Fendrich et al., (1990) reach a different conclusion about the contributory role of family environmental factors versus parental depression on offspring diagnoses, their analyses indicate that families with affective disorders have high levels of marital discord, parent–child conflict, and related risk factors. Downey and Coyne present several alternative models for further testing, in which the relations between depression, marital discord, and child outcomes indicate various causal paths with different theoretical and treatment implications.

The present investigation attempted at least a preliminary approach to some of the underexplored topics in the area of parent–child relations in families with affective disorder: Do the behaviors of depressed and nondepressed women toward their school-age children differ? Is there an association between maternal behaviors toward the child and the child's functioning? What contextual factors influence maternal interactions? What aspects of the child's functioning may be particularly affected by maternal dysfunctional interaction? What can we say about reciprocity in the interactions of children and their mothers?

Results of the Study

Children's Awareness and Perceptions of Maternal Disorder

Children were interviewed about their perceptions of maternal illness. We attempted to avoid any mention of maternal affective disorders, and we wondered if the children were aware of such conditions and what they perceived the consequences to be. Children were highly aware, for the most part, of their mothers' depression. In analyses conducted by Friedmann (1989), unipolar offspring were all aware of their mothers' depression, compared with about 75% of the children of bipolar and medically ill women. Moreover, the more aware children were, the more they tended to have negative reactions marked by anger, anxiety, and sadness. Children of unipolar depressed mothers reported that their mothers displayed more depression and saw more serious mood changes in their mothers than did children in any other group, including the bipolar group. Children of bipolar and medically ill women, on the other hand, were most likely to see their mothers as having significant anxiety. Interestingly, irritability was the change in their mothers that children most associated with the mother's depression, and the more they perceived that she became irritable when depressed, the more likely the children themselves were to experience depression. Children reported that they became anxious and sad when the mother was depressed or ill, but older children were particularly likely to report that they became angry. Overall, the results suggest that anger and irritability were salient features of family interactions involving a depressed or ill mother. Unipolar children in particular saw their mothers as frequently depressed and irritable.

Maternal Group Differences in Observed Interaction Behaviors

The present study was the first affective disorders offspring study involving school-age children (8- to 16-year-olds) of women with affective disorders who were actually observed in interactions with their mothers. Two tasks were selected for observation, representing an achievement situation and a conflict situation. In the former task, as described in Chapter 2, children were asked to perform a block-stacking task while blindfolded and coached by their mother. They were led to believe that most kids could stack 8 of the 10 blocks, although in reality it is a very difficult task and only a few blocks could be stacked without knocking over the whole design. Inducing an achievement orientation and subsequent "failure" was intended to elicit behaviors that would permit the testing of certain hypotheses about self-regulation. The second task involved selection of an area of common disagreement in the family and discussing the conflict while attempting to resolve it. Typical topics included bedtime, chores, and allowance. For each task the mother interacted with her child for 5 minutes; in cases where there were two children per family, separate observations were conducted.

The two tasks were intended to provide both semistructured and unstructured situations, and thus vary by situational characteristics as well as content, in order to give a wider representation of the "typical" interaction than a single task alone would give. However, it turned out that the achievement (Block) task was overly constrained by the situational demands, leading to low variability. In addition, some of the dyads responded to it less as an achievement situation than as a funny game not to be serious about. Therefore, we have less confidence in the results of this task, and only brief descriptions of patterns are reported.

The conflict discussion task, on the other hand, exceeded our hopes of capturing a valid sample of mother-child interaction. Six children refused the task, clearly anticipating that the ensuing conflict with their mothers, even about fairly mundane matters, would be too stressful. The dyads that did participate obviously forgot about the observation and appeared to engage in unrestrained discussion of the conflict, yielding a rich variety of responses. However, even though we witnessed on tape a great deal of conflict discussion, it is likely that the most distressed families were not included, and therefore the resulting data are based on a somewhat conservative sample for testing hypotheses about conflict.

The coding system that was the basis for most of the analyses presented here is described more fully in Chapter 2.

Mother Responses

Maternal interactions were analyzed by group based on one randomly chosen child per family in cases where two children participated (Gordon et al., 1989). Five summary scores were computed combining conceptually similar categories and analyzed as proportions of total utterances. These included two scores capturing task involvement: task-productive comments and off-task commentary. Three concerned affective quality of the communication toward the child: positive-confirmatory comments, disconfirmatory comments, and negative comments. Finally, negative self-directed comments were included as a separate category.

Table 6.1 presents the mean proportion scores for each type of comment by group. An overall multivariate analysis of variance indicated significant differences between groups ($F[6, 48] = 1.97$, $p < .01$). Specifically, univariate planned comparisons indicated that the unipolar group mothers were significantly different from the medical and normal mothers on the task-focused and affective dimensions (with the exception of disconfirmatory comments). Unipolar women were more negative (critical) and less positive-confirmatory; they engaged in fewer task-productive comments

TABLE 6.1. Verbal interaction behavior of four groups of mothers during a discussion task with their children.

	Proportion of total utterances during task								Significant contrasts		
	Unipolar mothers (Group 1) ($N = 12$)		Bipolar mothers (Group 2) ($N = 12$)		Medically Ill mothers (Group 3) ($N = 11$)		Normal mothers (Group 4) ($N = 23$)				
Verbal behavior	*M*	*SD*	*M*	*SD*	*M*	*SD*	*M*	*SD*	*Groups*	$F(1, 153)$	*p*
Task productive	.255	.114	.447	.240	.371	.120	.419	.143	1 < 2	8.55	<.005
									1 < 3	3.11	<.08
									1 < 4	8.60	<.005
Off-task	.210	.191	.002	.103	.083	.078	.084	.110	1 > 2	4.54	<.04
									1 > 3	5.40	<.02
									1 > 4	7.29	<.009
Confirmatory/positive	.046	.065	.088	.065	.113	.048	.095	.096	1 < 3	4.29	<.04
									1 < 4	3.12	<.08
Disconfirmatory	.063	.055	.052	.038	.054	.053	.059	.059			
Negative	.161	.132	.089	.084	.055	.068	.030	.037	1 > 2	4.54	<.04
									1 > 3	10.07	<.002
									1 > 4	21.04	<.0001
Negative toward self	.014	.025	.000	.000	.013	.034	.002	.008	1 > 2	2.84	<.09

Note: From "Observations of Interactions of Depressed Women with Their Children" by D. Gordon, D. Burge, C. Hammen, C. Adrian, C. Jaenicke, and D. Hiroto, 1989, *American Journal of Psychiatry*, *146*, 50–55. Copyright 1989 by the American Psychiatric Association. Adapted by permission.

and more off-task, irrelevant comments. In four of the six dimensions they also differed significantly from the bipolar women; the two latter groups did not differ on disconfirmatory comments or on positive comments. Interestingly, while the unipolar women made the most self-critical comments, the bipolar women made virtually no such remarks about themselves.

Overall, therefore, the communications of the unipolar women especially seem to be different from those of the other groups. Unipolar women's communications were relatively more critical and negative, less positive and supportive, and the women displayed patterns of lower involvement with their children on the task at hand.

Examples of Mother-Child Interaction on the Conflict Task

Several excerpts from the transcripts illustrate the kinds of mother and child dimensions that were scored: staying on task or not, dealing with the issues or evading them, criticisms or irritable interactions. In addition, however, there are many qualities of the interactions that cannot be captured in simple behavioral dimensions, such as being unassertive or being commanding, controlling or being helpless, being constructive or undermining the other.

The first example is a 10-year-old boy and his medically ill mother, and the issue is "not minding his father." This child is normal but has mild symptoms of anxiety at this stage of his life, and he takes an avoidant stance with his mother.

Much of the first minute is taken with the child stating that he doesn't want to be on camera or recorded, and his mother trying to get him to talk about the issue. Then,

M: Now let's talk about you and your father.

C: (silence)

M: When he tells you to stop bouncing the ball in the house and you don't . . . will you tell me why?

C: Because.

M: Come on, you can tell me. Now don't just whisper, talk out loud.

C: (whispers) But I don't want a recording.

M: (irritated) Come on.

C: Momma, I don't want a recording.

M: Do you hate your Daddy?

C: (disagrees quickly) Mmmmh.

M: Because some days you mind him real good, don't you?

C: (agrees) Umhum, 'cause he don't take the ball away.

M: (irritated) Don't whisper. Say it out loud.

[C–M exchange in which he restates request not to be recorded, and she insists, then he starts to tell why he doesn't mind his father]

M: That doesn't give you a reason for not minding him. Like when he tells you to stop doing something it's because you're doing something wrong, Billy.

C: Yes, Mamma.

M: Don't you ever stop to think that maybe it frustrates him and that he brings you in there to me and makes me feel upset too because you refuse to mind him, and tell him "I don't have to mind you. I wanna go mind Mamma"?

C: No.

M: Well, it does, Billy. Do you think that maybe you could start minding him and being a good little boy?

C: Yeah.

M: . . . and stop causing us problems. Billy, sit down and talk to me.

[M–C discussion of the equipment; child restates wish not to be recorded]

M: (insistent tone) But I want to know why you don't mind your father.

C: Bec . . . I don't . . . because.

M: Tell me how you feel when you don't mind him. What makes you say things like that?

C: Sometimes he gets mad at me at something else and he blames me.

M: He doesn't always blame you. Tell me one time you did something (he blamed you for). Come on son, look over at Momma. I gotta hear you and see you to understand what you're trying to tell me.

C: (crying)

[M insists that he give example, interrupts when he starts]

C: Like when Bobby gets in trouble and he sees that I'm outside playing, he goes and said I did something wrong.

M: What were you doing?

C: I was playing catch. I wasn't missing the ball.

M: Well, if you hit Annie with the ball . . .

C: I didn't. She hit my hand, and he said I did something to her, and I didn't.

M: Why didn't you just tell him?

C: I didn't because he was too mad, and then I saw he was sweating so I didn't tell him.

M: Billie, will you start minding him now?

C: Yes.

M: And stop telling him you don't have to?

C: Yes.

Adam, the 14-year-old son of a unipolar depressed mother, is very angry and sarcastic with her as they discuss the issue of his going to school regularly (he has a great deal of truancy):

M: School's coming up in about 3 weeks. Have you thought about it at all?

C: (shakes head, says nothing)

M: Are you worried about it at all?

C: (shakes head, says nothing)

M: You don't want to to this, do you? We get to go home in 5 minutes. Well, I've been thinking about it and I'm not worried about it, but I want to hope that we can get you to school every day and not miss so many days as you did last year. Do you think you can do that?

[M and C discuss his going to bed early so he will get up in time for school]

M: That worked out pretty well, don't you think?

C: I don't know. Yeah, OK (angrily).

M: OK, and in the morning you don't feel like you can go to school I want you to try and be able to tell me that you don't want to go rather than say you're sick or pretend to go and then come back home. I want you to be up front with me about it.

C: Yeah, then you just say "go to school" (sarcastically).

M: I'll probably try to talk you into it, yeah. 'Cause the more days you miss, the more you get behind and the harder it is to go back. You think I'm unreasonable in expecting you to go most of the time?

C: I don't know.

M: You'd just as soon skip it entirely?

C: I already know, Mother.

M: I'd like to work out a plan where you . . .

C: (interrupts) Yes, Dr. J—(sarcastically).

M: We're supposed to talk about this for 5 minutes, and I'm trying. When you do start school I'm hoping that we'll be able to keep regular hours. You'll be able to get to bed at 10 so you won't be too tired the following moring. That's what we did when you came home from the hospital last time and it worked pretty well, don't you think?

C: Whatever . . . yeah, OK. (angrily).

The next pair consists of a 14-year-old and her bipolar mother, discussing the topic of chores. At this point, the girl has had one major depressive episode, and within 6 months of this interview she had another.

[M and C discuss which topic to pick, and Mom decides on chores]

C: No, because you always got mad because I didn't do the chores, and I did just as many as you did! Now I can't even talk to you about chores because I'm afraid you'll be mad at me.

M: Okay, so that's a great subject. So . . . we think you don't do enough chores?

C: I think I do, uh, I do at least as much as you do.

M: You do?

C: Yes, and . . .

M: You do?

C: Yes, and . . .

M: (interrupts) I don't think so, I don't. I am going to start writing down the things I do, like besides picking up the dog doo, and weeding the garden and all those kinds of things, and changing . . . how many times have you changed a lightbulb?

C: I changed all of mine. I change all the ones that come into my path, Mom.

M: Well, that's good (sarcastically).

C: I don't just leave it undone!

M: Well, that's beautiful. But, you know, like I changed a light bulb the other night that had been blown for at least several days. Over the TV.

[M and C discuss the light bulbs. C did not know which ones were supposed to be on or not, or how to unscrew them]

M: Well, ask and I'll tell you.

C: Well, I don't know what I'm supposed to be asking about, Mom (defensive). I didn't even know anything about it, and you're telling me to ask about it?

M: You don't have to get defensive, it's OK.

C: I'm not . . .

M: It's OK, really, it's OK.

[M and C discuss other chores, with Mom questioning every statement the child makes, then:]

C: I don't clean out the toilet and I don't clean the shower, I know.

M: Yes, and I do, and those are dirty things to have to do, and I don't ask you to do them . . . What else?

C: I make your bed when it's not made.

M: (surprised) You do?

C: And I clean up the dog doo when I'm out there. And I wash all the laundry . . .

M: (interrupting) But wait a minute. I think that you think that you're doing a big deal when you pick up four piles, and I'm out there every week.

[They continue arguing about who does more]

M: But you see what I'm saying? In other words, I'm sick and tired of doing all those terrible and yucky things. They're not easier for me, just because I'm older.

[They continue, with the mother undercutting the daughter's accomplishments]

Children's Responses

Statistical analyses were performed by Burge (1990) on the major categories of children's interaction behaviors during the Conflict task. The mean responses are displayed in Table 6.2. It was expected that children of unipolar depressed women would engage in fewer task-focused, problem-solving responses, and that the affective dimensions would reveal that they engaged in more conflict (negative) responding, but they would be less likely to disagree openly and would display more evasion, appeasement, and whining (classified as immature).

TABLE 6.2. Means for children's interaction behaviors by maternal group.

	Maternal group					
Interaction behavior	Unipolar (n = 13) 1	Bipolar (n = 14) 2	Medical (n = 11) 3	Normal (n = 23) 4	Significant Contrasts	p
Task productive	.27 (.11)	.35 (.22)	.35 (.11)	.37 (.17)	1 < 4	.06
Off-task	.18 (.14)	.15 (.19)	.10 (.09)	.08 (.13)	1 > 4	.01
Questions	.06 (.05)	.05 (.04)	.07 (.05)	.10 (.11)	1 < 4	.02
Agree	.13 (.12)	.25 (.16)	.16 (.09)	.18 (.12)	1 < 2	.002
Disagree	.09 (.05)	.07 (.05)	.11 (.06)	.12 (.06)	1 < 4	.02
					1 < 3	.07
Negative	.16 (.16)	.03 (.06)	.09 (.10)	.04 (.06)	1 > 4	.002
					1 > 2	.002
					1 > 3	.08
Immature	.06 (.16)	.05 (.05)	.04 (.04)	.04 (.05)	ns	

Note: From Burge (1990). Sequential analysis of the interaction of depressed mothers and their children. Unpublished doctoral dissertation. University of California, Los Angeles. Numbers in parenthesis represent standard deviations.

A two-way multivariate analysis of variance (maternal group by child age [older vs. younger]) indicated a significant main effect of maternal group, $F(7, 46) = 2.19, p < .01$, and for age, $F(7, 48) = 2.86, p < .01$. The overall interaction effect was not significant. Of particular interest were the univariate planned comparisons between maternal groups. As predicted, children of unipolar mothers engaged in more off-task behaviors and tended to make fewer task-productive comments than did children of normal mothers. It could be said, therefore, that their conflict problem-solving skills were less effective than those of normal group children. Also as predicted, compared to the children of normal mothers, the unipolar group children were more negative (and significantly more than each of the other groups) but displayed fewer direct disagreements. They also asked fewer questions, but contrary to the prediction that they would engage in more "immature" behaviors, there were no group differences on this summary measure of evasion, whining, and appeasement.

The age differences that were observed appeared to represent expected developmental changes in interpersonal problem solving, in the sense that younger children were more likely to agree with their mothers than were older children (over age 12), and older children were more likely to make negative comments. Only one significant interaction of age and maternal group (asking questions) emerged, however; in the unipolar group the older and younger children were equal in question asking, whereas in all other groups the older children questioned the mother more than the younger ones did. Generally, since the groups were balanced with respect to children's age and gender, the maternal group patterns were not apparently distorted by differences in children's ages.

Perceived Interaction Style

The mothers and children completed a questionnaire report of their perceptions of the mother's behaviors toward the child. The Parent Perception Inventory (Hazzard et al., 1983), as described in Chapter 2, yields a score for the perceived frequency of positive behaviors, negative behaviors, and the overall balance (positive minus negative). The bipolar mothers rated themselves significantly higher ($p < .05$) on positive behaviors (Mean = 29.7) compared with all other groups (unipolar = 27.0, medical = 26.5, normal = 26.9). Bipolar women also saw themselves as displaying significantly fewer negative behaviors toward their children compared with women in the other groups (p values $< .05$). The other groups did not differ from each other.

Children's perceptions of their mothers, based on a random sample of one child per family, indicated no significant group differences. The single exception was that medical group children reported more negative behaviors than bipolar children ($p < .05$).

It is likely that the children's and mother's reports contain both accurate representations and socially desirable representations, and the overall correspondence of the subjective reports and observed interactions was relatively poor. The validity of the observations may be gauged in part by how well they correspond to children's actual functioning, to which we now turn.

Children's Outcomes Associated with Maternal Interaction Behavior

The interaction scores and sample employed in the Gordon et al. (1989) report were further analyzed to test the relationship between each interaction dimension and children's outcome variables. Four maternal interaction scores that had shown significant variability across the groups were included in regression analyses: negative/critical comments, positive feedback/confirmation, task-productive remarks, and off-task remarks. Hierarchical multiple regressions were computed, entering each of the four dimensions last in order to determine its unique variance contribution when the overlapping effects of the prior entries were controlled.

Children's Concurrent Outcomes

Children's diagnoses, maternal reports of behavior problems and social competence on the Child Behavior Check List (CBCL), academic rating, and Conner's teacher ratings of behavior problems were all obtained at about the same time as the maternal interaction task was conducted. Therefore, the direction of causality cannot be discerned, but it was clear that the interaction qualities were significantly associated with each of the children's outcome variables. Table 6.3 presents the amount of variance accounted for by the combined maternal behaviors, as well as the R^2 of any interaction variable that was significant when entered last. It can be seen from the rightmost column that all of the equations were statistically significant, indicating that the combined maternal interaction behaviors were moderately predictive of children's functioning. Additionally, it

TABLE 6.3. Hierarchical regressions to predict children's outcome (Conflict task).

Concurrent children's outcome variable	Maternal interaction dimension—incremental R^2				
	Task productive	Off-task	Confirm	Negative	Overall R^2
Affective diagnosis	.08				.28
Nonaffective diagnosis					.17
CBCL Behavior Problems				.21	.34
CBCL Social Competence			.07	.04*	.22
Academic Performance		.05*		.13	.31
Conners Teacher Rating	.09*			.08*	.31

* $p > .05 < .10$. Otherwise, all R^2 values are significant at least $p < .05$.

appeared that the variable representing maternal criticism was the most statistically *unique* predictor of functioning, contributing significantly or marginally significantly to four of the six outcomes (indicating more negative functioning, as reported both by the mother and school/teacher reports, associated with more maternal criticism). Social competence was uniquely associated with higher levels of maternal confirmatory remarks.

Prediction of Children's Outcomes at 6-Month Follow-Up

Burge and Hammen (in press) analyzed the predictive relationship between maternal interaction behaviors and children's subsequent functioning at the first 6-month follow-up. To test theoretically predicted links between aspects of maternal communication and children's outcomes, two summary scores of maternal interaction behaviors were computed. It was hypothesized that affective quality and problem-solving behaviors represent two distinct and potentially different contributors to children's adaptive development. Therefore, one index score, composed of the sum of positive feedback dimensions minus the negative feedback dimensions, represented positivity of the quality of interaction. The second is an index of task productivity, comprised of behaviors representing task-focused communications (e.g., giving directions, asking for information) minus off-task commentary. Both index scores were computed as proportions of total maternal utterances in the overall interaction task.

Four measures of children's functioning were employed as dependent variables in hierarchical regression analyses, representing diagnoses, school behavior and academic performance (based on rating scales discussed more fully in Chapter 2). For each outcome, two regressions were computed, each entering one of the two maternal interaction indices last. This method permits the evaluation of the incremental contribution of the last variable after the effects of the first are controlled. Table 6.4 summarizes the results.

Presence of depressive diagnoses during the follow-up was predicted significantly by the two maternal dimensions, yielding a multiple R of .45, accounting for 20% of the variance in affective diagnoses. Both positivity and task productivity made unique contributions to depressive diagnoses, although the latter was only marginally significant. Nonaffective diagnoses, on the other hand, did not appear to be significantly predicted by maternal interaction style as indexed in the two dimensions.

Ratings of school behavior during the 6-month follow-up indicated that they were significantly predicted by maternal communication indices; together the two dimensions accounted for 24% of the variance in school-related functioning (adequacy of discipline, peer and teacher relationships). Both of the maternal interaction dimensions contributed to school behavior ratings.

For academic achievement (grades, mastery of academic content), maternal communications predicted overall ratings significantly. How-

TABLE 6.4. Hierarchical regression analyses to predict children's outcomes at 6 months.

	Incremental R^2 when entered last		
Variable	Positivity	Task productivity	Overall R^2
Affective diagnosis	.08**	.05*	.20**
	$F(2, 55) = 6.88, p < .01$		
Nonaffective diagnosis	.06*	.00	.06
	$F(2, 55) = 1.87, p > .05$		
School Behavior Rating	.07**	.08**	.24**
	$F(2, 55) = 8.70, p < .001$		
Academic Performance Rating	.06**	.04	.16**
	$F(2, 55) = 5.25, p < .01$		

Note: From "Maternal Communication: A Predictor of Children's Outcomes at Follow-Up in a High-Risk Sample" by D. Burge and C. Hammen, (in press). *Journal of Abnormal Psychology*.
* = $p > .05 < .10$. ** = $p < .05$.

ever, only positivity of maternal communications was a significant unique predictor.

The results help bridge the gap between research indicating increased risk to children of women with affective disorders on the one hand and studies implicating impaired interactions in families with depressed parents on the other. The present results indicate that children's risk may stem in part from dysfunctional interactions between the depressed mother and her child. Both current and subsequent functioning in children were shown to be related to aspects of maternal communication. Such communications indicated that negative quality and impaired focus on the task at hand were associated with children's dysfunctions.

It would be inappropriate, however, to conclude that women with affective disorders are poor parents who directly cause impairments in their children. Such an unwarranted interpretation of the results ignores two important considerations: the context in which maternal interactions occur and the potential reciprocal effect that mothers and children have on each other.

Predictors of Maternal Interactions

As we argued in Chapter 5, maternal diagnoses of affective disorders reflect not just a potential "disease" process but also a statement about the person's functioning in various roles. Thus, as a predictor variable, diagnostic status is confounded with the commonly ongoing stressful conditions that are a contributor and consequence of depressive symptoms. Further, depressive symptoms can occur in individuals who do not receive diagnoses and may be absent for the moment in individuals who do carry diagnoses of recurrent affective disorders. Thus it may be entirely misleading to conclude that women with unipolar or bipolar diagnoses are impaired in parental interactions. It is necessary instead to attempt to examine the contributions of depressive symptoms and stress to maternal functioning.

To pursue the question of the predictors of maternal interactions with their children, current Beck Depression Inventory scores and the chronic stress total were entered in multiple regression equations. For simplicity, the two indices—positivity of communication and task productivity—served as dependent variables. Table 6.5 presents the results of the regression analyses originally reported by Burge and Hammen (in press). It appears that the two dimensions are predicted moderately well (multiple R values .46 and .42) by mood and chronic stress. Specifically, however, chronic stress uniquely predicts affective quality of communication and mood uniquely predicts task productivity. High levels of chronic stress appear to diminish the relative positive content of communications, possibly provoking more critical comments by reducing the parent's tolerance of unwanted actions and attitudes by the child. Depressed mood, on the other hand, seems especially to inhibit the mother's ability to be engaged with the child and to perform task-oriented effortful interactions.

Influence of Parent and Child on Each Other

Except for the Hops et al. (1987) observational analyses, few studies explored the role of children's behaviors on their depressed mothers or indicated that negative communications by the mother might be responses in part to dysfunctional behaviors by the child. The importance of studying the reciprocal patterns of interactions of parents and children has certainly

TABLE 6.5. Hierarchical regressions to predict maternal behavior in the communication task.

	Prediction of positivity of communication	
Variable	R^2 change	Significance of R^2 change at last step
BDI scores	.10	$t(56) = .90$, ns
Chronic stress	.11	$t(56) = 2.86, p < .01$
Overall $F(2, 55) = 7.47, p < .001$; multiple $R = .46$, $R^2 = .21$		
	Prediction of task productivity	
BDI scores	.16	$t(56) = 2.39, p < .05$
Chronic stress	.02	$t(56) = 1.06$, ns
Overall $F(2, 55) = 6.04, p < .01$; multiple $R = .42$, $R^2 = .18$		

Note: From "Maternal Communication: A Predictor of Children's Outcomes at Follow-Up in a High-Risk Sample" by D. Burge and C. Hammen, (in press). *Journal of Abnormal Psychology*.

been widely promoted but has not yet led to investigations in families of children at risk for affective disorders. Therefore, we approached the issue in two ways: analyses of maternal perceptions and interactions as a function of child behaviors and causal modeling analyses testing a bidirectional effect.

First, Conrad and Hammen (1989) pursued the question of whether maternal depression reduces tolerance for noncompliant behavior by the child. Previous studies had suggested that relatively depressed mothers of clinic-referred children might actually exaggerate the youngsters' problems because depression made them more critical and intolerant (e.g., Forehand et al., 1982). This is a version of the idea that depressed people exaggerate problems and overestimate the magnitude of negative events. More recent research, with nonclinical depression in mothers, suggested that both maternal depression and the child's own behaviors contribute to maternal negative judgments of children's symptoms (Brody & Forehand, 1986). Therefore, our initial goal was to evaluate whether maternal depression was associated with more negative evaluations of the children's problems, or the extent to which the evaluations were actually reactive to the child's true problems.

Conrad and Hammen (1989) compared mothers' ratings of both externalizing and internalizing child symptoms on the Child Behavior Check List, with objective indicators of those dimensions based on observer and teacher ratings. Hierarchical regression analyses were used to predict maternal ratings, entering first the actual objective ratings, then the maternal BDI score, and then the interaction of the two variables. For both internalizing scores and diagnoses of externalizing behaviors, the interaction of the objective score and maternal BDI was a significant predictor of maternal ratings. Figure 6.1 illustrates the interaction, dividing mothers at the median BDI score and children at the median internalizing score. Nondepressed mothers tended to make no distinctions between their truly symptomatic and nonsymptomatic children, whereas relatively depressed mothers rated their truly symptomatic children as having significantly more problems than their nonsymptomatic children. In other words, contrary to conventional perceptions, the depressed women were more accurate and did not appear to unduly exaggerate the symptomatology of their children. It was the nondepressed women who appeared to ignore or gloss over the symptoms of their children who were actually symptomatic.

The next goal of the study was to determine the implications of such perceptions: Do depressed women who perceive their children's actual problems interact more negatively with them in the conflict discussion task? Overall negative communication and overall positive communication proportions were computed by collapsing across relevant maternal interaction codes. Two-way analyses of variance (high–low maternal depression, high–low levels of children's actual symptoms) were per-

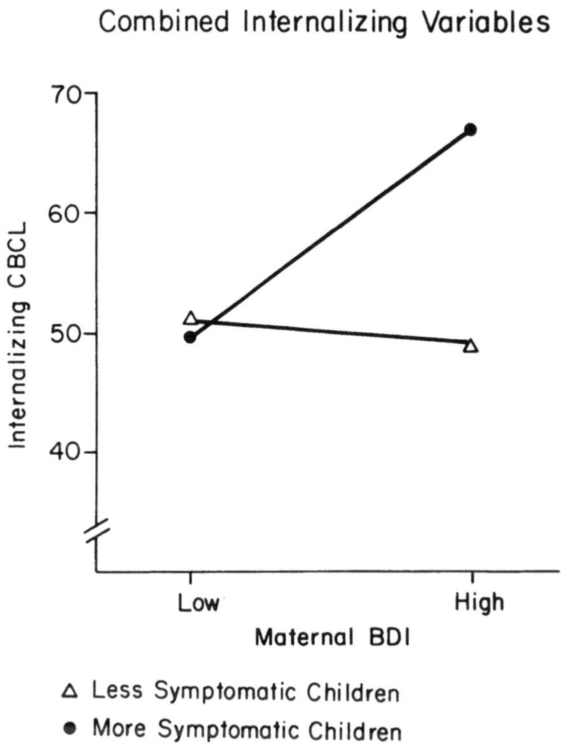

FIGURE 6.1. Maternal perceptions of child internalizing disorder as a function of maternal depression and symptomatology of the child. ("More symptomatic" children refers to those scoring above the median on a composite score of the Children's Depression Inventory and diagnosis of internalizing disorders. CBCL = Child Behavior Checklist. BDI = Beck Depression Inventory.) From "Role of Maternal Depression in Perceptions of Child Maladjustment" by M. Conrad and C. Hammen, 1989, *Journal of Consulting and Clinical Psychology*, *57*, 663–667. Copyright 1989 by the American Psychological Association. Reprinted by permission.

formed for the two composite scores. Table 6.6 presents the mean interaction scores by group for the analyses.

For children's internalizing symptoms, there was a significant main effect of maternal mood, $F(3, 51) = 9.07$, $p < .01$. Depressed women displayed higher proportions of negative/critical comments than did the nondepressed women. The expected difference between depressed and nondepressed mothers of relatively symptomatic children was significant ($p < .05$), indicating that more depressed mothers were more negative toward their depressed children than were nondepressed mothers. There were no differences on proportions of positive communications.

Table 6.6. Maternal communications as a function of child's behavior and maternal depression.

Maternal group	*n*	Proportion of communication: Negative	Proportion of communication: Positive
	Children's internalizing composite		
High composite			
Low BDI	10	.087	.117
High BDI	13	.203	.060
Low composite			
Low BDI	21	.103	.092
High BDI	12	.147	.084
	Children's externalizing disorders		
Diagnoses			
Low BDI	4	.112	.108
High BDI	5	.297	.050
No diagnoses			
Low BDI	27	.095	.100
High BDI	20	.149	.076
	Teachers' ratings of externalizing behaviors		
High ratings			
Low BDI	4	.035	.104
High BDI	8	.178	.065
Low Ratings			
Low BDI	13	.124	.118
High BDI	8	.139	.080

Note: BDI = Beck Depression Inventory. From "Role of Maternal Depression in Perceptions of Child Maladjustment" by M. Conrad and C. Hammen, 1989, *Journal of Consulting and Clinical Psychology*, *57*, 663–667. Copyright 1989 by the American Psychological Association. Reprinted by permission.

For children's externalizing diagnoses, there were significant main and interaction effects. Most relevant to our hypotheses, relatively depressed mothers directed more negative/critical comments toward their more symptomatic children than did nondepressed mothers (and more than toward their nonsymptomatic children). Again, the groups did not differ on proportions of positive communications. Finally, the groupings of children based on teachers' reports also supported the overall hypothesis of more negative comments directed by depressed women toward their symptomatic children (although the significance level was $p = .06$).

These results are consistent with the hypothesis that relatively depressed women are less tolerant of actual dysfunction in their children. There was no evidence that they were more hostile in general, for their negativity was directed only toward children who truly had problems, and not toward their nonsymptomatic children. Moreover, the relatively depressed women showed no evidence of distortion or exaggeration of perceptions of their children; if anything, they were more accurate than the nondepressed women. Finally, the depressed women seemed to display negativism and criticism when their children were symptomatic but did not differ from nondepressed women in proportions of positive communication.

This analysis does not establish the causal sequence between maternal depression, maternal criticism, and child maladjustment. However, it does suggest that at least once established, there is a reciprocal process in which children's actual maladaptive behaviors contribute to maternal criticism, and it is likely that a pernicious cycle of mutual negative effects is maintained.

To test this reciprocal model more fully, Hammen, Burge, and Stansbury (1990) used causal modeling statistical analyses to test several components of an interpersonal model. First, we predicted that maternal interaction behaviors would affect children's outcomes. This is the traditional view of risk for psychopathology in high risk samples. We used children's outcomes at the 6-month follow-up in order to enhance the logic of a causal relationship linking the temporally precedent maternal behaviors to subsequent behaviors. Second, however, we added a reciprocal component, linking maternal functioning and child characteristics; each of these variables was comprised of observed interaction behaviors as well as additional characteristics, noted later. This step suggests that while maternal communication style influences subsequent outcomes of children, maternal communications are reciprocally influenced by the child's communications during the interaction task. Next, to further emphasize that child's role, we included a causal path from child characteristics to child outcomes. Although this step might seem obvious, it is nevertheless left implicit or ignored altogether in most depictions of children at risk for psychopathology.

We also added contextual components to emphasize the larger, environmental ingredients that influence mother and child behaviors. Attempting to go beyond the traditional intrapsychic emphasis, we hypothesized that each member of the dyad would be influenced by personal-situational factors. For the mothers, we included depression level (BDI score) and social adjustment (SAS; Weissman & Bothwell, 1976), which indexes chronic strain in role functioning across various domains. We expected that such variables would be much more informative for functioning than psychiatric status as such and would influence the quality of communication directed toward the child in the Conflict Discussion task. For the children, we included two background variables that we also thought might influence their communication behaviors somewhat more generally than psychiatric status: age and self-esteem.

Figure 6.2 presents the predicted model and the statistical weights associated with the hypothesized connections between variables. The model provided an adequate statistical fit to the data, as indicated by a nonsignificant chi-square suggesting that the hypothesized and actual correlation

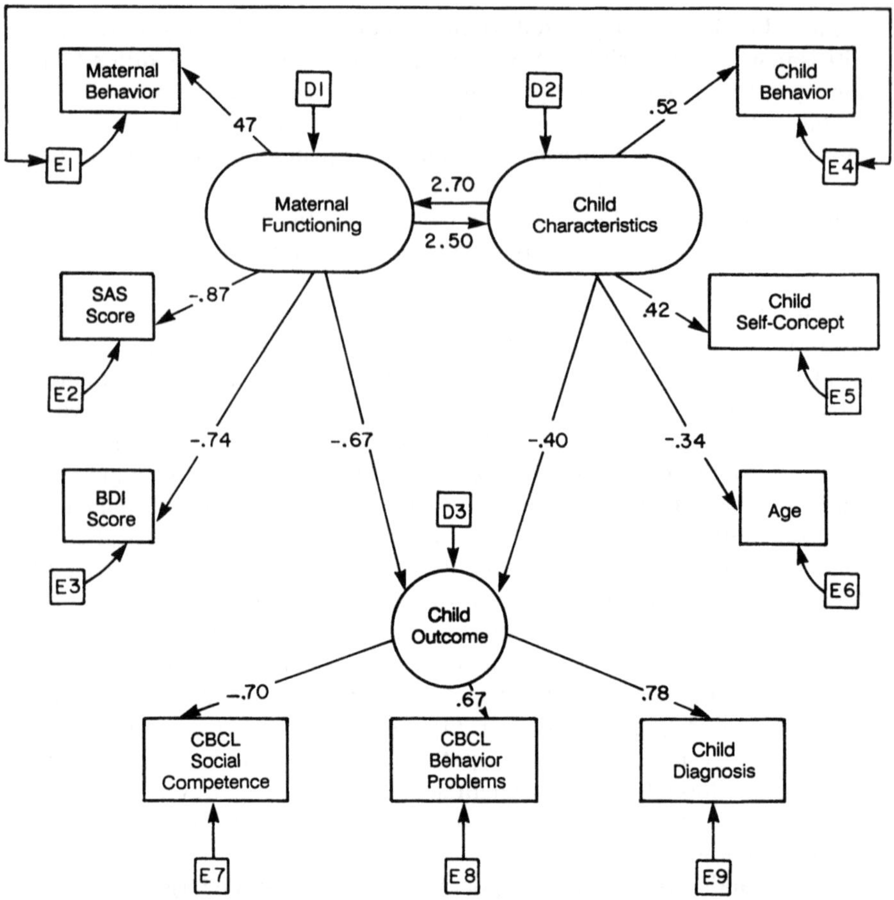

FIGURE 6.2. Causal modeling analysis of reciprocal mother–child effects and child outcomes. From "Relationship of Mother and Child Variables to Child Outcomes in a High Risk Sample: A Causal Modeling Analysis" by C. Hammen, D. Burge, and K. Stansbury, 1990, *Developmental Psychology*, *26*, 24–30. Copyright 1990 by the American Psychological Association. Reprinted by permission.

matrices did not differ and by a Bentler–Bonett normed fit index of .91. Alternative models that did not include both the mother and child paths to child outcomes did not fit as well, and it was concluded that the tested model was the best fit to the data.

A particular feature of this model is the apparent reciprocal relationship between maternal dysfunctional communication and having older children, with relatively negative self-concept, who were more negative and critical in their interactions with their mothers. Thus it is likely that both mothers and children contribute to each other's unhappiness and distress—rather than simply that "bad parenting" by the mother accounts for children's negative outcomes 6 months later.

SELF-CONCEPT AND NEGATIVE PARENT–CHILD RELATIONSHIPS

Since vulnerability in attitudes toward the self may be one path to depression (e.g., Beck, 1983; Hammen, in press-c), we speculated that one source of poor self-esteem might be critical/negative expressions by the mother toward the child. That is, to the extent that critical and negative commentary might reflect negative attitudes toward the child, the child might come to internalize a negative view of the self. Correlational analyses indicated that relatively poor self-concept on the Piers–Harris scale (Piers & Harris, 1969) and several other indicators of negative self-cognitions was significantly associated with quality of parent–child relations. As reported in Chapter 4 (see Jaenicke et al., 1987), children's perceptions of the quality of maternal behavior toward them on the Parent Perception Inventory and *actual* observations of critical/negative behaviors were associated with self-esteem. The causal direction cannot be determined validly in this cross-sectional analysis, but we speculate that one of the mechanisms of children's risk for psychopathology, especially depression, is self-esteem that is acquired in part through the reflected attitudes of the parents toward the child.

We had also wondered if children might acquire negative self-views by observing their self-critical mothers. In other words, modeling of negative cognitions might be one major way that children acquire vulnerable self-cognitions. A simple correlation between frequency of mother and child self-critical comments during the conflict discussion task failed to support such a prediction. Instead, however, there was a significant correlation between maternal criticism directed at the child and the child's self-critical comments, $r = .51$ (Jaenicke et al., 1987). This finding supports the hypothesis that a consequence of maternal negative quality of interactions with the child is poor self-regard. Negative self-concept in turn may contribute to subsequent depression and other maladaptive behaviors.

Additional Information on Family Interaction Processes

It is impossible in brief, somewhat constrained interactions processes, such as the Conflict Discussion task reported here, to capture complex, subtle, lifelong patterns in which the child has participated. For example, many of the families not only displayed somewhat critical, negative interactions in the brief task but actually reported ongoing, serious conflict through the follow-ups. Children and mothers reported physical fighting between them; several of the mothers threw the children out or sent them to live with fathers because of the high level of conflict. Children stole from their mothers, they ran away, they destroyed furniture and property at home; in turn, mothers, fathers, or stepfathers physically punished the youngsters. Indeed, it was necessary to report three families for suspected physical abuse of a child, where a parent or stepparent had used excessive force, or caused physical damage, while trying to "discipline" an errant child. Other evidence of dysfunctional family processes came from instances of reported sexual victimization of children: in one family the biological father exposed himself to his daughter, in another case the mother suspected sexual abuse of a daughter by her former husband, and in one instance a previous companion was suspected of physical improprieties with a child.

In the broader family context, there was an enormous amount of past and current marital difficulties in all groups, with extreme cases of women and children having to seek shelter from a physically assaultive husband/father or constant court battles over custody. At the other extreme, there were some children who never knew their biological fathers or had not seen them for many years. Some children were shuttled between parents, depending on who could cope with them at the moment. In one instance a child came home to his father only to be told to pack his bags to go back to the mother because the father was going into hiding to avoid prosecution for a fraudulent business deal. Siblings were sometimes divided between parents.

Overall, we know from the signals that emerged in the brief observation tasks of interactions, and from the stressful life events and circumstances reported over the course of the study, that serious breakdowns of family communication were not rare. They occurred frequently in the unipolar group, but they also existed—sometimes to severe degrees— in families in all of the groups. We formed clinical impressions of different kinds of family interaction pathology besides the conflict that we learned about. There were families in which the mother was overly dependent on her child, with inappropriate boundaries, intrusiveness, resistance to the child's separation and differentiation. Not just a few mother–child dyads, in which a single mother was raising a single child, raised some concerns about overinvolvement and enmeshment. Since we did not collect systematic information on dynamics of the relationships in the family, however, we were left simply with impressions and concerns that there were many forms of interaction dysfunction that ought to be investigated in future studies.

Finally, lest the impression be given that many of the mothers were uncaring or inept, it is important to emphasize our strong impression that the vast majority of the mothers of all groups cared very deeply about their children. They were concerned about their welfare, highly aware and worried about the effects of their disorders or illnesses on the youngsters, and making valiant attempts to juggle their own and their children's needs—often in the presence of daunting environmental stressors and limited supports.

Summary and Directions for Further Research

The results of direct observations in the present study indicate that children of unipolar depressed mothers seem to be especially subjected to negative and avoidant interaction styles shown by their mothers. The mothers displayed critical and disconfirmatory communications with their children and engaged in behaviors during the Conflict Discussion task that reflect low involvement and resistance to task-focused resolution of the conflict. In turn, such negative and withdrawn patterns are associated with diagnoses and dysfunction in the children, both in the short term and at 6-month follow-ups, suggesting that they may be fairly typical and general styles of interaction that have enduring consequences. Maternal difficulty in sustaining positive, noncritical, and involved behaviors appeared to be related to chronic stress and depressive symptoms. Depressive symptoms seemed to interfere with sustaining involved, task-focused responding (also interpreted as avoidance of conflict), while chronic stress appeared to contribute to criticism and diminished expressions of praise and support. Since depressive symptoms and chronic stress occur widely in the population, their pernicious consequences are not limited to clinically depressed individuals, and we cannot conclude that depressive illness is itself the cause of dysfunctional parenting.

The present study also suggests that mutual mother–child relationships require further analyses, and that each participant in the interactions influences the other. Relatively depressed mothers do not appear to be indiscriminately negative toward their children or to exaggerate the symptoms of their children. Instead, they appear to agree with external sources about their children's symptoms to a greater extent than do nondepressed women, and their interactions with their children are shaped by characteristics of the children. We can speculate that reciprocal patterns of critical/negative interactions prolong and deepen the distress of both mothers and children. The vicious cycle of nonsupportive communication probably serves to perpetuate maternal depression and to contribute to children's further maladaptive behaviors. Indeed, in Chapter 7 we continue to explore the mutual effect of mother and child symptomatology on each other.

There seems to be an especially direct link between negative quality of mother–child relationship and poor self-regard on various measures of children's self-cognitions. As indicated in Chapter 4, negative self-concept is predictive of depressive symptoms in children.

Although the present study has attempted to address many of the gaps in existing research on parent–child relationships and risk for depression, it is clear that the results provide only general conclusions. As our limited discussion of research indicated, there are numerous specific questions to be posed, which will engage the efforts and talents of developmental, clinical, psychiatric, and sociological researchers for years to come. At this stage we know little about the specific aspects of maternal interaction that negatively influence children, and we know little about the specific ways in which children are influenced, how their behaviors and self-representations are affected.

7
Familial and Parental Clinical Characteristics

In this chapter the characteristics of both parents are explored, and associations between features of the clinical disorder and children's dysfunction are examined. Factors such as greater severity or chronicity of maternal disorder, as well as earlier age of onset, may indicate a more pernicious course that is likely to influence risk to children. The characteristics of first-degree relatives of the parents also are considered. Evidence of "loaded" family pedigrees may imply different outcomes for children. Finally, characteristics of the biological fathers of the children in the study are explored and discussed in relation to children's outcomes.

Much of the literature that is reviewed here has had at least an implicit genetic orientation, suggesting that more loaded family pedigrees for disorder predict earlier onset or more severe childhood disorder, or that earlier onset of parental disorder (suggestive of an illness process) is associated with more childhood pathology in offspring. On the other hand, a psychosocial interpretation is also possible. Evidence of severe course and early onset, as well as dysfunctional families of origin of ill parents, implies disruption in development and problems with the skills of the parents. Such impairments could contribute to disorder in their children. In the final analysis, when lacking genetic markers for affective disorders, it is impossible to distinguish between genetic and psychosocial hypotheses. The present chapter attempts, therefore, to present the information descriptively. Although the genetic basis for affective disorders remains a strong hypothesis for at least some forms of disorder, as we shall see, the question is almost totally confounded with psychosocial influences.

Research on Parental Characteristics and Children's Outcomes

Severity and Chronicity

Research from the original high risk schizophrenia offspring projects attempted to relate children's outcomes to characteristics of parental psychopathology. Indeed, as noted in Chapter 2, most studies found that parent diagnosis did not lead to differential outcomes in the youngsters. Instead, chronicity and severity of impairment, regardless of parent diagnosis, were related to children's adjustment (Harder, Kokes, Fisher, & Strauss, 1980; Kauffman, Grunebaum, Cohler, & Gamer, 1979; Sameroff et al., 1984; Wynne, Cole, & Perkins, 1987). Richters (1987), for instance, presented assessments of parental premorbid adjustment and number of hospitalizations/days in hospital, based on schizophrenic, unipolar, and bipolar samples. He found that poor premorbid parent adjustment was related to peer and teacher ratings of offspring adjustment in childhood, although hospitalization information was largely unrelated to children's outcomes. Social/occupational adjustment of the offspring in young adulthood was also related to parental premorbid adjustment. Although Richters used indirect measures of parental severity/chronicity of disorder, it is noteworthy that they were related not only to children's outcomes but also to offspring ratings of home life and characteristics of their parents. Richters concludes that offspring adjustment was related not to diagnosis (or genetic transmission) but rather to chronic stress associated with a parent who functioned poorly.

Relatively few studies specifically of the offspring of affectively ill parents have attempted to relate characteristics of the parents' disorder to that of the children. Of the few that do so, nearly all concern unipolar depressed parents. The one study of bipolar families indicated no association between severity of parental disorder (defined as the difference between bipolar I and other bipolar disorders) and children's outcomes; the samples were relatively small, however (Kuyler et al., 1980).

Among unipolar high risk studies, Keller et al. (1986) identified 37 families in which at least one parent had a past or current depressive disorder and children were between the ages of 6 and 19. Actual parental disorder was quite mixed; the majority of parents had past or current major depressive disorder (MDD), although some had only minor depression or dysthymia and had additional RDC diagnoses. There was also heterogeneity of current depression; 14 of the 37 families had currently depressed parents and the others had past depression. The authors constructed seven indices of severity and chronicity of parental depression (e.g., total duration of MDD, number of episodes of MDD, times hospitalized for MDD) and found that all were significantly associated with greater impairment of functioning in the child except for number of hospitalizations. Similarly, the same six indices were associated with presence of increased rates of diagnosis in children (current or past). Of the 72 children, 17 had a history of major depression, but it was unclear if such diagnoses were specifically associated with severity/chronicity of parental disorder. Keller et al. also report that children's adaptive functioning and diagnosable disorders were related to impaired marital adjustment and to lower social class. The authors further noted that all of the major depressive episodes in the children, and the majority of other DSM III diagnoses, occurred after the onset of parental depression. Keller et al. call for further studies of both the heritability and "exposure" effects of parental affective disorders on children.

Orvaschel, Walsh-Allis, and Ye (1988) studied the 6- to 17-year old offspring of 34 parents with recurrent major depression (at least three episodes) and 29 control families. They found no associations, however, between number of parental episodes or severity of current depression and children's diagnoses. On the other hand, Weissman, Leckman, Merikangas, Gammon, and Prusoff (1984) in their initial indirect study of children of depressed parents found that number of parental episodes of depression was higher for children who experienced major depression. However, there was no association between children's rates of disorder and age at exposure or number of years of exposure to parental depression.

Rutter and Quinton (1984) studied offspring of parents with diverse psychopathology and showed that it is the persistence of disorder rather than diagnostic specificity that predicted significant impairment in children. Parents who had chronic ongoing personality disorders were especially likely to have children with chronic or recurrent major dysfunction.

Overall, the data suggest that severity/chronicity of parental disorder is probably related to severity of children's disorder. The sole apparent exception (Orvaschel et al., 1988) may have been limited by the restricted range of episodes in the parents, since all had recurrent disorder with at least three major episodes. However, there are several unanswered questions: Are the children specifically at risk for depression if their parent had recurrent depression? Does the effect also hold true for offspring of bipolar parents? Most important, can we account for the mechanism of the effect of severity? Exposure to and timing of parental episodes need to be explored more fully.

Age of Onset of Disorder

Age of onset of disorder in the parent may be an index of severity/chronicity of the disorder, a sign of greater genetic risk, and an indicator of greater exposure of the child to parental dysfunction. From any of these perspectives, early onset would appear to increase children's risk for psychopathology.

Only one study of unipolar parents examined parental age of onset in relation to child's psychopathology. Orvaschel et al. (1988) found that parents' age of onset for depression was significantly associated with depression in children. Depressed parents with a depressed child had an earlier age of onset than depressed parents whose child did not (yet) display depressive disorder.

Most of the research on age of onset has examined child's age of onset as related to parental disorder. Weissman, Gammon, et al. (1987) examined age of onset of depression in offspring of depressed and normal parents and found that children of depressed parents had significantly earlier onsets (around age 12 or 13) than depressed children of normal parents (after 15). There was no specific comparison between age of parental onset and that of children in the sample. However, the results are consistent with previous studies of depressed adults indicating earlier onset of depression associated with higher incidence and earlier onset of depression in first-degree relatives (Weissman, Leckman, et al., 1984; Weissman, John, et al., 1986). Also, Puig-Antich et al. (1989) found that children with early (preadolescent) onset of major depression were likely to come from families with higher rates of major depression (and alcoholism and anxiety disorders), compared to families of normal children.

Family studies of bipolar probands have also indicated higher prevalance of affective disorders in relatives of early onset manic depressives (e.g., Gershon et al., 1982; Rice et al., 1987). Recently, Strober et al. (1988) examined the families of bipolar I adolescent patients. Those with childhood onset of significant symptoms had significantly higher aggregations of bipolar I disorder in their relatives than did those with adolescent onset of symptoms.

Overall, such studies suggest that earlier onset of affective disorders reflects a more pernicious familial pattern.

Family Pedigree Studies

Analyses of family patterns of psychopathology have consistently indicated elevated rates of affective disorder. Specifically, unipolar probands have been found to have families with increased rates of unipolar disorder (typically ranging from around 11 to 18%) and low rates of bipolar disorder (Andreasen, in press; Goldin & Gershon, 1988). On the other hand, bipolar patients show elevated rates of both unipolar and bipolar disorders in their first-degree relatives (e.g., Andreasen, in press).

Analyses of possible genetic transmission of unipolar depression appear to be especially hampered by the heterogeneity of depression. Both in its manifestations and in its origins, there are likely to be various types of unipolar depression. Winokur (1979) proposed a subtype of "depressive spectrum disease" with early age of onset and a family history of alcoholism and sociopathy, compared with "familial pure depressive disease" with a family history of depression but not alcoholism or sociopathy. The depressive spectrum disease type has been found to have certain characteristics: more life events, divorce, and other indicators of a stormy lifestyle, along with early age of onset and possible personality disorder features (Zimmerman, Coryell, & Pfohl, 1986; Zimmerman, Coryell, Stangl, & Pfohl, 1987).

Bland, Newman, and Orn (1986) proposed a distinction between recurrent and nonrecurrent depression and early versus late onset depression.

They found that the recurrent–early onset depressives had significantly higher rates of depression in relatives than did the other groups. Weissman, Gershon, et al. (1984) also found that relatively earlier onset depressives had higher rates of depression in family members. It should also be noted that recent studies (reviewed in Goldin & Gershon, 1988) have shown a birth-cohort effect, in that depressed persons born after 1940 appear to have earlier ages of depression onset than do those born earlier.

Taken together, the genetic family history data suggest familial transmission of bipolar disorders and unipolar disorders. In view of the heterogeneity of the latter, however, the search for specific subtypes of depression may aid in the determination of which factors may be genetic and which environmental. In the present study, the unipolar women are, by selection criteria, early onset and multiple episode cases, and therefore are likely to have high rates of disorder in family members. They may also possibly fit criteria for depressive spectrum disease. Rather than consider this to be a genetic subtype, however, it is likely that early onset, multiple episodes, and family psychopathology are probably correlated with stormy lifestyle and stressful events including divorce. The pattern represents a severe psychosocial dysfunction, and the genetic versus environmental factors are intertwined.

Characteristics of Fathers (Spouses) in Offspring Studies

Although many of the studies of children of parents with affective disorders have included both mothers and fathers as the patient parent, the bulk of the samples have been women. Only a few investigations compared the effect on children of having an ill mother versus an ill father. Keller et al. (1986) found no effect of ill fathers on children's outcomes, and Orvaschel et al. (1988) found no association between ill parent sex and child diagnosis. With respect to bipolar disorders, Klein et al. (1985) found that bipolar women were more likely to have children with disorder (any, or affective) than were bipolar fathers. The discrepant findings may be due to the very small sample size of families where only the father was the depressed patient.

On the other hand, a much larger sample (125 children of 56 depressed parents) was reported by Weissman, Gammon, et al. (1987), who found no differences between children's outcomes as a function of parent sex. These results need to be qualified, however, by analyses of the same sample reported by Merikangas, Prusoff, and Weissman (1988) examining the effects of parental concordance for disorders on children's outcomes. Merikangas, Prusoff, and Weissman found that 69% of the spouses of the depressed parents met criteria for major depression, anxiety disorder, or alcoholism. Complex patterns of children's outcomes emerged, depending on the gender of the parent and the combination of disorders in the spouses. However, the overall conclusion was that paternal diagnoses exerted weaker effects than did maternal diagnoses.

Merikangas, Prusoff, and Weissman (1988) also note that having two ill parents substantially increased the likelihood of disorder in the children, a finding that has been reported elsewhere (e.g., Weissman, Gammon, et al., 1984). However, studies of bipolar families do not show this effect, as reported by Nurnberger et al. (1988) and Kuyler et al. (1980).

Increased risk due to two ill parents is especially noteworthy, because Merikangas and colleagues (e.g., Merikangas, Weissman, Prusoff, & John, 1988) have noted the high incidence of "assortative mating" in patients with affective disorders. That is, persons with depression and manic depression tend to marry others with psychiatric disorders. Moreover, the authors argue that the spouse disorders are not due to psychopathology in reaction to the ill partner, because family history of psychopathology in their own relatives is high, suggesting a familial, rather than marital, origin. Additionally, Merikangas, Prusoff, and Weissman (1988) reported that the marital relationship and aspects of current functioning were worse in couples with concordance for major disorders. Taken together, such findings greatly complicate the search for simple genetic contributions to children's disorders. Instead, it is important to examine the spouse's adjustment and family loading for psychopathology, as well as the environmental consequences of two maladjusted parents.

Rutter and Quinton (1984) also observed substantial rates of disturbed parents married to spouses with psychiatric disorders; ill women tended to be married to men with personality disorders, while ill men tended to have wives with affective disorders. Overall, 25% of husbands of women with disorders had disorders themselves, and 41% of wives of men with diagnoses had disorders themselves. Rutter and Quinton argue that although some of the disorders may indeed reflect assortative mating, two other associations are apparently present: those who develop disorder in response to difficult spouses (and marital conflict), and conditions in which both psychiatric disorder and marital conflict may be caused by prior conditions.

Comorbidity in Parents with Affective Disorders

Not only do most offspring studies neglect to evaluate or report on the existence of disorders in the spouse of the proband parent, but they also generally fail to report the presence of psychiatric disorders that coexist with the affective disorders. Recently, however, Merikangas, Prusoff, and Weissman (1988) have drawn attention to the frequency of comorbid diagnoses in parents with affective disorders (and their spouses). For example, 89% of those with unipolar major depression also had lifetime diagnoses of anxiety disorders, and 23% had secondary alcoholism. Moreover, fully 40% of the marital couples consisted of dual mating for depression and/or anxiety disorders, while 40% had only one affected member. Noting that a substantial number of spouses also had current or past alcoholism, even in the normal group, only 19% of all couples had no disorders.

Coexisting disorders along with major depression in the proband parents appeared to increase the risk of disorder in offspring (Merikangas, Weissman, et al., 1988). These authors suggest that the combination of major depression and anxiety disorders was especially aggregated in families. Indeed, these authors speculate that anxiety symptoms may constitute an early form of expression of affective disorders. More specifically, Weissman, Leckman, Merikangas, Gammmon, and Prusoff (1984) found that depression plus panic disorders and agoraphobia in the parent increased the risk of finding depression and anxiety in the children. Generalized anxiety disorder along with depression in the parents did not appear to increase the risk to children for disorders. Leckman, Weissman, Merikangas, Pauls, and Prusoff (1983) reported results of a family study of depressed patients; they found that depression plus panic disorder was associated with significantly increased family loading for psychiatric disorders. Subsequently, Weissman, Merikangas, et al. (1986) suggested that major depression with anxiety disorders (or secondary alcoholism) may constitute a more homogeneous subtype of major depression in terms of its increased association with family loading for major depression in relatives.

A discussion of parental comorbid disorders and their effects on children would be incomplete without considering Axis II disorders. Recently, Downey and Coyne (1990) emphasized the problem of comorbid Axis II disorders in studies of offspring of parents with affective disorders. They noted, for instance, that Shea, Glass, Pilkonis, Watkins, and Docherty (1987) reported that 35% of patients with major depression also had a personality disorder. Such combinations are found to be associated with younger age of onset, more hospitalizations and longer episodes, a family history of alcoholism and antisocial personality disorder, and a poorer recovery at hospital discharge (Black, Bell, Hulbert, & Nasrallah, 1988). At the very least, the Axis II diagnosis appears to be a marker of chronic dysfunction associated with many of the kinds of risk factors likely to have a negative impact on children's outcomes even apart from the parental diagnosis of major affective disorder.

Methodological and Conceptual Limitations of Recent Research

Strides have been made in identifying variations in parental disorder that affect the type, severity, and likelihood of offspring dysfunction. The greatest gap remains a lack of attention to parent variables besides diagnostic status. However, the existing studies have generally also been handicapped by small sample sizes and by nonstandardized measures of parental severity and chronicity of disorder.

By far the greatest gaps in methodology stem from conceptual limitations. Most of the offspring research assumes a genetic vulnerability to the disorder in question, and it is often assumed that parental factors such as family loading, age of onset, assortative mating, and comorbidity are indicators of the genetic risk. However, as Walker, Downey, and Nightingale (1989) ably pointed out, the risk factors are nonorthogonal—that is, correlated. Alterations in our designs and statistical methods are required to address them. For instance, there are many kinds of intercorrelated factors within the context, within the family, and within the individual (Walker et al., 1989). Within-family risk factors that are typically correlated with genetic diathesis include assortative mating likely resulting in nonoptimal parenting, gene–environment interactions such as greater pathology associated with parental dysfunction, and the effects of family members on each other. This nearly overwhelming array of correlated risk factors requires large samples with multiple measures, subjected to multivariate statistical methods. In the final analysis, we could all welcome the development of accurate genetic markers for affective disorders, as tools to help sort out the role of the correlated psychosocial risk factors that might mediate the expression of genetically influenced disorder in children.

Results of the Study

Severity of Maternal Disorder and Children's Outcomes

The chronicity and severity of maternal disorders and their association with children's disorders were analyzed. It seems logical to expect that women who have more severe and more numerous episodes of affective disorder will be more disruptive to their children's development. This question of "exposure" was tested in several ways: effects of lifetime history of disorder, number of depressive episodes specifically, effects of current symptoms, and maternal course of disorder during the follow-up observations as related to children's symptoms.

Maternal Lifetime History of Disorder

An overall index of the severity of the mother's past history of affective disorder, counting frequency and treatment of severe episodes, was described in Chapter 5. The highest ratings on the 7-point scale referred to recurrent, severe major depressions with hospitalization; mid-range scores indicated a single major depression or some degree of intermittent depressed mood with some level of impairment of functioning, and low scores indicated mild, transient depressed moods. Hammen, Adrian, et al. (1987) reported hierarchical regression analyses based on all maternal groups, testing the separate contributions of severity of lifetime history ratings, current depressed mood, and chronic stress on children's outcomes. The contribution of maternal lifetime severity ratings of disorder as a unique predictor, after controlling for the effects of the other two variables, was significant only for one outcome. Children's own lifetime history of any disorder was uniquely predicted by that of the mother, along with chronic strain as a unique predictor. In all of the other child outcome analyses, it was current mood and chronic stress that tended to emerge as significant unique predictors.

Since the foregoing analyses included all families in the sample, it is important to test the hypothesis of maternal severity of disorder and child outcomes more specifically only for the affective disorders families. Therefore, variability in the lifetime disorder outcomes of the children in the unipolar and bipolar families was examined as a function of variability in maternal history. Using the random sample of one child per family, children were classified into two groups: those who had no psychiatric history or only mild, nondiagnosable symptoms and those who had one or more diagnoses of significant disorder. A *t*-test comparison of the two groups was performed on the mothers' number of lifetime episodes of affective illness (mania or major depression), and a few mothers with "too many to count" were omitted from the analyses. Despite this relatively conservative test, there was nevertheless a significant difference between the child groups, $t(21) = 2.05$, $p = .05$. As expected, children with more severe histories of past diagnoses had mothers with more past episodes ($M = 10.9$, $SD = 8.1$) than did children with no or mild symptoms ($M = 5.6$, $SD = 4.4$).

Examples of Women's History of Affective Disorders

The unipolar women all had multiple episodes of major depression as a criterion for entry into the study, and the majority of them had been hospitalized at least once. The bipolar women also had many episodes. In the following vignettes, a few cases are presented of women who have not been described elsewhere, emphasizing only their clinical history.

Mrs. M. says that she was depressed since age 13, and over the years has experienced—by her report—at least 14 episodes of major depression. She was hospitalized for a suicide attempt when her child was a toddler, and notes that her child was "depressed" since about age 2, displaying withdrawn behavior and not talking. She had a period of significant drug and alcohol abuse in her early 20's, and continues to have generalized anxiety and panic attacks, punctuated by major depressive episodes.

Mrs. N. has had about 6 hospitalizations for depression since the age of 17, mostly for suicide attempts. She continues to be intermittently depressed and anxious, and we might speculate that she would also carry an Axis II diagnosis of borderline personality disorder.

Mrs. O. believes that she was depressed since childhood, with apparently diagnosable symptoms at least by adolescence, and recalls being suicidal before age 18. She reports that she had a period when she was not depressed at about age 26 during therapy, but felt continuously depressed since about age 33, reporting drug use during a 5-year period. There apparently was a great deal of irritable behavior, and histrionic scenes during a protracted divorce and custody dispute in the past few years, and she states that now is the first time in her life that she has felt truly normal.

Mrs. P. has a history of many problems that were initially not recognized as a bipolar disorder, but with the passage of time in following her, and in consideration of her family history of maternal manic depression, she came to have the diagnosis of bipolar disorder, probably bipolar II. She reported behaviors since age 7 that she believes suggested hypomania and depression, but her first treatment at age 16 was hospitalization for visual hallucinations, which led to a diagnosis of schizophrenia. However, it was also a period of intense drug abuse that had started at about age 14, and she continued drug use sporadically into her 20's with a cocaine abuse problem at about 26. In the setting where she was first identified for the study, her initial presenting problem and diagnosis was for bulimia, with later diagnoses of major depressive episodes, and eventually as atypical bipolar disorder.

Mrs. Q. was not formally diagnosed as manic depressive until about age 30 when she had grandiose delusions (believing she was a famous rock star) and was spending money and gambling excessively while also experiencing intense periods of perceptual acuity. However, it was clear that she had had earlier symptoms of significant mood swings, dating from early childhood. She described cycles of being an A-student, energetic and active, and then going into 6 months of depression during which she felt worthless, guilty, hopeless, and had many accidents. Currently, despite medication, she seems to have fairly continuing cycles of mania lasting around 2 months followed by depressions of around 3 months.

Mrs. R. has had 4 distinct manic episodes, the first at age 16, and about 6 major depressive episodes with a total of 5 hospitalizations. Her depressions are the worst problem for her, leading to suicidal feelings. As a child she was also troubled by depression, recalling that around age 13 she had a lengthy period of school refusal, and feared leaving the house and had many physical symptoms. Her parents forced her to attend school, but she recalls the entire period of her youth as one of feeling unhappy, sullen, and socially withdrawn.

Effects of Current Maternal Symptomatology

Despite the apparent effect of past history of maternal disorder on past history of child disorder, the regression analyses conducted by Hammen, Adrian, et al. (1987), noted earlier, with one exception indicated that past maternal history failed to emerge as a significant predictor of current outcomes when current maternal mood and chronic stress were entered in the equation. That is, although there appears to be a general association between child and maternal maladjustment in the past, it may not be the genetic predisposition that we find contributory. Instead, a strong case can be made that it is the current expression of maternal disorder that affects the child. Specifically, maternal mood scores on the Beck Depression Inventory were by far the most significant and pervasive influence on a variety of children's current outcomes. Across all the families, current mood was likely associated with children's current diagnoses, reported behavior problems, social competence, and school behaviors. Such findings suggest that whatever occurs *when* the mother is depressed—not the latent presence of an affective disorder—exerts negative influences on children. Unipolar and bipolar women who were not currently depressed therefore had children with better outcomes, whereas medically ill and normal women undergoing stressful and demoralizing conditions contributing to elevated BDI scores had children with more negative outcomes.

Again, pursuing this matter more specifically in the unipolar and bipolar families, we explored whether children's severity of symptoms would be related to those of their mothers. Using a randomly selected child in each of the unipolar and bipolar families, we first compared mothers' and children's self-reported depression scores at each 6-month follow-up. The sample sizes were limited, owing to missing data, so that only four follow-ups could be used. The correlations between maternal BDI and child CDI ranges from −.14 to .27, but none were statistically significant.

Next, each of the three follow-up years' diagnoses of the mother and children were scaled independently for comparison with each other. A 4-point scale was employed, similar to those used in other aspects of the study: 0 = none, 1 = mild but nondiagnosable symptoms, 2 = minor disorder, mild in severity or brief in duration, 3 = major disorder. There were 36 affective disorders mother–child pairs in Year 1, 30 in Year 2, and 22 in Year 3. Correlations ranged from .34 ($p < .02$) in Year 1 to .33 ($p = .07$) in Year 3.

Whereas the positive association in Year 1 was expected, it is surprising to see a nonsignificant but noteworthy negative association in Year 3. Several factors shed light on this negative finding. First, the patterns of maternal episodes for the unipolar and bipolar women are somewhat different, and second, as noted in Chapter 3, the outcomes for unipolar and bipolar offspring are very different. The bipolar youngsters were relatively free of major disorders compared to the unipolar offspring over the course of the follow-ups. The unipolar women had higher rates of major depression. Number of major episodes divided by number of months observed yielded an index of .038 for unipolar women, which was twice the rate of that for bipolar women (.02). Of the 16 unipolar women, 14 (88%) had at least one major depressive episode during the follow-up period, compared with only 4 of 12 bipolar women (33%). The bipolar women, of course, also experienced manic episodes and hypomanias, but their major depressions appeared to be less frequent compared with unipolar women. Thus it may be that the unipolar and bipolar samples represent different patterns of mother–child association of symptoms, owing to differences in maternal pathology but possibly also to children's resilience. What is needed, however, is a more fine-grained examination of the timing of disorders in the affective illness samples, to which we now turn.

Timing of Mother–Child Disorders

We propose that it is not just the severity of maternal affective disorder that shapes children's risk for psychopathology; more precisely, it is the effect that the symptoms have on disrupting the adaptive interactions in the family. Therefore, we would expect to see an association in the *timing* of the episodes of mothers and children. As discussed in Chapter 6, the quality of the interaction between the mother and her child may be significantly affected by depression; in turn, quality of interaction predicts the child's adjustment. Moreover, the reciprocal nature of the interactions was emphasized, indicating the need to consider the mutual influence of the child and the mother on each other.

Following from this perspective, as noted in Chapter 5, Hammen, Burge, and Adrian (in press) performed hierarchical multiple regression analyses to predict children's depression level at follow-up, entering maternal symptoms, child stress, and the interaction of the two. We found that maternal symptoms, regarded as a stressor experienced by children, predict children's depressive symptoms. Also, the interaction of maternal symptoms and children's own stressful events predicted severity of depression. We speculated in Chapter 5 that high levels of maternal symptoms render the mothers unavailable to children to help buffer the effects of their own negative events.

In the same article, Hammen, Burge, and Adrian (in press) explored the timing of the experience of symptomatology of mothers and children. First, definite diagnoses in Year 1 of the follow-up were inspected and tabulated with respect to their temporal relationship with each other. Table 7.1 presents the associations, where diagnoses occurred either overlapping in time or within 1 month of each other. Many of the disorders were intermittent and ongoing, so that exact onset was impossible to determine, and such episodes are indicated in the table. There did not appear to be a specific association of onset–onset or chronic–chronic diagnoses. However, if temporally close diagnosable conditions were collapsed into

Table 7.1. Distribution of mother and child definite diagnoses in year 1.

	Child		
Mother	Onset	Chronic/intermittent	None
Onset	4	3	8
Chronic/intermittent	7	5	4
None	2	4	38

Note: Diagnosis onset occurred within at least 1 month of each other; "none" means no disorder, or none within a month of the other's episode. From Hammen, Adrian & Burge (in press). The relationship between mother and child episodes in a longitudinal study of risk for depression. *Journal of Consulting and Clinical Psychology*.

categories of present versus absent, the overall association of mother and child disorders was statistically significant, $\chi^2(1, n = 75) = 16.50, p < .001$. Thus children and mothers were strongly concordant for occurrence and timing of diagnoses. Out of 25 diagnosed children, only 6 had diagnoses that were not temporally associated with maternal diagnoses. Regarding the temporal precedence of those diagnoses considered to be child onsets, about half occurred during chronic maternal conditions, and the other half indicated a varied picture of whose symptoms started first.

Looking specifically at timing of children's *major depressions* over the full 3 years of follow-up, we found that there were 11 children with definite major depression onsets. Only 1 of these occurred in the absence of maternal symptoms. Five appeared to occur in the context of maternal chronic/intermittent depression; 3 followed onset of maternal minor depression, and in 2 cases the mothers had major depression that followed the onset of the child's episode (in both cases the child was hospitalized and the mothers became depressed).

These analyses underscore the significance of the interpersonal context of depression, suggesting patterns of mutual responsiveness of mothers and children to each other. Obviously, we are not suggesting that each is the necessary and sufficient cause of the other's symptoms. Also, we are not clear about all of the mechanisms that are involved in the expression of depression that might have an impact on others. Nevertheless, the present results suggest that whether or not the propensity for depression is genetically transmitted, the course of disorder in both children and mothers needs to be explored beyond mainly descriptive associations between severity and outcomes, to include the psychosocial processes that account for the unfolding of symptoms.

Age of Onset of Disorders in Mothers and Children

One feature of maternal psychopathology that might be related to children's disorders is maternal age of onset of disorder. Whether reflecting a severe family situation or genetic loading for disorder, the presence of an early age of onset of disorder in the mother is likely to be predictive of greater risk to her children. In the combined unipolar and bipolar groups of children, 20 of the 40 experienced major disorder (the others experienced minor disorders, nondiagnosable symptoms, or no symptoms and were excluded). The ages of onset of first diagnosable disorder of the mother and her child were compared, yielding an overall nonsignificant correlation coefficient ($r = .18, p > .05$). Separate analyses for the unipolar and bipolar groups were very similar, and they were nonsignificant. Thus there was no evidence of an effect of early maternal age of disorder on age of onset for the children. It needs to be noted, however, that the relatively restricted ranges of ages of onsets in the present sample and the small sizes of the group may limit the reliability of the findings.

Next, the possibility that earlier maternal onset might be associated with more severe pathology in the children was examined. Children with major onsets were compared with those having mild or no disorders in terms of age of maternal onset of disorder. For the unipolar children, the two groups did not differ, $t(20) = 1.32$, ns. The same comparison for the bipolar children was also nonsignificant, $t(16) = 0.0$, ns. The severity of children's diagnoses across the 3 years of follow-up evaluations was examined with respect to maternal age of onset. A 4-point severity scale for each year was used to make the ratings comparable, and an average across the 3 years (or length of available follow-up) was computed. This average severity score was then correlated with age of maternal onset of disorder. For unipolar children, the association was negligible ($r = -.01$, ns); the same occurred for the bipolar group ($r = -.07$, ns). Thus it appeared that overall, maternal age of onset was not related to children's age of developing symptoms or severity of symptoms. It is likely that the ranges of ages of onset were too restricted, and possibly that our samples were too small to permit sensitive tests of the question. It is certainly possible that the women were not accurate or reliable reporters of their ages of first disorder. Although we attempted to gather as much information as possible from the women and from their medical records, such retrospective information is problematic.

Maternal Disorder During Infancy

Another factor of children's age of onset of disorder might be the severity of maternal symptoms during their infancy, a period assumed to be critical to the development of attachment and healthy development. Unipolar children were divided into groups based on age of onset: diagnosable disorder prior to age 12 ($n = 13$), onset at age 12 or later ($n = 4$), or no diagnoses ($n = 5$). Maternal episodes of depression and hospitalizations were dated with respect to the child's first 2 years. Four unipolar women were hospitalized during the child's first 2 years; 3 of these were in the early onset group, and the other was in the no diagnosis group. Of 13 unipolar group children in the early onset group, 10 had mothers who had definite or probable major depression or dysthymia during their first 2 years. Of 4 in the late onset group, 3 had mothers with definite or probable depression in the first 2 years. In the nondiagnosed group of 5 children, 3 had a mother with a definite or possible depression in the first 2 years. Overall, there was no apparent association between maternal episodes in the child's infancy and timing of child's disorder. In general, unipolar mothers tended to be chronically or intermittently ill from the child's earliest years.

Similar analyses were performed for the bipolar group children. Seven had an early onset (below age 12) of significant disorder, 4 had later onset, and 5 had no symptoms or minor symptoms. Three mothers were hospitalized within the child's first 2 years, and 7 mothers had major episodes within this period. However, there appeared to be no association with these episodes and children's onset of disorders.

These analyses do not support the idea that exposure to severe maternal pathology at an early age is itself prognostic of early onset of disorder in children. That is not to say that early exposure is not a significant risk factor; the present sample does not permit necessary comparisons. In the present sample, the women were persistently or recurrently symptomatic, so that early exposure is confounded with chronic/episodic exposure, and therefore the effects of the former cannot be evaluated by themselves. Studies of larger and more heterogeneous samples would be welcome to address such issues more fully.

Characteristics of Fathers

Paternal Diagnoses

Diagnoses of the biological fathers were based on Family History RDC interviews of the mother. Every effort was made to obtain specific behavioral information, rather than just the woman's opinion. Obviously, there were some cases where the biological father was long gone, and the ending of the marriage may have left angry feelings so that the mother attempted to discredit him by emphasizing problematic behaviors. The most difficult category was antisocial personality; we attempted to use this category only when there was a substantial history of antisocial acts, including legal violations and jail. A few of these cases were predominantly drug-related, but others included histories of violence, occupational instability, and legal infractions. The method of diagnosing was fairly conservative, so that mild symptoms or traits were not included. The distributions of our best-guess paternal diagnoses are presented in Table 7.2.

Overall, it is apparent that the fathers displayed substantial rates of psychopathology, especially including alcohol abuse and antisocial personality disorders. The rates of disorder were higher in the husbands of unipolar and bipolar women, but the medical and normal groups also included pathology. If we compute percentages based only on the fathers for whom information was known, 36% of unipolar, 50% of bipolar, 50% of medical, and 63% of normal families had fathers without diagnoses.

Assortative Mating

This technical term for the tendency of persons with psychiatric problems to marry each other appeared to apply in the present sample. Obviously, as Table 7.2 indicates, the majority of unipolar and bipolar women had indeed at some point been married to men with psychopathology, primarily alcoholic and sociopathic men, as other studies have also found. Including the entire sample of couples across all groups, women were

TABLE 7.2. Biological father diagnostic status by group.

Diagnostic status	Maternal group			
	Unipolar	Bipolar	Medical	Normal
No diagnosis	5 (31)	7 (47)	5 (36)	15 (60)
Alcohol abuse	5 (31)	3 (20)	2 (14)	2 (8)
Antisocial	2 (13)	2 (13)	1 (7)	4 (16)
Unipolar	0 (0)	0 (0)	1 (7)	0 (0)
Bipolar	0 (0)	1 (7)	0 (0)	1 (4)
Other (schizophrenia, pedophilia)	1 (6)	0 (0)	0 (0)	1 (4)
Nondiagnosable symptoms (personality disorder, single major depression)	1 (6)	1 (7)	1 (7)	1 (4)
	—	—[a]	—[b]	—[a]
No information	2/16 (13)	1/15 (7)	4/14 (29)	1/25 (4)

Note: Numbers in parentheses represent percentages.
[a] Includes family with 2 children in study who have different fathers.
[b] Includes 3 unknown biological fathers of adopted children.

categorized for presence or absence of history of depression (3 women in the medical group had past major depression, along with all the unipolar and bipolar women). Men were categorized for presence/absence of diagnosable conditions. Table 7.3 presents the resulting distribution, and $\chi^2(1, n = 68) = 3.77$, $p = .05$, indicating a significant pattern of assortative mating.

It is of interest to note that the family pedigrees of the biological fathers (obtained from the mother) indicated that diagnosable men typically came from families with at least one first-degree relative diagnosable. For instance, using conservative behavioral indicators of pathology and including only definite diagnoses of relatives, 85% of ill fathers in the unipolar and bipolar group had at least one ill relative, whereas only 40% of nondiagnosable men had ill family members. According to Merikangas, Weissman, et al. (1988), therefore, the data suggest true assortative mating in the sense of psychopathology "preexisting" in the man rather than simply resulting from marriage to an ill woman (or in response to other circumstances).

TABLE 7.3. Distribution of diagnosed biological parents.

Mother diagnosed	Father diagnosable	
	No	Yes
No	22	12
Yes	13	21
Total	35	33

Association of Father Disorder with Child Disorder

Three indices of children's diagnostic status were examined: presence of any diagnosis prior to the beginning of the study, presence of any affective diagnosis prior to the study (both variables rated on a 0 to 3 scale of severity), and average severity scale rating across the follow-up period by year.

Analyses of variance by group and father diagnosis were computed for the total sample and for the random sample of one child per family. The results were virtually identical, and means for the random sample analyses are presented in Table 7.4.

The presence of any lifetime disorder in the children showed significant main effects of diagnosis group, $F(3, 62) = 6.3, p < .001$, and father diagnosis, $F(1, 62) = 11.0, p < .002$. Note, however, that there was also a significant interaction of the independent variables, $F(3, 62) = 4.48, p = .007$. Inspection of the means indicates that for all groups except the unipolar, having a diagnosable father was associated with much higher rates of disorder in the child. For the unipolar group, however, it was reversed.

The same pattern occurred for the lifetime history of depressive diagnoses, with a significant interaction indicating the anomalous pattern for the unipolar families, $F(3, 62) = 2.97, p < .05$. Finally, for the average severity rating across years of the follow-up, there was no longer a main effect of father illness, but the interaction term was still significant, $F(3, 62) = 5.78, p = .002$.

It makes sense that having had a father with diagnosable disorder might contribute to worse functioning in the child—which is what happened in all groups except the unipolar. But why would the unipolar children appear to have less severe psychopathology with ill fathers compared to non-ill fathers? Part of the explanation may lie with the status of the

TABLE 7.4. Children's diagnostic severity ratings by group and father psychopathology.

		Child			
Child outcomes		Unipolar	Bipolar	Medical	Normal
Any diagnosis					
Father	Diagnosis	2.0	1.9	2.0	1.3
	No diagnosis	2.8	.3	.5	.2
Affective diagnosis					
Father	Diagnosis	1.8	1.3	1.7	1.1
	No diagnosis	2.4	.3	.4	0.0
Average in follow-ups					
Father	Diagnosis	1.3	1.2	1.6	.8
	No diagnosis	2.8	.9	.6	.2

Note: Higher scores indicate more disturbance.

father's presence in the family. A good many of the unipolar (and bipolar) women were divorced from the child's biological father, and it is possible that diagnosis and divorce are somewhat confounded. Therefore, we turn next to a consideration of father absence/presence and its association with children's outcomes.

PRESENCE/ABSENCE OF THE BIOLOGICAL FATHER AND CHILDREN'S OUTCOMES

Analyzing children's diagnostic severity ratings as a function of maternal group and father presence/absence yielded a consistent pattern. Analyses of children's previous (lifetime) diagnoses indicated significantly worse functioning as a main effect of both group status and father absence. Father absence was signficantly associated with worse functioning for all the groups, $F(1, 88) = 5.54, p < .05$ for any diagnoses, and $F(1, 88) = 3.89$ $p = .05$ for affective diagnoses. The interactions were not significant but suggested that the unipolar group children fared slightly worse when their fathers lived at home, whereas all other youngsters did better when he was at home.

By the time of the follow-ups, however, father presence/absence did not make a difference in children's functioning, $F(1, 88) < 1$, $p = .38$. It would seem that lifetime (past) diagnoses may indeed have been affected by the father's absence; some children may have reacted with disorders during parental conflict or divorce, others may have adapted poorly early on in the absence of a father who left home early. By the time of the follow-ups, however, actual paternal presence did not seem to influence functioning. By that time, level of disorder might best be predicted by past adjustment and by current relationships with the mother and stressful events in the child's life. Many may have adapted to the absence of the father as such.

Finally, the question of the separate and interactive effects of paternal presence and diagnostic status were examined. Table 7.5 presents means for two-by-two analyses of variance that were performed on the children's severity of diagnosis ratings as before. For any lifetime disorder in the child, there were no significant main or interaction effects, although post hoc t tests indicated the expected pattern: when the father lived at home, those with diagnosable conditions had children with worse diagnostic status ($p = .05$, one-tailed); if he didn't live at home, his diagnostic condition made no difference. Additionally, if the father had no diagnosable condition, his absence was associated with significantly worse functioning than if he was at home, and if he had a diagnosis, it didn't matter whether he was at home or not in terms of children's outcomes. For severity of depressive disorders in the children, there was a nearly significant interaction effect, $F(1, 85) = 3.63$, $p = .06$. The patterns were the same as described previously: absence made a difference if the father had no diagnosis but not if he did; and if he was at home, having a diagnosis was

TABLE 7.5. Children's outcomes as a function of father diagnosis and presence.

Father diagnosis	Father present	Father absent	Overall
	Mean lifetime diagnosis rating of children		
Not ill	.57	1.44	.75
Ill	1.60	1.60	1.60
	.70	1.57	
	Mean affective diagnosis rating of children		
Not ill	.29	1.22	.48
Ill	1.40	1.13	1.16
	.43	1.16	
	Mean follow-up diagnosis rating of children		
Not ill	.55	1.56	.75
Ill	1.18	1.01	1.03
	.63	1.11	

Note: Higher scores indicate more disturbance.

worse for the child, but if he was not at home, presence of a diagnosis made no difference. Finally, the analyses for severity of disorders during the follow-up also indicated a significant interaction, $F(1, 88) = 3.82$, $p = .05$, with patterns in the means similar to those described previously.

Overall, despite small samples, the data consistently point to the psychosocial rather than the genetic impact of paternal disorder. Father absence was associated with worse functioning in the children, and if he was absent, it didn't matter whether he was ill or not. That is, the presumed genetic contribution of the father's illness did not appear to be additive; its effect when he was gone from home was no different from that attributable to his absence. On the other hand, if ill fathers lived at home with their children, the youngsters were definitely worse off than those living with non-ill fathers. These interpretations are of course compatible with a psychosocial explanation of the consequences of dysfunctional parents.

Association of Child Functioning with Number of Ill Parents

Finally, we turn to the question of the effects of having two ill parents and whether the effects are significantly worse than having one ill parent. The analyses of children's severity of diagnoses all showed a similar pattern, illustrated by the effects on the presence of any lifetime disorder. For children with two normal parents, the mean severity rating was .37; having one ill parent was associated with a rating of 1.44; and with both parents ill the rating was 1.78. Although there was a linear trend, the planned comparison between one- and two-ill parent groups was nonsignificant, $t(65) = 1.28$, $p = .21$. Thus the effect of having two ill parents was not significantly worse than just having one ill parent.

Next, we specifically considered the relative impact of maternal versus paternal pathology. Two-by-two analyses of variance permitted comparing mother-only and father-only as well as the other combinations. Any diagnosis and affective diagnosis ratings of children are presented in Table 7.6, and both indicated separate main effects of presence/absence of father illness and mother illness but no significant interaction. However, these cell means indicated worse but nonsignificant differences in functioning in the ill-mother-only than in the ill-father-only conditions. For the variable measuring children's functioning in the follow-up years, there was a significant interaction effect, $F(1, 88) = 5.23, p = .025$. The planned t-test comparison of mother versus father indicated significantly worse functioning for children of ill mothers compared to children of ill fathers, $t(30) = 2.49$, $p < .05$. Thus it appeared that in the children's earlier years dysfunction occurred when either parent was symptomatic. However, during the follow-ups it was far less significant to have an ill father. It is likely that by the follow-up observations most of the divorces were long since completed and the psychological influence of the father was less relevant to the child than that of the mother. The same patterns occurred when the analyses used more restrictive criteria for parent illness.

Association of Paternal Disorder with Dysfunction in Normal Group Children

In view of the apparent association of paternal disorder and children's functioning, we hypothesized that the children in the normal group who displayed maladaptive outcomes despite normal mothers might actually be affected by their dysfunctional fathers. Thus we divided the normal group children on the basis of their father's diagnostic status and compared their

TABLE 7.6. Children's outcomes as a function of maternal and paternal diagnostic status.

Mother diagnosis	Father not diagnosed	Father diagnosed	Overall
	Child's mean lifetime diagnosis rating (prior to follow-up)		
Not diagnosed	.44	1.47	.77
Diagnosed	1.58	1.95	1.81
	.75	1.74	
	Child's mean affective diagnosis rating		
Not diagnosed	.13	1.00	.40
Diagnosed	1.42	1.47	1.45
	.48	1.26	
	Child's mean follow-up diagnosis rating		
Not diagnosed	.36	.87	.52
Diagnosed	1.81	1.27	1.48
	.75	1.09	

Note: Higher scores indicate more disturbance.

own diagnostic ratings. There were significant differences in the predicted direction on all three child outcomes, $t(36) = 3.19$ for any diagnosis, $t(36) = 2.95$ for affective diagnosis, and $t(33) = 1.85$ for average in the follow-ups, all p values $< .05$, one-tailed. Thus the "mystery" of dysfunction in children of normal mothers can be explained in terms understandable for all the other groups: Exposure to maladaptive parenting, from both mothers and fathers, appears to increase children's risk for disorder.

Maternal Family History of Psychopathology

The intergenerational transmission of dysfunction is a matter of enormous scientific curiosity, as well as practical significance. Evidence of family loading for psychopathology in the first-degree relatives of diagnosed women can be taken as evidence of genetic liability (to which their children are also susceptible). On the other hand, three-generation patterns can be taken as evidence of psychological transmission of the consequences of dysfunctional parenting and psychological maladaptation. In this section we describe the family pedigrees of the women in the study and then explore their correlates.

DESCRIPTIONS OF FAMILY LOADING FOR PSYCHOPATHOLOGY

The Family History RDC information on the mothers' families was reviewed, and the patterns are quite striking—although consistent with genetic family studies. Table 7.7 summarizes the major observations.

The unipolar women were strikingly likely to come from dysfunctional families, in that 14 of 16 women (88%) had at least one diagnosable parent. The rate of major depression is very high; it includes 1 mother who com-

TABLE 7.7. Psychopathology in maternal first-degree relatives—Definite diagnoses only.

Parents	Unipolar ($n = 16$)	Bipolar ($n = 14$)	Medical ($n = 14$)	Normal ($n = 25$)
Unipolar, treated	6	0	2	4
Unipolar, untreated	5	0	2	2
Bipolar	0	3	0	0
Suicide	1	0	0	0
Alcohol abuse	4	5	4	4
Antisocial personality	0	1	0	1
Mean weighted score[a]	11.6	7.2	7.8	5.7
	(7.0)	(7.5)	(9.1)	(7.7)
Mean number of affected relatives (siblings, parents)	2.0	1.6	1.2	.6
	(1.0)	(1.2)	(1.1)	(.6)

[a] A score of 10 for each parent diagnosis of alcohol abuse, antisocial personality, and untreated depression; 15 for treated depression; 20 for hospitalized or suicidal conditions.
Note: Standard deviations are in parentheses.

mitted suicide and 2 who were hospitalized for depression. All of the depression was in the mothers, and 3 fathers and 1 mother were alcoholic. (There were several additional cases of dual diagnoses and minor disorders that are not indicated in the table).

The bipolar women also came from dysfunctional families, although not at quite as high a rate as the unipolar women. Nine of the women (64%) had at least one ill parent, and the rate of bipolar disorder is notably high with 3 of their own mothers diagnosed as manic depressive. All of the alcoholism and psychopathy were in the fathers.

The medically ill women and the normal women were represented by depression and alcoholism in their families, with 43% of the medically ill women having at least one parent diagnosable, and 40% of the normal women affected by parent illness.

Two indices of family loading were used to compare the groups. First, number of afflicted maternal first-degree relatives (siblings, parents) was counted, and the overall comparison between groups was highly significant, $F(3, 95) = 9.95, p < .001$. Post hoc group comparisons indicated significant differences between the unipolar and other groups except the bipolar group; the bipolars differed from the normals, and the medically ill group differed from the normals (p values $< .05$).

A second index was based on maternal *parents* only, and weights were assigned for degree of parent illness. Although the weightings were rationally derived, they attempted to distinguish between treated and untreated parents and to assign weights to each parent as indicated. Scores of 10 were given for each case of alcoholism, sociopathy, and untreated depression, with 15 for treated depression and 20 for hospitalized or suicidal depression. As seen from the means in Table 7.5, the average unipolar woman had a higher loading than any other subject. Overall, the groups differed significantly, $F(3, 95) = 2.71, p < .05$. The unipolar women differed significantly from the normal women ($p < .01$) and marginally

TABLE 7.8. Correlations between indices of maternal family psychopathology and mother and child attributes.

	Number of mother's ill first-degree relatives	Maternal "loading" index for parent diagnosis
Severity of child diagnoses		
Any lifetime	.38	.34
Lifetime affective	.46	.29
Average in follow-ups	.28	.16, ns
Index of maternal function		
Positive Quality of Interaction	−.20*	−.19*
Task Productivity in Interaction	−.46	−.21
Chronic Stress Index	−.43	−.24
Lifetime Severity of Depression	.41	.17*

* $p < .10$. All other values significant at $p \leq .05$.

from the bipolar women ($p = .08$). The other groups did not, however, differ from each other.

The next question that arises is whether a woman's severity of disorder is related to the extent of her family loading of psychopathology. The 7-point scale of severity of lifetime affective disorders was correlated with the two indices of family pathology. Number of family members diagnosable was significantly correlated with the woman's severity of disorder, $r = .41$, $p < .001$, and the parent loading variable was marginally correlated, $r = .17$, $p = .085$. In general, therefore, it could be argued that family history of psychopathology in the parents and siblings was associated with women's tendency to experience affective disorders. Such results are, of course, consistent with genetic family study data showing more severe pathology with increased family loading for disorder.

Associations of Maternal Family Pathology with Child Disorder

What are the implications of increased familial pathology for children's own outcomes? It might be hypothesized that women with more loaded family pedigrees might have children at higher risk for psychopathology. Indeed, that appears to be the pattern: correlations between number of maternal first-degree relatives with disorder and children's diagnostic outcomes were significant. Table 7.8 displays the correlation coefficients; severity of any lifetime disorder ($r = .38$, $p < .001$), severity of affective disorders ($r = .46$, $p < .001$), and average severity of diagnosis during the follow-ups ($r = .28$, $p = .01$) were all related to number of ill relatives on the mother's side. Similar associations were observed when the family pathology variable was the loading index based on mothers' parents' diagnoses, $r = .34$, and .29, for any disorder and affective disorder (p values $< .05$).

Although the present study cannot separate the genetic-biological transmission effects from socioenvironmental effects, it is instructive to consider whether extent of maternal family pathology might be associated with *dysfunctional parenting*. That is, it is likely that having been raised in a family with or without parental psychiatric impairment has an effect on the skills and attitudes that the woman acquires with respect to her own parenting. Therefore, correlations were computed between observed interaction behaviors in the Conflict Discussion task between the mother and child (described in Chapter 2; also see Chapter 6) and the extent of maternal family pathology. Two interaction indices were computed, as discussed in Chapter 6: overall positivity of quality of interactions (the proportion of positive minus negative comments to the child) and the task productiveness of the interaction (the relative proportion of task-focused minus off-task utterances, reflecting the mother's involvement with the child during the discussion and her willingness/ability to discuss the conflict). The lower portion of Table 7.8 presents the correlations. Positive quality of comments was marginally related to maternal family psychopathology; less positive commentary was associated with higher rates of, or more severe, family disorder. Task productivity was especially strongly and significantly related; lower involvement and task focus were associated with more dysfunction in parents and family members.

It should be noted that maternal chronic stress was also significantly related to family psychopathology, in that higher levels of ongoing difficulties and strains were associated with higher rates of disorder in maternal relatives. To the extent that the chronic stress index taps into aspects of the woman's skills and characteristics that generate stressful conditions or fail to resolve them through coping efforts, it might be argued that being raised in a dysfunctional family adversely affects such attributes. Indeed, we argued in Chapter 5 that unipolar mothers are especially likely to experience stressors that they have at least partly caused, many of which were interpersonal difficulties (see Hammen, in press-a). Elsewhere, in a study of male and female unipolar depressed outpatients, Hammen, Davila, Brown, Gitlin, and Ellicott (1991) found that parental disorder was linked to more severe patient relapse episodes, through the mediation of chronic and episodic stressors. That is, having psychopathology in parents predicted increased stressors in the person, which in turn predicted depressive symptoms, according to a causal modeling analysis. In Chapter 9 more will be said about a three-generational model of depression vulnerability.

Maternal Comorbidity of Anxiety and Substance Abuse

In view of the observations of Weissman, Leckman, et al. (1984; Merikangas, Prusoff, et al., 1988) that comorbid anxiety disorders (especially panic disorder) might increase children's risk for depression and anxiety, we explored the patterns in our sample. Overall, there did appear to be associations between mothers' and children's comorbidity of anxiety and depression. There were 24 mothers in the study with anxiety of some magnitude, and 54% of their children also had anxiety (separation anxiety, overanxious disorder) with or without other disorders. To express this another way, 13 of 25 children with anxiety disorders (52%) had mothers with anxiety disorders.

Looking specifically at patterns in the unipolar families, there were 8 women with diagnoses of comorbid panic disorder, and 5 of their 9 children also had significant anxiety disorders (among the other 4, two had other disorders, and two had no disorders). There were 5 women with generalized anxiety disorder, and 5 of their 6 children also had anxiety disorders. Overall, however, 65% of the offspring in the unipolar group had some level of anxiety with or without other disorders. This suggests that anxiety is highly likely, along with depression, to be an outcome of children of unipolar women (see also Kovacs, Gatsonas, Paulauskas, & Richards, 1989).

Secondary alcohol or drug abuse in the depressed parent is also thought to be associated with increased child risk for disorder (e.g., Merikangas, Weissman, et al., 1988). There were 15 women in the study with such histories (mostly past substance use), but only 3 of their children also had substance use diagnoses. To put this another way, 3 of 10 children with such diagnoses had mothers with substance use disorders. Thus there did not appear to be specificity for substance use. From another perspective, substance use disorders in the mother slightly increased children's risk for any disorder, in that 80% of offspring of such mothers had diagnoses, compared to 73% of mothers who had other disorders but not alcohol/drug abuse. The effects are too small to have confidence in their reliability, however, and much larger samples are needed to explore the issue of comorbidity more fully.

Maternal Personality Disorders Characteristics

The question inevitably arises about concurrent Axis II disorders in the women with affective disorders. As Downey and Coyne (1990) suggested, personality disorders co-occur frequently with depressive disorders; therefore, maybe it is these psychopathologies, rather than affective disorder, that account for children's negative outcomes. One difficulty with this suggestion, however, concerns the validity of the construct and diagnoses of personality disorders. What are they? And even if we diagnosed them, what would they give us—possibly little more information than a description of the severity and chronicity of maternal disorders. Until more is known about the dimensions of defect that such disorders imply, they may in fact provide no additional information.

In the present study, no formal Axis II diagnoses were performed. However, it was clear that many of the women's medical charts had noted varieties of personality disorders, and our observations of them would confirm the applicability of such descriptive terms.

What we *do* have, however, is some indication of the dimensional characteristics of personality functioning as measured by a short form of the MMPI. In terms of descriptive attributes of the women, analyses of variance on separate MMPI *T* scores revealed that the unipolar women scored highest on the validity scale (defensiveness) *K*, Hypochondriasis (*Hs*), Depression (*D*), Hysteria (*Hy*), Psychopathic Deviance (*Pd*), Paranoia (*Pa*), Psychasthenia (*Pt*), and Social Introversion (*Si*). They differed significantly from the normal women on all scales except Hypomania (*Ma*) and Social Introversion (*Si*), and they differed from the medically ill women on *F*, *K*, *D*, and *Pd*. The bipolar women scored highest on *F* (a validity scale), *Sc* (schizophrenia), and *Ma*, although they did not differ from the unipolar women on any scales (all p values $< .05$).

The other question was whether the elevations on scales were related to children's outcomes. Correlations were computed for mothers' scores and the random sample of one child per family's diagnostic and school ratings. In general, the patterns suggested the following: significant moderate correlations between most scales and Academic Performance Rating, non-affective diagnoses in the first follow-up and lifetime affective disorders. In general, the first four clinical scales, *Hs*, *D*, *Hy*, and *Pd*, were most strongly predictive of children's (negative) functioning. The results probably yield no surprises and confirm the overall findings of the project that symptomatic functioning in the mother, rather than diagnosis as such, appears to be related to children's maladaptive outcomes.

Summary and Directions for Further Research

The results of the present study support, extend, and clarify descriptive findings from offspring and genetic family studies in the literature. Several such studies, for instance, have suggested that parent diagnosis is less relevant to children's outcomes than severity and chronicity of the disorder. Our results confirm this for the most part, but they go further to suggest that it is the active manifestations of the maternal disorder that are disruptive to children's functioning. Specifically, current mood and stress were especially related to children's current outcomes and those at a 6-month follow-up. Moreover, diagnosed women who were not currently depressed may have had children functioning well while relatively depressed but nonpsychiatric women may have had children with problems. Additionally, there were statistically significantly linked temporal patterns of symptomatology and episodes in mothers and their children in the longitudinal course. The impact of impairment and symptoms in one appeared to increase the likelihood of disorder in the other. For mothers and children the patterns suggested mutual impact, and one particular pattern could be inferred from analyses of children's reactions to their own stressful life events: When the child experienced high levels of stressors *and* the mother was currently symptomatic the child became more depressed than if he or she experienced high levels of stressors but the mother was not symptomatic. The implication is that when symptomatic, the mothers are unavailable to support their children and bolster their coping responses in the face of adversity. Depression appears to be the outcome.

One of the great curiosities, which is also an often-ignored confound in high risk studies, concerns the tendency of dysfunctional parents to marry others with diagnosable conditions. Not surprisingly, the current study also found evidence of this "assortative mating"—a pattern that greatly obscures the search for pure genetic patterns. The unipolar and bipolar women in our sample were especially likely to marry men with alcohol/drug problems or antisocial personalities. Not too surprisingly, such women were frequently divorced from those men who were the biological fathers of the children in the study.

Prior research has been somewhat ambiguous about the impact of ill fathers, with some studies suggesting less impact than if the mother is ill and others suggesting equal impact. In the current study we found evidence for patterns that may help clarify the inconsistency. Paternal diagnoses were indeed related to children's outcomes, and in the child's earlier years they apparently were as potent an effect as were the mothers' diagnoses. However, during the longitudinal phase of our study the mother's, but not the father's, diagnoses were related to severity of disorder in the children. We suspect that this means that some of the earlier disorder in the children may have been related to the divorce of the ill fathers, which had now been resolved for most youngsters. Once such disorder is resolved, the child's ongoing relationships with the mother and contemporary events were especially significant.

This confounding of father diagnosis with father absence/presence was further explored and indicated that father absence is related to poorer outcomes in children (until their later years). Moreover, having an ill father in the home was associated with worse functioning than was having a non-ill father at home. When he was gone his diagnostic status didn't matter, and such patterns are compatible with a psychosocial rather than genetic pathway explaining the association between negative child outcomes and paternal diagnosis.

Characteristics of the father's psychopathology also shed some light on the "mystery" of child dysfunction in the normal families of the study. We had previously observed that maternal depressed mood, even in normal women, and chronic stress were associated with negative outcomes of the children; we also observed that paternal diagnosis was associated with the diagnostic status of children in the normal group. These factors—divorce, paternal psychopathology, chronic stress, and maternal depression—are good examples of the nonorthogonal risk factors operating in families (Walker et al., 1989).

Finally, our results concerning maternal family history of illness clearly were in accord with previous family pedigree studies. All the women in the sample, especially the unipolar and bipolar women, showed increased likelihood of diagnosed relatives if they had a history of depression or manic depression. The more "loaded" a woman's family tree, the more she had a severe history of recurrent episodes. Although this finding is compatible with a genetic transmission theory, the psychosocial alternative model was also explored within the limits of possibility in the study. We proposed that a woman who came from a family with psychiatric disorder was likely to have been impaired in her own functioning as a result of the family disruption. In turn, her failure to acquire adaptive skills and personal resources would be likely to contribute to her own generation of, and coping with, stressful circumstances and increase the likelihood of maladaptive relationships with her own children. In the present study we did indeed find significant relationships between psychiatric impairment in the mother's family and her own level of ongoing chronic stress and in her relatively negative and dysfunctional communications with her child observed in the Conflict Discussion task.

Although the correlational nature of the data limit our certainty in drawing causal connections between family factors and child outcomes, they at least allow us to build theories and hypotheses about the impact of psychosocial factors in the families at risk. In future studies, we can look forward to genetic markers that can help us to properly evaluate the contribution of biological diatheses as they are shaped and challenged by the powerful interpersonal impact of dysfunctional family members on each other. Considerable work is needed to assess the presumed psychological mechanisms that we have hypothesized and to more precisely elaborate the relations among them that we have postulated in only simplistic terms.

Finally, much larger samples of unipolar and bipolar women are needed to provide greater variability in their clinical characteristics. The current findings concerning maternal age of onset and severity of pathology were limited by having women specifically selected to have early onset and recurrent episodes. Larger samples would also help to further clarify the differences that might exist between unipolar and bipolar diatheses and their interactions with psychosocial variables in the family members.

8
Risk and Resilience

The high rates of impairment and dysfunction in the children in families of the present study are sobering. Various chapters, each detailing a specific form of adverse condition, have attempted to relate such risk factors to children's diagnoses and dysfunction in general. In the present chapter the focus is on *individual differences* in outcomes.

Just as the negative outcomes in children are sobering, the differences *between* children are astonishing. In certain instances there are extraordinary differences between families suffering similar adversities, or even differences between children in the same families. A more complete understanding of the consequences of high risk conditions must also, therefore, include exploration of factors that determine variability of outcomes. Thus we discuss and examine certain constructs that have been termed "protective" or "resilience" factors. We also examine how certain risk factors, aggregated over different domains, affect individual outcomes in children.

Resilience in the Face of Adversity

This phrase, borrowed from Rutter (1985), has explicitly or implicitly guided the thinking of researchers in the fields of life stress and depression, as well as high risk, where it originated. However, the focus has not been on "resilience" as such; rather, researchers in stress and depression have attempted to understand why one person will react with symptoms to an objectively minor event when someone else might not become depressed even in the face of apparent major loss and disruption. For instance, stress researchers—noting the statistically significant but small correlations between life changes and symptoms—have accomplished major conceptual and methodological advances since the mid-1970s in attempts to improve the predictability of this relationship. Cognitive processes in the form of appraisals of the meaning of events along with the contextual realities affecting magnitude of threat and personal and environmental resources have been increasingly integrated into complex models (see Hammen, 1985; 1988a, for reviews). Similarly, depression researchers have increasingly expanded models to identify individual "vulnerability," capturing depressive reactions to circumstances varying in individual meaning as well as in coping capabilities (Hammen, 1988a; in press-c).

High risk researchers, from a different perspective, have been especially active in stimulating analysis and discussion of factors that determine children's variable outcomes in the face of negative conditions such as parental psychiatric illness. Risk researchers have specifically addressed the matter of "invulnerabilty," or resilience in the face of adversity. Anthony (1974) presented the well-known doll analogy to describe his concepts of invulnerability. He used the image of three dolls, made of glass, plastic, and steel, each exposed to the same blow of a hammer. "The first doll breaks down completely, the second shows a dent that it carries permanently, and the third doll gives out a fine metallic sound" (Anthony, 1987b, p. 10).

Anthony (1987b) identified four categories of individual reactions to stresses. There are the hypervulnerables, who react even to ordinary and expected stress; the pseudoinvulnerables, who are actually vulnerable but come from an overprotective environment and are relatively unchallenged (but do break down when the environment fails them); the invulnerables with acquired resilience, who become increasingly resilient with each trauma to which they are exposed and "bounce back" from; and the nonvulnerables, who are robust from birth and who continue to thrive within any "average expectable environment." Anthony would also argue that these categories may be modified by acquired coping and competence skills. Anthony's vulnerability continuum assumes a variety of primary (e.g., biological/constitutional) vulnerabilities and secondary (learned) vulnerabilities.

As Rutter (1985) points out, the concept of invulnerability was often misunderstood as a stable, constitutional, unvarying toughness. Therefore, the concept of resilience is commonly used in preference, conveying the idea that resistance to stress is relative rather than absolute, based on both biological and environmental factors, and varying over time and circumstances.

Garmezy (1985) reviewed studies of children and adults raised under adverse conditions, including divorce and family instability, war, poverty, perinatal stress, and parental psychopathology. He concluded that there are three recurring categories of variables that appear to account for resilience: personality predispositions of the child (including temperament, high self-esteem, and autonomy), a supportive family (including warmth, cohesiveness, and order), and external supports that encourage the child's coping capabilities (see also Masten & Garmezy, 1985). As Compas (1987) points out, however, this approach typically focuses on relatively stable characteristics of the child or environment, rather than on what it is that the child *does*.

Rutter (1985) postulates the operation of "protective factors" and "interactive processes" to help understand individual variation in responses to chronically stressful conditions that affect children. Protective factors "refer to influences that modify, ameliorate, or alter a person's response to some environmental hazard" (p. 600). These are not necessarily positive experiences, and they may not even be detectable in the absence of stressors. Interactive processes refer to the kinds of effects variables may have on each other, including multiplicative, synergistic, effects apparently due to one factor when the other variables have been taken into account, or effects on other independent variables. Such processes may occur over time, not just at one point in development.

Added to the definitional difficulties are issues of whether risk and resilience factors are conceptually distinct, or whether they are opposite sides of the same coin. Is the absence of a protective factor a risk factor? One can think of examples where these relationships may or may not exist. The conceptual issues and their resolution are not a focus of this chapter; instead, each of several concepts is discussed briefly and the contribution of each to understanding children's variable outcomes in the face of adverse conditions is considered. Rutter (1985; 1990) and others (e.g., Lewis, Dlugokinski, Caputo, & Griffin, 1988) have identified a number of domains of risk and resilience effects, stemming from constitutional/biological and environmental sources. In the following section, evidence for the impact of such factors is briefly reviewed, chiefly with respect to children of psychiatrically ill parents.

Risk/Resilience Factors in Children at Risk

Child-Based Factors

Lewis et al. (1988) distinguish among factors that are qualities of the child, those that are characteristic of the family, and broader environmental factors.

Biological/Constitutional Factors

Genetic factors are, of course, suggested as major variables determining whether a child will or won't succumb to the psychiatric illness of the parent. The evidence for genetic risk for unipolar and bipolar disorders has been reviewed elsewhere (e.g., Chapter 7), leaving us with the conclusion that genetic bases of unipolar disorders are far less clear than those of bipolar disorders. Even if the genetic basis were established, however, two enormous complications limit our ability at this point to predict a child's outcomes. One is that we don't know what it is that is transmitted in affective disorders. For instance, there could be a dysregulation in cortisol mechanisms affecting stress reactivity and recovery from emotional reactions, or it might have to do with some other biological deficiency that determines the vegetative symptoms of the syndrome depression once negative appraisals activate depressed mood. There are numerous such possibilities. It is therefore difficult to specify the nature of the genetic risk factor and thus also impossible to determine genetic resilience characteristics that might override the effect. It is also possible, of course, that genetically based characteristics having little to do with the underlying depressive predispositions might be protective. For instance, we can imagine that sociability, a heritable trait, might be "antidepressive." At any rate, the genetic bases of risk and resilience factors may be presumed to be important, but we don't yet know enough about what they are to invoke their significance at this time.

Other biological risk/resilience factors such as gender, age, and temperament may play some role in children's outcomes. Most research on developmental psychopathology has indicated higher risk for boys than girls for emotional and behavioral disorders (e.g., Rutter & Quinton, 1984). However, the present investigation has not found significant sex differences (see Chapter 3; Pelligrini et al., 1986, also did not find sex differences in their resilient/nonresilient sample of children of bipolar parents). Nor have most investigations including the present one identified age as a major individual difference in outcome. Most of the children in the present study experienced onsets in mid-childhood, around age 10 to 12, but there was no evidence that children exposed to maternal disorder during infancy were at greater risk or earlier onset risk. In general, children were more likely to experience diagnosable disorders as they grew older, presumably as a function of increasing exposure to their mother's chronic and episodic depressions (see Hammen, Burge, Burney, & Adrian, 1990; Chapter 3).

Temperamental characteristics of the child may play an indirect role in children's outcomes after exposure to parental psychopathology. Rutter and Quinton (1984), for instance, found that temperamentally "difficult" children had worse outcomes in families with parental psychopathology and were often the target of parental irritability and criticism. Certainly a child who is relatively demanding or irregular in eating and sleeping patterns may challenge depressed parents who are low in energy and motivation. Certainly the "fit" between child temperament and parent characteristics, expectations, and attitudes may play a strong role in parent behaviors. Indeed, an infant who is more "difficult" than expected or whose behaviors fail to conform to the parents' knowledge and expectation may even be a source of depression for the parent (e.g., Carey, 1986; Cutrona, 1983). In turn, low self-esteem and depression in the parent may influence her reactions and interactions with the infant (e.g., Cohn et al., 1990; Field et al., 1990).

We need more information on "shared" environments; such shared family conditions have led genetics researchers to hypothesize genetically transmitted psychopathology as evidenced in family patterns. However, shared environments, such as those studied in genetic family studies, also include the influence of shared psychological environments covering behaviors, events, and conditions to which all children in the family may be exposed. However important the shared environments might be, Plomin (e.g., Plomin & Daniels, 1987) argues that the *nonshared* environments might be even more influential than the shared environments. Thus characteristics of siblings that indicate differences between them might be highly informative for the study of risk and resilience in the face of putative genetic risk. This topic has not been explored in children of families with parental affective disorders, and it will be pursued more fully in the results of the present investigation. Other biological factors include physical health of the child, both birth-related factors and later disease and injury. Weissman, John, et al. (1986), for instance, reported that children from families with a parent who was depressed had more negative perinatal events and experienced more childhood convulsions, head injuries, and operations requiring hospitalization than did children from other families. In addition to their generally poorer health, such children were seen as achieving developmental milestones in infancy significantly later than infants of nonpsychiatric parents. Although the direction of the causality is unknown, it is likely that parental depression puts children at greater risk for pregnancy complications and health risks and that such difficulties and ill children contribute to parental mood disorders.

Competence

Competence factors within the child are an important determinant of individual differences in outcomes after exposure to adverse conditions. Indeed, competence is a topic of specific focus in the search for protective factors. This work is complicated, however, by the various definitions of the construct. According to Caplan, "Most researchers define competence as a system of learned attitudes and aptitudes, manifested as capacities for confronting, actively struggling with and mastering life problems through the use of cognitive and social skills, and involving a capacity for resilience and perseverance in the face of emotional frustration and cognitive confusion" (1980; p. 671). From a different perspective, Cole (in press) recently offered an alternative definition of competence, viewing it as the responses of others. The feedback a child receives determines "objective" competence across various domains. In contrast, *internalized* competence refers to the child's own construction or perception of personal competence. Cole describes the development of actual and internalized competencies, and their consequences, over time. The implication of this approach for risk/resilience is that children who have received positive feedback across a variety of domains are likely to face adverse conditions with positive self-regard and a belief in their efficacy that permits them to maintain positive mood, motivation, and adaptive problem solving. Yet another approach to competence has focused on unusual gifts and talents children at risk might display, distinguishing them not only from children of ill parents who do not fare as well, but also from competent normal children from normal families (e.g., Kauffman et al., 1979; see also early views of Rutter, (1978) and Anthony (1974). Finally, competence has sometimes been viewed as an outcome in which the effects of stressors are mediated by various personal and family conditions (Masten et al., 1988). In view of the many approaches, a variety of constructs, such as self-concept (self-esteem), intellectual ability and academic accomplishment, coping and problem solving (including affect regulation), and social skills and their association with children's outcomes, are discussed.

Self-esteem, an evaluative judgment about one's worth and value, figures into most constructions of resilience. A positive view of one's self and one's self-efficacy typically implies an ability to appraise a stressful situation as relatively less threatening, with a belief in one's efficacy to obtain desired outcomes or minimize negative consequences, contributing to motivation and persistence (e.g., Bandura, 1982; Brown & Harris, 1978; Rutter, 1985). Indeed, as Rutter notes, although much has been written about good coping strategies, what may be important is not so much the specific coping behaviors but the existence of a coping process at all. That is, it may be essential for the adult, or child, to have enough positive regard for the self and belief in personal efficacy to undertake coping activities.

Self-concept is a complex and multifaceted construct (e.g., Hart & Damon, 1986; Harter, 1983; 1986), evolving over a developmental course, constructed from different areas of functioning on different levels of self-awareness and self-understanding. Self-esteem, the evaluative part of self-concept, is highly associated with mood: indeed, when self-regard is negative, its very presence helps to define the depression syndrome. In children, the correlations between self-esteem and depression are significant (as reviewed in Chapter 4). Not only as an overall, evaluative view of one's worth is self-concept related to depression, but also the specific facets of the self-concept, such as social competence and intellectual ability, may be related to mood status. Therefore, a child who is proficient in particular domains of functioning (and who receives positive feedback for such qualities) may be relatively protected—although the propensity for depression to be associated with distortion in self-evaluation may actually mitigate against protective effects of compensatory skills. Linville's (1987) notion of self-complexity may also be relevant to resilience; individuals who have a variety of areas of self-definition, rather than a single or overly dominant role, may be relatively more able to withstand threats to self-esteem stemming from challenges to a particular role by obtaining gratifications and feelings of self-worth from other realms. Thus strength of self-esteem as a protective factor against adversity probably requires not just evaluative judgments, but also the number and diversity of actual and perceived competencies, as well as their meaning and significance to the individual.

Intellectual and school competence are specific competencies that have been suggested as protective factors that assist children, both by providing accomplishments that bolster self-esteem and by enhancing problem-solving abilities. Anthony (1987a) found that while children of psychotic (manic depressive and schizophrenic) parents in the St. Louis Project who functioned well in school were less vulnerable, IQ itself did not differentiate between resilient and nonresilient children. Pelligrini et al. (1986) also failed to find vocabulary-based IQ differences in resilient/nonresilient offspring and controls, although Worland, Weeks, and Janes (1987) did find that lower verbal IQ was a predictor of mental health difficulties in children in the St. Louis Risk Research study. Weintraub et al. (1986) found that children of schizophrenic and affectively ill parents were rated by their teachers as less cognitively and academically competent than their normal peers in the Stony Brook High Risk project. The teachers tended to rate the children of unipolar depressed parents as most deviant of all. Various studies have assessed the relationship between depressive symptoms in children and actual and other-rated academic achievement. Generally, the studies are consistent in reporting significant relationships between academic performance and mood (reviewed in Cole, in press). However, while relatively dysphoric children may be performing poorly in school, it is unclear whether good academic performance serves as a protective factor, compensating for the ill effects of stressful circumstances.

Unusual talents, creativity, and aptitudes have been found to distinguish certain children of ill parents who have survived without display of major symptomatology (e.g., Anthony, 1974; Rutter, 1966). Kauffman et al. (1979), for example, compared the 6 most and 6 least competent children of schizophrenic and psychotic women with affective disorders. The most competent children had talents, but they also had superior social skills in forming friendships and relating to others. Moreover, they excelled compared to normal competent children and were more creative according to the measures used to study them. Interestingly, most of the competent youngsters were children of schizophrenics, and most of the least competent offspring were children of depressed women. Kauffman et al. note the negative impact of maternal depression, associated with low levels of positive involvement with the children, as a factor in children's outcomes.

Children's *coping behaviors* represent a different approach to understanding resistance to stressful conditions, because the emphasis here is on what the child does, rather than on enduring characteristics or attributes of the child or the environment. Coping responses are usually defined as effortful or purposeful reactions to stress (e.g., Lazarus & Folkman, 1984). Compas (1987), in his review of child and adolescent coping, emphasizes that coping cannot be characterized only by descriptions of the individual's skills and resources but must include the relationship between the child and the environment. In this view, Compas includes discussions of infant attachment and responses to separation, social support, interpersonal cognitive problem solving, and other constructs in his approach to child coping. His review indicates that both emotion-focused and problem-focused coping behaviors have been shown to be important in dealing with stress, but little research has addressed the questions of what kinds of skills serve best for what kinds of situations. Compas also notes the need for more and better measures of coping in children and for distinctions to be drawn between the effortful coping behaviors and the stable and automatic, or nonvolitional, features of adaptive responses such as temperament.

Coping as *problem solving* is discussed later, with specific respect to social problem solving, resolution of interpersonal conflict, and other cognitive representations of the social environment. An additional area of interest in children's coping concerns emotion regulation. Zahn-Waxler, Cummings, McKnew, & Radke-Yarrow, 1984, and Zahn-Waxler et al. (1990) have observed the behaviors of children of affectively ill women, as well as their responses to semiprojective techniques, and have noted a variety of problematic and unusual responses to conflict. These authors conclude that the high risk children have difficulties in the experience and representation of emotions and in the regulation of affect.

Social skills and social cognitive development represent a complex area with strong implications for children's resilience. Just as adults appear to be protected against depression in the face of adversity if they have supportive relationships or a close confiding relationship with another adult (e.g., Brown & Harris, 1978; Dean, Lin, & Ensel, 1981), so too do children appear to benefit from positive relationships with others. In the section to follow, family relationships and attachments are discussed as risk/resilience factors. In this section, the focus is on peer relationships and general social competence.

Children appear to display relatively stable individual differences in social competence from toddlerhood (Howes, 1987b). Youngsters' immature, withdrawn, and aggressive behaviors are likely to elicit negative reaction from peers, and sociometric status of children appears to be a relatively stable predictor of various adaptive and maladaptive behaviors in later years. Impaired peer relationships are predictive of dysfunction in children, with evidence generally indicating that children with externalizing problems such as aggressiveness and antisocial conduct are especially likely to be rejected by peers (see Hartup, 1983, review; Strauss, Lahey, Frick, Frame, & Hynd, 1988). Recently, research has begun to demonstrate that depressed children, like depressed adults, exhibit certain impairments in social skills and are less popular than nondepressed children (e.g., Altmann & Gotlib, 1988; Blechman, McEnroe, Carella, & Audette, 1986; Kazdin, Esveldt-Dawson, Sherick, & Colbus, 1985). Indeed, in a study of ratings of hypothetical peers who were depressed or not, Peterson, Mullins, and Ridley-Johnson (1985) found that children showed patterns of rejection of the depressed child similar to those shown by others in studies of depressed adults (e.g., Coyne, 1976; Hammen & Peters, 1978). It appears, however, that clinically depressed children tend not to be disliked or rejected to the same extent as children with externalizing disorders or mixed depression–externalizing disorders (Asarnow, 1988). Overall, evidence supports the association between depressive symptoms and impaired social skills and negative social outcomes (e.g., reviewed in Cole, in press). However, the cause–effect relationship is unclear, since impaired social functioning may be a consequence, as well as a cause, of depression. The role of compensatory social skills in protecting a child from adverse conditions is unclear.

Quality of family interactions undoubtedly affects the child's acquisition and demonstration of social competence, although such processes are likely to be enormously complex. For instance, the quality of parenting and socialization practices appears to be related to social skills (e.g., reviewed in Maccoby & Martin, 1983) and to social cognitive skills (e.g., Putallaz, 1987). More specific paths between parental attitudes and practices, social problem solving, and peer status and social competence have been explored by Pettit et al. (1988). However, much of the research has not elaborated specific mechanisms linking parental practices and child social competence, and virtually no research explores these links in families at risk for children's depression.

Both social cognition and peer relationships may be impaired in children of psychiatrically ill parents. For instance, children of affectively ill and of schizophrenic parents are less popular with peers and more aggressive in their interactions than children of comparison parents (e.g., Weintraub et al., 1986; Zahn-Waxler, Cummings, McKnew, & Radke-Yarrow, 1984). Barocas, Seifer, and Sameroff (1985) reported overall reduced social functioning associated with maternal mental illness in the Rochester High Risk study. An earlier report on children of psychotic mothers supported this idea, finding that relatively more overall competent children appeared to be more socially skilled than their less competent counterparts who were also children of ill mothers (Kauffman et al., 1979). Downey and Walker (1989) explored social cognition in children of maltreating (referrals for suspected physical abuse) or psychiatrically ill parents and of control parents. They examined children's performance on an interpersonal problem-solving competence task and also assessed attributional analyses of hypothetical situations involving an aversive event by a peer. They found that peer rejection was significantly related to lower interpersonal problem-solving competence. However, parental psychopathology was not related to peer rejection, whereas parental maltreatment was. Nor was social cognition associated with parental risk status, suggesting that social problem solving did not mediate the association between child maladjustment and parental maladjustment. Instead, however, children with high levels of social competence appeared to function better with peers, regardless of parent status. Downey and Walker concluded that social cognitive skills may help children at risk *compensate* for being raised by maltreating parents.

Beardslee, Schultz, and Selman (1987), on the other hand, argued that social cognitive skills do mediate between parental illness and child outcomes. Although like Downey and Walker's (1989), their study is cross-sectional, they found significant associations between offspring adaptive functioning and "interpersonal negotiation strategy" (INS; Selman, Beardslee, Schultz, Krupa, & Podorefsky, 1986). Adolescent offspring of parents with affective disorders or normal parents completed the INS measure consisting of eight interpersonal dilemmas. Responses were scored for level of ability to coordinate the perspectives of the protagonist (the adolescent) and the significant other in the story, in order to resolve the conflict. Not only was the adolescent's adaptive functioning related to the level of mutuality in social problem solving, but also the INS scores were correlated negatively with duration of parental illness. However, some of the children in the high risk group showed discrepancies between INS level and actual functioning; for instance, there tended to be girls with high social competence but relatively impaired current functioning. The authors interpreted the findings overall to suggest that high levels of interpersonal mutuality may help protect children at risk.

"Social engagingness"—having qualities that elicit positive responses from others—was one of three protective factors identified by Radke-Yarrow and Sherman (1990) in their sample of children at risk due to affective disorder in *both* parents. Above-average intelligence and having a characteristic highly valued by the parents were additional protective factors; the study is discussed more fully in the section on family relationships.

Pelligrini et al. (1986) studied disordered and nondisordered offspring of bipolar parents and controls on a variety of presumed personal resource characteristics. A composite score based on social problem solving, self-esteem, and internal locus of control showed that resilient offspring had much higher competencies than all the other groups, including normal offspring of normal parents. Also, high levels of social support were associated with children's outcomes. Lack of a supportive relationship with a best friend was associated with greater risk for disturbance in children, whereas perceived availability of good relationships with siblings, peers, and non-ill relatives was associated with good outcomes (see also Kauffman et al., 1979). Support from nonrelative adults was characteristic of offspring of ill parents who were themselves diagnosed. The authors suggest that the superior social and psychological resources of the nondisordered high risk (resilient) youngsters might have made them adept at finding and maintaining good relationships with others, but clearly the direction of causality is unclear.

Evidence linking the quality of parent–child interactions with social skill development is relatively sparse, especially in high risk families. However, several highly suggestive articles indicate the importance of pursuing this question. Goodman and Brumley (1990), for instance, examined the association between toddler social behaviors and maternal behaviors in samples of women with schizophrenia or depression and control women. Schizophrenic women were markedly withdrawn and emotionally uninvolved with their children during observations, and depressed women's behaviors were generally midway between the schizophrenic and normal women's scores. Maternal responsiveness and involvement were significantly associated with children's social behaviors. The authors speculate that maternal responsiveness is a critical variable shaping and rewarding children's social competence. Interestingly, an earlier study by Kaufmann et al. (1979) found that the "superkids," competent offspring of ill mothers, were more likely to be children of schizophrenics, whereas few children of depressed women were among the competent, resilient children, because of lack of maternal involvement and warmth. Thus it is apparent that maternal behavior with the child, not maternal diagnosis, is the important contributor to outcome, including resilience.

Family Relationship Factors

Research on both adult and childhood depression has consistently pointed to the negative quality of the parent–child relationship as a risk factor (see Chapter 6), as indeed it is for almost any child maladjustment. Children with impaired attachment or those who experience families with high levels of discord, criticism, and rejection are likely to display maladaptive outcomes. In turn, it is presumed that such family disruption is a product of parental psychopathology (in this case depression), varying in severity of effects as a function of severity and chronicity of parental symptoms (see Chapter 7). However, because of the problem of "nonorthogonal risk factors" (Walker et al., 1989), further work is needed to establish that dysfunctional child-rearing is due to depression rather than to stressful conditions or poor parenting skills arising from the parent's own dysfunctional background (Rutter, 1990; see also Chapter 7).

With respect to protective/resilience factors, it is likely that variations in children's outcomes stem from variations in parental severity and chronicity of symptoms. As discussed in previous chapters, both the chronicity and timing of maternal disorders had an impact on children's symptoms. Also, Hammen, Burge, and Adrian (in press) showed that high stress-exposed children had more positive outcomes if their mothers were not symptomatic at the time (a stress-buffering effect).

Other research has suggested that presence of relatively high levels of family cohesion predict better outcomes for children of depressed parents (e.g., Holahan & Moos, 1987). There is some evidence that a good relationship with one or more parents is a protective factor (Fisher, Kokes, Cole, Perkins, & Wynne, 1987; Rutter, 1989), and this effect may extend to other significant relatives or adults, but further studies are needed. Unfortunately, also, many families with affective disorder in a parent also find that the other parent is likely to have a diagnosable condition—or that divorce has disrupted the contact with the father (see Chapter 7).

The quality of the relationship with the parents, especially the ill parent, may be an additional complication. On some occasions the parent may use the offspring as a confidant and source of comfort, as reported by Radke-Yarrow, Richters, and Wilson (1988) of women with their daughters. This kind of enmeshment may have mixed outcomes, encouraging maturity and responsibility on the one hand but portending significant problems in the family structure on the other. Anthony (1987a) has suggested that children may be protected by being *less* psychologically involved and identified with their ill parent. Citing data from the St. Louis High Risk Project, he argued that children of affectively ill parents may be acutely sensitive to the feelings of others (presumably as a function of their experience with an ill parent), but the resilient youngsters were able to be objective and dispassionate about their parents' disorders. In contrast, children of schizophrenic parents were seen as more involved with parents, to the point of symbiosis. Overall, the less vulnerable children were seen as those who could distance themselves psychologically from the parent's psychosis and from being caught up in overinvolvement with the ill parent. Somewhat similar findings were reported by Beardslee and Podorefsky (1988) on a small sample of 15 resilient offspring of parents with major affective disorders (e.g., Beardslee et al., 1985). A characteristic of these youngsters was "self-understanding," which included a profound awareness of their parent's illness along with an ability to remain separate from it and free of self-blame. They were empathic with their parent's plight, and 11 of the 15 had major caretaking roles in the family; however, despite such involvement, they were sufficiently psychologically separated so as to have come to some realistic understanding of their parent. Most of them had major involvements in school or job activities. Although the clinical methods employed in the study are not adequate for systematic evaluations, they capture the flavor of important ingredients that might be associated with resilience to effects of parental psychopathology: empathic understanding of the parent illness but psychological separateness, and involvement with meaningful roles outside the home. Implicit is the idea that parental criticism or blame of the child may contribute to enmeshment of the youngster, making it difficult for him or her to maintain self-confidence and avoid self-blame for parental difficulties. A major difficulty with such formulations, nevertheless, is the clarification of cause–effect relationships. The symptomatic child by definition is not resilient, but such children may contribute to parental distress—and to blame and criticism directed toward the child—thereby involving the child in a dysfunctional family system that is difficult to escape.

A recent study by Zahn-Waxler, Kochanska, Krupnick, and McKnew

(1990) suggests that guilt and self-blame processes may be distorted in children of depressed mothers. Five- to nine-year-olds responded to interviews and semiprojective vignettes to elicit their narratives about themes concerning interpersonal conflict and distress. Whereas children of non-ill mothers made adapative responses, children of depressed women displayed aberrant responses. For example, younger children of depressed women showed overarousal and exhibited high levels of responsibility and involvement, whereas older children displayed patterns that were interpreted as extreme or distorted reactions suggestive of extreme guilt or defense against guilt. The authors suggest that early exposure of children to maternal depression may overinvolve them in ways that are burdensome and that overtax their ability to deal effectively with feelings of responsibility. Moreover, it is speculated, such intense arousal and overinvolvement may draw them away from appropriate resolution of developmental tasks of attachment and separation–individuation.

Radke-Yarrow and Sherman (1990) compared the children in 25 families with both parents having affective disorders as well as highly adverse conditions to a sample of children from normal families. They identified three hypothesized protective factors, intelligence, social charm, and what they termed a *match* between a child characteristic and a core need in one or both parents that this child fulfills. Thus in one family simply being a boy was highly desired; in another the child was especially healthy and sturdy, qualities greatly prized by the mother. From these factors, the authors speculate, the child obtains a sense of importance and worth, experiences a warm relationship with the parent(s), and is able to perform competently in school and thus obtains positive feedback from teachers and peers. Of the 25 older children in the high risk group, 5 children had all of the protective factors and only 1 had a diagnosable disorder (separation anxiety); of the remaining 20 who were not "protected," only 4 were functioning well in all areas. Additionally, the authors note that many of the children who appeared to be survivors paid certain costs for their survivorship, such as denial or unwillingness to show emotions. This provocative study stimulates interest in complex and interrelated family and child characteristics that predict resilience.

Theoretical and Methodological Shortcomings in Research on Resilience

As previously noted, a major difficulty is definitional: What is the relationship between risk and resilience? Is the absence of a protective factor a risk factor, or is the absence of a risk factor a protective factor? Is an average amount of a coping capability sufficient to be a protective factor, or does an unusual amount of the quality have to be present to protect against adverse consequences? It is likely that some variables of relevance to children's outcomes fall on a continuum with a linear relationship to outcome, while others may not be so related. To some extent this is an empirical matter (and a semantic issue), but there may be ways in which a fuller resolution of the definitional questions could lead to theoretical elaboration of risk and protective factors that have yet to be identified.

A related conceptual/methodological matter is the potential confounding of dependent and independent variables. Sometimes the line between a protective factor (or risk) and an outcome might be a fine one. For instance, social competence could be a protective factor against negative outcomes as well as a measure of outcome. Academic performance might be both an indicator of symptomatic outcome and a risk factor predicting negative outcomes. The concept of "coping" is a difficult one, with the potential for confounding the symptoms with the behaviors. Additionally, the concept of positive or negative outcomes may itself obscure important qualitative differences in how a person might react to stressful circumstances. It has been noted, for example, that some individuals who may appear to be immune to stressful conditions, in the sense of non-diagnosable reactions, may nevertheless have maladaptive defenses—sociopathic or overly distanced and defended in ways that impair intimacy (see Anthony, 1987a; Rutter, 1985).

The mechanisms of resilience or protection have been elaborated only minimally. Among the many obstacles to a comprehensive theory and empirical validation of protective factors are the complexities of the concepts. As Rutter (1985) noted, the effects occur over time, operate indirectly (often through interpersonal interactions), and are modified by personal differences such as cognitions about meaning and the timing of occurrence. He concludes, for instance, that many traditional views of personality development need to be transformed: "The infancy years are not determinative; cognitive processes play a major role in emotional and behavioural responses; temperamental features are influential, but operate through interactions as much as individual reactivity; much behaviour is context-related; many of the links in development are social rather than individual; continuities over time are usually indirect rather than direct; and fluidity in functioning continues right into adult life" (p. 606).

Related to the need for further elaboration of the complex processes involved in resistance to stressful conditions is additional clarification of processes. For instance, stress buffering and stress inoculation (or "steeling") represent two different mechanisms by which a child might resist the negative impact of stressors. In the former, attributes of the person or the environment might serve to diminish the impact of a stressor—either by preventing its impact or by mitigating its consequences. In the latter, stressful circumstances might provide a cumulative inoculation effect, such that prior exposure might reduce the impact of subsequent exposure. Stress-resistance processes are not limited to these possibilities, and considerable development of theories is needed.

The complexity of the resilience/protective process certainly raises the need for multiple variables to be studied over longitudinal courses (Lewis et al., 1988). Additionally, assessment procedures and method development are tasks of high priority. For example, the assessment of social cognition and social competence behaviors is complex owing to the multiple dimensions that determine the effectiveness of interpersonal relationships. However, this is an area of likely important contributions. Studies variously consider observed behaviors, sociometric ratings of peer status, and self- or parent- and teacher-rated social competence, as well as social cognitive measures of perceptions and imagined solutions of hypothetical social dilemmas. The development of instruments and the evaluation of their roles in children's peer relationships are likely to become significant in future research—indeed, such activity has already begun. Measures need to not only consider ability to generate quantities of solutions to hypothetical situations but also evaluate their quality (e.g., Fischler & Kendall, 1988; Selman et al., 1986). Such capabilities, of course, vary with developmental level. Moreover, the ability to think about social situations and solve interpersonal conflicts and the actual behaviors that children display in such situations are likely to differ, and research must attend to the relations between social cognition and interpersonal behavior, as well as between each and children's peer status and objective social functioning in various contexts.

Results of the Study

Resilience/Risk Factors and Children's Diagnostic Outcomes

Throughout this book various risk factors have been analyzed with respect to children's outcomes. These have included maternal psychiatric history and current mood, chronic and episodic stress, cognitions that imply vulnerability to depression including self-concept, and family interactions and relationship qualities. In the present context, however, the goal is to examine these and additional variables from the opposite perspective—as protective factors when they occur in ways that imply superior functioning. Also, in this section the risk/resilience factors are analyzed in the aggregate and with respect to the strength of their relationship to outcomes.

Seven variables were identified to be analyzed for their roles as potential protective or resilience predictors or that, when absent or minimal, could constitute risk factors. The selection was based on the review of relevant research literature suggesting likely predictors of risk/resilience. These included self-concept (Piers–Harris), paternal diagnosis, presence of the father in the home, maternal current mood (Beck Depression Inventory score at the initial evaluation), level of ongoing difficulties or chronic stress

TABLE 8.1. Correlations between risk/resilience factors and child outcome—Entire random sample.

Measure	Diagnostic rating: Lifetime affective disorder	Diagnostic rating: Average any follow-up diagnosis
Self-concept[a]	−.39	−.38
CBCL Social Competence[a]	−.44	−.41
Academic Performance[a]	−.40	−.53
Maternal BDI (Initial)	.50	.33
Chronic stress[a]	−.55	−.37

Note: All r values are significant at $p < .01$ or $p < .001$.
[a] Higher scores are more adaptive functioning.

TABLE 8.2. Correlations between risk/resilience factors and child outcome—High risk children only.[a]

Measure	Diagnostic rating: Lifetime affective disorder	Diagnostic rating: Average any follow-up diagnosis
Piers–Harris Self-Concept[b]	−.33	−.37
CBCL Social Competence[b]	−.51	−.42
Academic Performance[b]	−.45	−.56
Maternal BDI (initial)	.45	.21**
Chronic stress[b]	−.24*	−.07, ns

Note: All r-values are significant at $p < .01$ or $p < .001$ unless noted.
[a] Children of normal, nonpsychiatric women have been excluded.
[b] Higher scores are more adaptive functioning.
*$p < .05$. **$p < .10$.

(based on maternal social functioning, work, financial, and health status), social competence (Social Competence *T* score on the Child Behavior Check List), and academic performance. (All of these variables were described in Chapter 2.) Tables 8.1 and 8.2 present the simple correlations between the variables and two measures of children's diagnostic status, the scaled rating of affective disorder (lifetime) rated at the initial evaluation and the average diagnosis rating across all follow-up contacts. Paternal diagnosis and presence of father in the home are not included in the correlation tables since these are not interval-scaled variables.

Table 8.1 includes the random sample (one child per family) for all four maternal groups; Table 8.2 includes only the children considered to be at risk owing to maternal illness (affective disorder or chronic medical condition). As expected, all of the risk/resilience variables were significantly correlated with both measures of children's diagnostic outcome for the entire (random) sample. Similarly, among high risk children only, the variables are also predictive, with two minor exceptions: measures of maternal mood and chronic stress are not significantly related to children's diagnoses in the follow-ups, probably reflecting the more restricted ranges of the variables in the high risk samples.

The next analysis involved examination of the association between children's outcomes and the number of protective (risk) factors to which they were exposed. Each of the seven protective factors was dichotomized at the point thought to represent relative "protectiveness": Piers–Harris self-concept score of 65 or over (corresponding to approximately the 85th percentile of normative samples), a father without diagnosable conditions, father living at home, mother not currently depressed, relatively less family chronic stress (median split), social competence CBCL scores one standard deviation or more above the mean, and academic performance reflecting good-to-superior grades in school.

Table 8.3 presents the correlations between number of protective factors and children's diagnostic outcome ratings for the random sample of children from all groups and for the children in the three high risk groups only. For both sets of children, presence of more protective factors is significantly associated with lower diagnostic ratings. The relationships are stronger for the contemporaneous measures (of risk factors and current/recent diagnosis) than for follow-up diagnoses, but the associations are nonetheless highly significant.

To explore the nature of the statistical association between number of protective factors and diagnostic status, trend analyses were conducted. Children were assigned to one of four groups having 0–1, 2–3, 4–5, or 6–7 protective factors. The four resulting groups were subjected to an analysis of variance with a test for linear trend. For average diagnosis across the follow-up periods, the linear effect was highly statistically significant, $F(1, 53) = 20.95$, $p < .0001$, and $F(1, 56) = 46.36$, $p < .0001$ for lifetime affective disorders for the entire random sample. Very similar highly significant linear trends occurred for the sample of high risk children only. Figures 8.1 and 8.2 are graphic representations of the relationship between number of protective factors and diagnostic ratings for the high risk children only. It should be noted that only 4 children had the highest number of protective factors; nevertheless, the figures suggest that the more protective factors available, the less likely the child is to receive diagnoses.

To examine the relative contributions of the protective factors, given their intercorrelations, two exploratory multiple regression analyses were

TABLE 8.3. Correlations between number of protective factors and outcome.

Sample	Diagnostic rating: Lifetime affective disorder	Diagnostic rating: Average any follow-up diagnosis
Entire random sample	−.67	−.53
High risk sample	−.54	−.39*

*$p < .01$; all other $p < .001$.

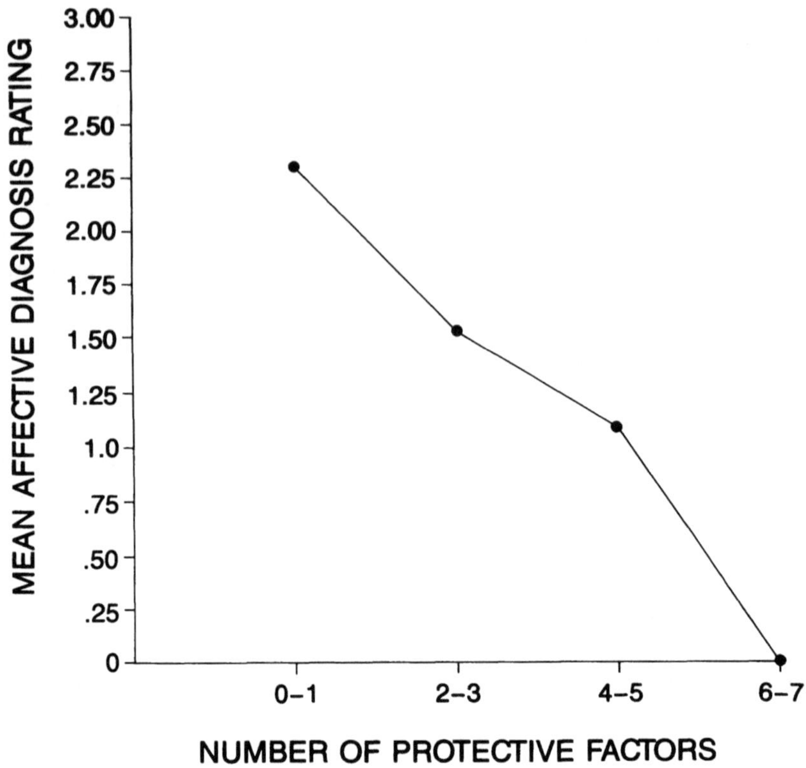

FIGURE 8.1. Lifetime affective disorder ratings by number of protective factors (high risk random sample; excludes children of normal mothers).

performed. The first, based on the entire random sample, entered chronic stress first to see which variables would contribute incrementally beyond that "basic" factor. Low chronic stress (R^2 = .13) and high academic performance (R^2 = .19) appeared to be the significant contributors to children's healthy functioning, measured by the average diagnostic rating over the follow-ups. Both variables were statistically significant, but no other variable entered the equation.

The second analysis was based only on the high risk groups, omitting the normal family children. A stepwise multiple regression indicated that only academic performance was distinctively related to average diagnosis over the follow-ups, yielding a multiple R of .47, $F(1, 42) = 12.21$, $p = .001$.

Examination of Nonshared Environments: Sibling Pairs

One way to identify possible protective factors is to explore the child's competencies and relationships that are unique to the child, even if living

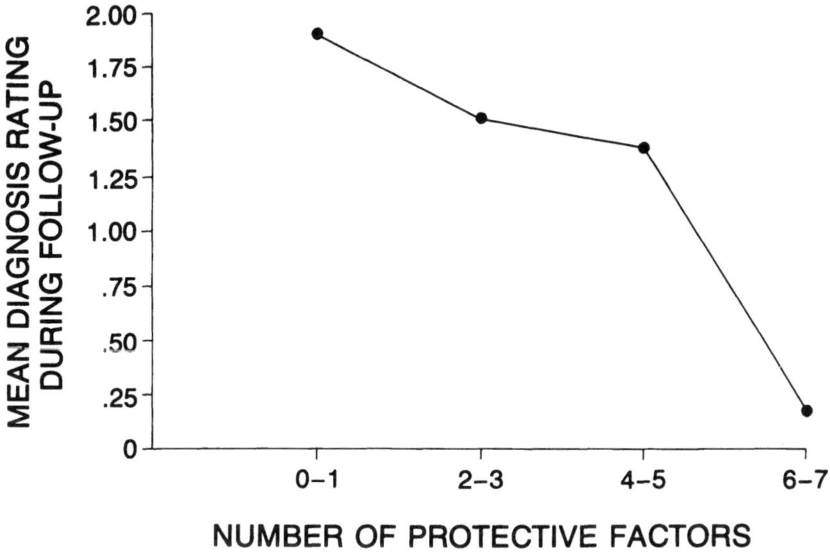

FIGURE 8.2. Average diagnosis rating during follow-ups by number of protective factors (high risk random sample; excludes children of normal mothers).

in the same environment as a sibling. Of the 28 families contributing two children to the study, 10 sibling pairs were identified in which one child experienced significant diagnosable disorder (lifetime) while the other did not. The other 18 pairs were concordant, 4 with both diagnosed and 14 with neither diagnosed. Anderson and Hammen (1990b) used this sample of siblings with different outcomes to examine their "nonshared environment" individual differences that might be associated with protection from negative outcomes.

Of the 10 pairs that were discordant for outcomes, we first examined demographic factors and found that none were noteworthy. Four pairs were children of unipolar mothers, 1 pair had a bipolar mother, 3 pairs were children of medically ill women, and 2 sets were children of highly chronically stressed nonpsychiatric women. There were 2 girl pairs, 2 boy pairs, and 6 mixed pairs, and although 8 of 10 diagnosed children were boys, the gender effect was nonsignificant. Birth order was not an apparent significant factor, in that 5 of the diagnosed members of the pairs were firstborn children, compared with 3 of the nondiagnosed children. Age was a significant predictor, however, in that the diagnosed child was older (M = 14.03 years, SD = 2.4) than the nondiagnosed child (M = 11.3, SD = 2.2), $t(9) = 3.12$, $p < .01$. It did not simply seem to be the case that the diagnosed child had had a longer time in which to develop symptoms, since the diagnoses all had onsets in the child's younger years (and may be continuing), while the well siblings were not only not diagnosed in the past but did not develop diagnosable conditions during the follow-ups. Thus, although it may be true that the older sibling has more time to become ill, the well sibling seemed to be truly resistant over time.

The two sets of nonshared environmental variables most likely to constitute protective factors concern children's competencies and their family relations. Each of these was explored.

Children's Competence

Three scores were available that directly or indirectly tap competence domains: self-concept, mother-rated social competence on the CBCL, and children's academic performance (based on school records and interview data, rated on a 5-point scale, described in Chapter 2). Table 8.4 displays the means for the sibling pairs on these variables.

In each case, the nondiagnosed sibling displayed higher perceived or other-rated competence. One-tailed *t* tests indicated that the effects were statistically significant for the Piers–Harris Self-Concept, $t(9) = 1.86, p < .05$, CBCL Social Competence, $t(9) = 2.23, p < .05$, and Academic Performance, $t(9) = 2.54, p < .05$. Thus competence constructs seemed to distinguish clearly between the ill and not-ill siblings, although the direction of causality cannot be determined from the correlational nature of the data.

Family Relationships

It was also predicted that the nondiagnosed children would enjoy a more positive, less negative relationship with their parents, and two sources of data were used to test this hypothesis. Mother–child interactions in the Conflict Discussion task (described in Chapter 2) yielded various dimensions of communication content. Three variables were combined to form a total of positive comments, and three combined for a total of negative comments. The positivity of the overall interaction was indexed by subtracting the negative from the positive totals and dividing the result by

TABLE 8.4. Mean competence scores of sibling pairs and matched normal controls.

Measure	Diagnosed sibling	Nondiagnosed sibling	Matched control
Piers–Harris Self-Concept	57.6	66.5	73.7
	(9.9)	(7.3)	(3.6)
CBCL Social Competence	38.8	50.0	46.0
	(12.1)	(14.2)	(5.8)
Academic Performance Rating	2.8	3.9	4.3
	(1.4)	(1.1)	(0.5)

Note: Standard deviations are in parentheses. From "Disturbed and Nondisturbed Siblings in High Risk Families: Correlates of Vulnerability" by C. Anderson and C. Hammen, 1990-b, unpublished.

the total utterances. The proportion of the negative total was also examined. Additionally, children reported their subjective perceptions of the mother's behavior toward them on the Parent Perception Inventory (see Chapter 2) in a positivity summary score across the various items of specific behaviors, subtracting perceptions of negative behaviors from the positive. The PPI was completed separately for mothers and for fathers (where available). The means are presented in Table 8.5.

On actual observed interactions, mothers appeared to be more negative toward the child who was the diagnosed member of the pair. For the relative positivity balance, the one-tailed t test was statistically significant, $t(7) = 2.13$, $p < .05$, and the proportion of negative utterances was also significantly higher for the diagnosed child, $t(7) = 1.96$, $p < .05$. (In two of the pairs one or both children refused the interaction task.)

For the subjective perceptions of parent behavior, the effects were not statistically significant. However, the nondiagnosed children tended to see their parents more favorably than did the diagnosed member of the pair.

Overall, Anderson and Hammen (1990-b) found some support for the possibility that more positive relations with the mother, as observed in the Conflict Discussion task, may be associated with children's relative resilience to disorder even under high risk conditions. Again, however, the direction of causality cannot be established from the data available.

Examples of Different Sibling Outcomes in High Risk Families

In the S. family, the older child, a 16-year-old girl, has had a history of significant conduct disorder, drug use, major and minor depression, and anxiety, and was hospitalized during her teens. During the follow-up period she had no significant

TABLE 8.5. Mean scores for family relationships of sibling pairs and matched normal controls.

Measure	Diagnosed sibling	Nondiagnosed sibling	Matched control
Observed maternal behavior			
Positivity balance[a]	−.20	−.09	−.03
	(.18)	(.17)	(.08)
Negative comments[a]	.26	.16	.09
	(.14)	(.17)	(.08)
Perceived parental behaviors			
Positive balance, Mother	14.0	21.0	24.7
	(11.1)	(5.6)	(5.4)
Positive balance, father	12.2	21.2	23.2
	(16.5)	(5.5)	(6.5)

Note: Standard deviations are in parentheses. From "Disturbed and Nondisturbed Siblings in High Risk Families: Correlates of Vulnerability" by C. Anderson and C. Hammen, 1990-b, unpublished.

[a] Proportions of total interaction comments.

conduct problems but had one major depressive episode and milder, minor depressions. She's into a "hippy" look and considers herself artistic, accompanied by labile moods and somewhat unstable relationships. She is failing in school and has low self-esteem. Her stressful events during the follow-up period included frequent serious fights with her mother and fights with her boyfriends. She and her mother have a very conflicted relationship, and the girl has a great deal of difficulty with anger toward her mother, describing her as "sick, weak, and bitchy."

In contrast, the younger child, a 12-year-old boy, has had relatively mild symptoms—of occasional anxiety or depression—but not marked enough to be diagnosable. This pattern also continued over the 3-year follow-up. He is doing quite well in school, is seen as sociable and competent, and has a self-concept score in the 90th percentile. He worries about his mother and feels guilty when she accuses him of contributing to her problems or of making her angry. Although he appears to be fairly resilient, we learned that 2 weeks before a follow-up interview he was so upset by declining grades and by a best friend ignoring him that he tried to cut his wrists with a bottle cap. His mother indicated that it was manipulative, to get attention from her and his friends. Thus, although he never developed major symptoms, he clearly has some difficulty dealing with the chaos in his family, and his behavior may portend problems ahead.

The mother reported that she had been depressed since age 16, and had abused drugs, and had panic attacks periodically. Although her past history was one of "double depression," she was relatively symptom-free during the follow-up period, although her mood shifts and chaotic relationships gave a flavor of borderline personality disorder. She appears to be extremely intrusive and overinvolved with her children, as inferred in her follow-up reports of family life, as well as by our observation during the Conflict Discussion task. She also seems to demand a lot of caretaking of herself from them. However, the fact that she did not have major symptoms of depression during the recent years of the younger child's life may have played some role in his relative resilience.

Mrs. K. was introduced in Chapter 5 as an example of high numbers of stressful events and ongoing difficulties. It is probably not surprising, therefore, that she experienced marked depression over the follow-up observations. Indeed, she reported that she had been depressed since adolescence, but her parents refused to get help for her. She got pregnant and married at age 16 to a man who turned out to be alcoholic, and she was divorcing him at the time the study started.

Despite this enormously troubled environment, the older child, a boy of 12, has had no symptoms, and does very well in school. He appears to be gifted with high intelligence, and has been placed in special classes. His mother says that the way he copes with the family difficulties is to withdraw, denying that the events have any impact on him. It appears that he and his younger sister are being shuttled back and forth between the parents. This may provide some protection from the worst of Mrs. K.'s mood difficulties, but apart from high IQ, denial, and his Dad, it is hard to capture the basis of his resilience. Indeed, his self-esteem appeared to be relatively low at the initial testing.

His younger sister has fared poorly. She is 10 and has already been hospitalized for somatization and anxiety problems. As a small child, she had significant conduct problems, including fighting, stealing, and firesetting, and the mother notes that she has been "easily upset" since early childhood.

Are Resilient Siblings More Competent than Normal Children?

An issue that is frequently overlooked in risk/resilience research is whether children who emerge from high risk situations appearing to be functional actually are possessed of extraordinary talents that shield and protect them in some fashion. Do they have unusual self-confidence or academic or social gifts? One way to examine this question in the present study was to compare the well siblings in the discordant pairs with children who were *not* at risk, who had no diagnoses, and who would be judged to be normal children of normal parents. To reduce confounding factors, Anderson and Hammen (1990-b) matchcd the nondiagnosed siblings in sex, and as closely as possible in age, with a child of normal parents. The mean age of nondiagnosed high risk children was 11.3 (SD = 2.2), and it was 11.9 (SD = 1.9) for the comparison children.

The right-hand columns of Tables 8.4 and 8.5 present the mean scores of the matched comparison children. They did not differ significantly on two of the three competence measures, Social Competence and Academic Performance. However, the normal group children had higher Piers–Harris Self-Concept scores, $t(9) = 3.24$, $p < .01$. Thus if anything, the nondiagnosed but high risk siblings escaped psychopathology without having extraordinary competencies beyond those of normal children, and with significantly less self-confidence.

Also, the two groups did not differ on three of four family relationship variables, although normal group children had consistently more positive scores. A two-tailed t test indicated a marginally significant difference favoring the normal group children on the PPI total score for perceived relations with their mothers, $t(9) = 1.85$, $p < .10$. Again, therefore, the siblings at risk who "survived" did not appear to be protected by unusually strong positive relations with their parents compared to normal group children, and they tended toward somewhat less favorable relationships.

Who Are the Resilient Children from High Risk Families?

Our final approach to understanding resilience and risk was to identify who the relatively resilient children were, from unipolar, bipolar, and medically ill families. Children were operationally defined as "resilient" if they had no symptoms or only mild, nondiagnosable symptoms. This included both lifetime diagnoses obtained in the initial evaluations and all follow-up evaluations. There were 7 of 22 such children of unipolar mothers, 7 resilient children of bipolar mothers out of 18, and 12 of 18 resilient children of medically ill mothers.

Several two-way analyses of variance were conducted to compare the resilient versus nonresilient children within each group, to learn if different charcteristics defined resilience under different maternal circumstances. Analyses of the competence indicators, CBCL Social Competence, Academic Performance ratings, and Piers–Harris Self-Concept scores all indicated significant main effects for resilience but no group differences and, most important, no interaction of maternal group and resilience status. There was a tendency for the children of bipolar mothers to score higher on these indicators, but in general the major significant effect was that in all groups the relatively resilient children scored higher.

The effects of age, sex, and presence of the father in the home were also explored. There were no significant effects of age or gender. While boys and girls were about equally likely to be resilient or not within the different groups, an exception was the unipolar offspring. Only 1 boy was in the resilience group, while girls were equally divided (a suggestive but nonsignificant effect). Presence of the father was nonsignificant, although suggestive ($p = .10$). Of the resilient children overall, nearly half had fathers at home, whereas only a minority of nonresilient children (21%) had fathers at home.

Finally, children's reports of social supports were examined. During the initial follow-up evaluations, children were interviewed about their friendships and their confidants in difficult situations. The majority of children reported that they had a "best friend" confidant, who provided support they were satisfied with, had other adults they considered supports, and could go to their parent(s) when necessary. Comparison of the resilient and nonresilient children in each high risk group shows slight but nonsignificant differences. In the unipolar group, 2 resilient children but 7 nonresilient youngsters reported some gap in their social supports (e.g., 4 of the latter either had no best friend or were dissatisfied with the friend, 4 had no adult supports). In the bipolar group, only 1 resilient child reported some dissatisfaction with a friend's support, but 4 of the nonresilient children made such complaints, and 3 had no adult supports. In the medical group, there were no noteworthy patterns. Overall, therefore, there is a hint that the children who fared less well had fewer close companions or less access to supportive adults than did the resilient children. However, the effects were nonsignificant, and reliance on children's own reports may obscure the completeness of the picture of their social resources.

Examples of Relatively Resilient Children

Children from the S. and K. families of unipolar mothers were previously discussed, and in at least one of those cases a somewhat overinvolved mother had a child who had heretofore escaped major symptoms. Yet another example of a resilient-appearing child occurred in the N. family.

Diana N. is the younger of two children; she is now 12, and her mother feels blessed to have her. The mother's older child was "kidnaped" by his biological father at an early age, and has little contact. Thus Diana has grown up with just her mother, and she is a very pretty, articulate child. The mother feels she "saved her life," by helping her have a reason for living despite numerous suicidal bouts in her earlier life. The mother says that she is determined not to let her illness rub off on the child, and so she makes considerable effort to be a good parent—and indeed, they seem to have a solid, affectionate relationship.

This child is an example of the kind of "specialness" that may facilitate resilience, as discussed by Radke-Yarrow and Sherman (1990). However, as those authors and others note, there remains a concern that the mutual dependency and involvement may eventually exact a toll. While it may help a child in the short run to experience special attention and acknowledgment from the parent, future difficulties with separation, and forming new intimate relationships, may appear. This, of course, is a topic for further study.

Summary and Directions for Further Research

The results of the present investigation of risk and protective factors are fairly consistent in showing that *competence* factors and variables indicating maternal functioning, including quality of interactions with the children, help to distinguish between children who have negative outcomes and those who do not. Even within the same family, these differences were observed; siblings who fared better were more academically and socially successful, had higher self-regard, and had more positive interactions with their mothers than did their less fortunate siblings. However, we did not see evidence of "superkids," those with unusual talents who overcame adverse conditions by virtue of the strength of their winning personalities or extraordinary intellectual or creative gifts. This is not to say that such talents do not exist; they may indeed emerge. Even more likely, however, is the unfortunate prospect that children who may not have evidenced difficulties up to now may nevertheless experience problems later on. The period of young adulthood, for instance, involving separation from their families and establishing intimate relationships with others, may be a time that taxes their capabilities. Beyond the academic and peer challenges faced in childhood, adult requirements for independence, responsibility, intimacy, and the like, may pose additional strains on the capabilities of children at risk. It would be highly desirable especially to follow youth from teenage years into young adulthood to observe such adaptations.

The major interpretive difficulty with the present results is that the direction of causality is obscured. It is unclear whether the relatively resilient children were always more "competent" and treated more favorably, or whether children experience difficulties that cause them to function less well interpersonally and academically. Is competence a protective factor, or is it an outcome? Does maternal behavior toward an ill sibling reflect the child's "difficultness," and does the mother treat more successful children better because they are more agreeable? In the final analysis, without longitudinal studies that follow high risk children from early ages to elucidate the causal directions, such issues cannot be resolved. For now, we conclude that children's ability to do well in school, to get along successfully with others, and to have supportive relationships with parents and friends are protective against future difficulties—and are consequences of unknown personal and family characteristics operating since infancy.

Finally, it is important to acknowledge that our present quest for protective and resilience factors has only touched the surface. We explored variables that had been identified in the previous research literature as likely prospects, but since the present study was aimed primarily at risk and negative outcomes, we are unlikely to have done justice to the more subtle or complex processes that might help children to shine in the face of adversity.

9
Summary and Implications: Understanding Depression in Families at Risk

Nearly 1000 interviews of mothers and their children were conducted in this study: for each youngster, countless questionnaires, reports by teachers and therapists, observations, and school records were obtained over a 1- to 3-year period. It is safe to say, therefore, that all of us who were connected with this study have a perspective on the family context of depression and a new sense of what it means that "depression runs in families."

The goal of this final chapter is to briefly summarize some of the main findings and discuss their implications. One implication is a new model of depression in children at risk; the parameters, hypotheses, and results of a test of the model are presented. This is followed by a discussion of the limitations of present study, noting the methodological as well as conceptual gaps. The things we wish we had done—or done differently, or hope to do in the future—will perhaps encourage others who are already embarked on related studies or are moved to do so by the prospects of the rich yield of information still to be tapped.

Results of the Study

The first question that guided the development and initiation of the study was whether, when improvements were made in the design and methods of offspring research, we would find children to be impaired. We asked whether the apparent risk to offspring of parents with affective disorders would be observed when compared to children in families exposed to similarly disruptive conditions of parental medical, rather than psychiatric, illness. We also asked if the dysfunctions would be observed in direct diagnostic interviews, and across a variety of domains of functioning besides psychiatric disorder, and using multiple and diverse methods of assessment. We further asked whether disorder would be observed when children were assessed when the mother was not in an acute episode, and whether the effects would be stable—or develop—over a longitudinal follow-up.

The answer to all of these questions is, unfortunately, yes. Under improved methodological conditions, there was overwhelming evidence of significant psychiatric disorder as well as impairment of functioning in social, academic, and mother–child relationship spheres in children of unipolar depressed mothers. The children of medically ill mothers had moderate rates of diagnoses and psychosocial dysfunction, but they was lower than those of the unipolar offspring. Moreover, although we were somewhat surprised at the outcome, the children of bipolar mothers revealed significantly less severe disorders and more adaptive psychosocial functioning than the unipolar children. In many cases, except for elevated rates of relatively mild disorders, the bipolar children and the children of normal mothers did not differ markedly. Of course, the bipolar children had not yet passed through the risk period: they may continue to be at risk for affective disorders as they grow older. The most striking difference between the unipolar and bipolar offspring, however, is the level of impairment in adaptive social and academic functioning. The children of manic depressive mothers appeared at least to have mastered certain essential competencies that could help to stabilize their lives in the future. Sadly, only for a few of the unipolar offspring can we make similar observations.

Many of the children of medically ill women had difficulties in terms of diagnosable conditions, school and academic problems, and conflicted relationships with their mothers. The majority of such children fared relatively well, however, even under the adverse conditions affecting the entire family. When there were difficulties for the children, they seemed related to the same kinds of risk factors that determined the outcomes in the unipolar families, including chronic stress in addition to medical stress, maternal depressed mood, and family disruption. Similar conditions occurred in the psychiatrically normal families, with similar negative outcomes for the children. Thus it appeared that the conditions conducive to children's dysfunction were not unique to women with affective disorders: clearly they can affect children in families demoralized by various stressful conditions.

The second major goal of the study was to explore cognitive, stress, and mother–child relationship characteristics. In an attempt to close the gap in the psychological aspects of the causes of children's risk for psychopathology, study of these three areas was guided by the methods and concepts that were available at the start of the study in the early 1980s. Additionally, certain characteristics of the mother and of her disorder were explored to see if they related to children's outcomes. It was assumed, of course, that many of these psychosocial and personal history factors cut across diagnostic groups, occurring with considerable variability both within and between groups.

The yield of the tests of psychosocial hypotheses exceeded even our most optimistic hopes. Although we never attempted, nor would it be possible, to discredit genetic theories of family transmission of affective disorder, clear, consistent, and strong evidence of the importance of psychological and social factors emerged. *Cognitions* presumed to index vulnerability to depression were indeed more common in the youngsters of women with affective disorders, with suggestive evidence that they are acquired not so much by observational learning as by negative interactions, including criticism and noninvolvement by the depressed mother. Not all hypothesized negative cognitions appeared to be vulnerability markers for onset of depression, however. Children's depressive attribution style did not predict future depression (although it was related to nondepressive diagnoses), whereas negative self-concept was a significant predictor of future depression. Further, children's self-schema content helped to refine the relationship between stressors and depression: those children, in particular, for whom interpersonal functioning was cognitively salient—and who experienced negative interpersonal events—became more depressed.

Stress—both as chronic, ongoing difficulties in various areas of living and as episodic negative events—is significantly elevated in high risk families. The unipolar women, and also their children, were especially likely to be exposed to higher levels of stressful events and conditions than any other group. In turn, just as previous studies have found for adults, children's depression was associated with stressors. Not only did this study develop contextual threat assessment of children's stressors, but we were also able to show that maternal disorder itself is a stressor for children contributing to symptoms. Moreover, children who experienced high levels of stressors were significantly more likely to become depressed if their mother was also symptomatic during that period than were high stress youngsters with nonsymptomatic mothers. Our interpretation was that maternal symptoms make the mother unavailable to help children cope with the ill effects of their own difficult events. In the absence of such buffering, children become symptomatic.

Not only do stressful events precede depression, but we also found evidence of the other direction of causality: depressed or depression-prone people *cause* events. Both unipolar depressed women and children of depressed women appeared to generate events (or were at least partly responsible for their occurrence). This was particularly pronounced for interpersonal events. The role of stress-generation is discussed further in discussions of the model of high risk outcomes to be presented.

There was ample evidence of interpersonal impairment, and it was nowhere more marked than in the relationships between the unipolar mothers and their children. Even a brief observation of a Conflict Discussion task revealed that unipolar women were particularly likely to be irritable and critical of their youngsters and less positive, and they were also likely to have difficulty staying focused on constructive problem solving in the task with the child. These patterns were mirrored in the children's own interactional behaviors. We interpreted the patterns to reflect the difficulty that depressed people have in being involved as well as their tendencies toward irritability and (ineffective) avoidance of conflict. Not surprisingly, such patterns by the mother were predictive of children's relatively impaired functioning and diagnoses during the follow-up period. The patterns suggested an association between poor quality of relationship and maladaptive behaviors in the child and indicated that the patterns that were observed in the brief interaction task were typical and enduring ongoing interactional problems. Indeed, inspection of the mothers' and children' reports of stressful events over time revealed serious conflicts between them.

It is important not to conclude, however, that bad parenting somehow is a trait of depressed women. Throughout, we emphasized that communication quality is strongly related to the amount of chronic stress and current depressed mood a woman experiences. Thus her difficulties in sustaining supportive, positive, and engaged interactions with her child are understandable as consequences of environmental conditions and mood state. Therefore, women with affective disorders in remission may function quite adequately, whereas chronically stressed and demoralized nonpsychiatric women might have considerable difficulties in relating to their children.

Moreover, quality of the relationship between the mother and child is not unilateral. It would be most misleading to view children as hapless victims of impaired mothers, when in reality the children were sometimes extremely difficult themselves, clearly overtaxing the abilities of well-meaning mothers to deal with them. This mutuality, or reciprocity, was demonstrated in several ways. The timing of depressive episodes in mothers and children revealed statistically associated patterns. Over the course of the follow-ups, there were clear indications that aspects of the mother–child relationships, including the other's symptomatology, could trigger an episode. Mother-then-child and child-then-mother episodes occurred with about equal frequency, suggesting the impact of each on the other. It was also observed in statistical causal modeling analyses that mutual relationships between the mother and child in their style of interacting contributed to the overall predictability of subsequent child outcomes. We saw that depressed women were not universally negative toward their children; they tended to behave significantly differently toward sibling pairs where one was symptomatic and the other was not. Overall, the depressed women had more negative relationships with children who were truly dysfunctional than with those children who were not. The nondepressed women, on the other hand, seemed to fail to acknowledge disorder in their children who were truly dysfunctional. Consistent with this, they appeared to differ little in the quality of interaction with disturbed and nondisturbed children. We speculate that depressed women are less tolerant of their truly difficult children than nondepressed women are, but that they accurately discriminate children's problems and tend to have more negative interactions when their children actually have difficulties.

Women's own personal histories were highly varied. Different histories resulted in significantly different children's outcomes. Not surprisingly, severity of past history (multiple episodes) predicted worse functioning in children. Also, women with affective disorders, as expected, had elevated rates of psychopathology in their families of origin. Intriguingly, women who had more pathology in their parents and siblings also showed higher rates of dysfunctional communication with their children. This small "missing link" is hardly surprising, but it indicates an important focus for understanding the intergenerational transmission of depression: In dysfunctional families women may acquire maladaptive interactional skills that make it difficult for them to sustain positive and effective communications with their children. It was also not surprising to find significant assortative mating in the biological parents of the high risk children. Unipolar women in particular were likely to have married men with apparently diagnosable conditions (especially conduct and substance abuse problems), who came from their own families that were "loaded" with psychopathology. The high rates of divorce and marital turmoil in the unipolar families was therefore understandable. Yet both father absence and father psychopathology were contributors to children's risk for negative outcomes. However, the findings were more consistent with a psychosocial than a genetic explanation, in that children who had a psychiatrically diagnosable father who lived at home and those with non-ill fathers who were absent were similarly subject to negative outcomes.

Throughout the analyses, we noted the presence of "nonorthogonal risk factors," a term used by Walker et al. (1989) to characterize the rather tragic aggregation of negative factors in high risk families. Such correlated ingredients terrorize researchers whose mission is to separate and analyze the relative impact of multiple co-occurring variables. Nowhere is this problem of confounding more pernicious than in the diagnostic status itself. A major logical error is committed repeatedly when offspring outcomes (or other characteristics) are attributed to the parental diagnostic status itself, instead of to separate ingredients which are confounded with it. A psychiatric diagnosis—especially of a recurring disorder—entails a history of disturbance over time determining degree of impairment, a degree of ongoing stressful conditions that are either consequences or causes of the symptomatic state and its recurrences, and the degree of current symptomatology that affects immediate circumstances independent of past history of disorder. Thus, for women with affective disorders, severity of their prior history of disorder, chronic stress affecting social, financial, and occupational realms, and current dysphoria are separable ingredients, each of which may have somewhat different correlates and consequences.

Implications of the Results

Implications for Understanding the Experience of Clinical Depression

"Depression affects lives." This statement is either a silly truism or a profoundly significant departure for development of research strategies and treatment programs. Although this statement is doubtless true of all disorders, it may be uniquely true of depression, in that the impact of the symptoms and behaviors of the depressed person is to generate conditions that increase the probability of impairment, recurrence, and aversive relationships. The findings of the present study contribute strongly to the growing awareness that depression occurs in a social and environmental context, that it is extremely debilitating with a grave toll on functioning in various roles and in self-regard. Depression that is severe and recurrent provokes stressful events and contributes to the cause of—or at least the inability to resolve—chronic stressful conditions. In these ways, it can be self-perpetuating. Thus it is not surprising that for most people who experience major depressive episodes, it is a recurrent disorder. Although other kinds of calamities—other psychiatric disorders, for instance, including bipolar illness or chronic life difficulties such as medical illness—certainly strain and impair the affected person and those around him or her, it may be that depression is especially detrimental. A person who is depressed is also lacking in energy and positive motivation to cope with difficulties, and the hopelessness, passivity, and withdrawal serve to perpetuate symptoms as well as potentially alienate and distress those around one.

Depression is also a family disorder. It runs in families, at least in large part because all members are potentially affected by the depressive symptoms and behaviors of the depressed member. Coyne et al. (1990) have written about the aversive consequences of depression on others who in turn reject the depressed one, and in the family context such patterns may perpetuate the symptoms. Moreover, the family members themselves may experience symptoms and distress (e.g., Coyne, Kessler, et al., 1987). When the child as well as the mother or another member of the family is depressed, the potential for conflict, resentment, disappointment, and feelings of abandonment is multiplied.

Thus clinical interventions need to deal with these realities: impairment, recurrence, and family context. Impairment means that the depressed individual cannot sustain supportive relationships in a mutually satisfactory way, cannot find the energy or cognitive capabilities to perform work tasks and solve problems effectively, cannot perform typical roles at the optimal level of functioning. It is hardly surprising, therefore, that persons with clinical depression seem to have as many difficulties in functioning, if not more, than persons with debilitating major chronic medical illnesses (e.g.,

Wells et al., 1989). Clinical depression is likely to be recurrent at least in part because the person provokes the environment to respond in aversive ways that cause additional depression. Impaired functioning due to the depression, as well as the scars and aftermath of major depression, are likely to affect a person's behaviors and the ways people view themselves, others, and the world. Recurrence of depression needs to be anticipated clinically: therefore, methods that give people the tools to alter their expectations and behaviors and thereby to prevent depression are urgently needed to supplement the focus on immediate symptom reduction.

Finally, the entire family is disturbed when one member has clinical recurrent depression. If there is a depressed parent, there are probably depressed children and impaired relationships throughout the family system. To the extent that the depressed patient has a family history of psychopathology and depression, the interpersonal impairments may be magnified. Thus clinical interventions aimed solely at intraindividual change—treating the illness within—do not go far enough in considering the consequences for other family members or the conditions that create relapse.

Implications for Theories of Depression

Limits of Previous Research

The point has often been made in recent years that simple, unidirectional theories of depression cannot accurately capture the complexity of the phenomenology of depression, and that the context must also be studied (e.g., Billings & Moos, 1985b; Brown & Harris, 1978; Coyne et al., 1990; Hammen, 1985; 1988). Whether the focus is on a neurochemical process, a genetic defect, a score on a questionnaire of cognitions, a checklist of negative events, a bad mother—all such simple models are doomed to failure if the complex psychological context of depression is ignored. Failure is marked by an inability to account for much of the variance in depression, by inability to find processes universally accounting for etiology, maintenance, recurrence, and recovery, and by limited application across the broad band of variants of depressive subtypes or demographically different groups. This does not mean, however, that it is time to renounce a cognitive focus, since cognition is central to understanding the ways in which the past is represented, the environment is experienced and given meaning, and actions and strategies are undertaken. A simplistic focus on interpersonal processes would be severely limited, moreover, without some consideration of people's schemas about relationships and some mechanism to account for how depression, rather than some other debility, might be the consequence or cause of distinct patterns of relating. In short, integrative models would seem to be a requirement of future advances in psychology (Hammen, 1990; in press-b, c,).

For similar reasons, another implication of the present work is that studies of depression in analogue populations, with mild symptoms or no history of depression, do not represent clinical depression. Demoralization and misery are usually transitory, normal experiences, and they do not necessarily have histories or futures, or impair the functioning, self-views, and relationships of the afflicted person. As noted earlier, the striking features of clinical affective disorders are impairment, recurrence, and family aggregation, and such conditions are only randomly present in high-BDI-scoring undergraduates. That is not to say that adolescent and young adult depressions are not of interest in their own right. They are, to be sure, and there are intriguing questions to be posed of this group over longitudinal studies. But the great majority of temporarily or mildly dysphoric students can do little to inform us of the processess of real depression

Thus far the perspective presented emphasizes phenomenon-driven research, suggesting the need to be faithful to the experience of depression as it is lived in people's environments. However, the extreme of this point of view—purely descriptive research—is also limited in its contribution, just as purely theory-driven research may be. It seems essential to the vitality of the field of clinical psychology to develop and test theories and to use clinical populations to weed out the weak and infirm among theoretical contenders. Further advances require the judicious development and testing of theories to elaborate the processes and mechanisms that account for the depressive syndrome and its sequelae and must be informed by knowledge of the clinical realities of affective disorders. Some of the more obvious gaps in the field and in this study will be noted later.

Genotype–Environment Correlation

Most of the original research on offspring of parents with affective disorders (or other psychopathology) was at least implicitly guided by genetic hypotheses. The present work, however, strongly implicates psychosocial factors contributing to children's outcomes. Lest we seem to be arguing, therefore, that the psychological determinants of offspring risk are *stronger* than the biological risk, it is time to recall Plomin's (1986) discussion of the genotype–environment correlation. Although the present methods were not suitable to test the nature of such correlations in the sample studied, these concepts are vitally important as ways of thinking about the relationship between potential genetic and environmental contributions. This is an area of enormous potential contribution, possibly helping to reintegrate the somewhat polarized nature versus nurture positions in high risk research.

Plomin (1986) reminds us of his earlier distinctions among passive, reactive, and active genotype–environment correlations in the example of the child of musically gifted parents. For argument's sake we will assume the ability is genetically transmitted. The musically gifted child will be exposed to a musical environment by the parents. Even if the parents did nothing about the child's abilities, the child might be identified as gifted at school and given special opportunities and experiences with music. Even if the parents and school did nothing at all, the child might seek out musical environments, looking for musical peers and listening to the radio and records. In the first instance, the parents have a double influence on the child, both by passing along the genes and by providing an environment that encourages musical talent. This is "passive" correlation in the sense that the child passively inherits environments correlated with his or her genetic predisposition. As Plomin notes, this is a relatively commonly studied phenomenon in behavioral genetics but not often considered by developmentalists. I would add that it is rarely even acknowledged in high risk offspring studies. For instance, in the present case, the child of a unipolar or bipolar parent not only acquires any genetic components of the disorder that may occur (itself an unresolved matter) but also in effect acquires the family environments. This means, for most cases of recurrent or chronic affective disorder, disruption, exposure to stressful conditions, and exposure to parental behaviors that interfere with adaptive parenting. This is distinct from whatever the child might learn about expression of emotion and emotional regulation, coping and problem solving, self-representation based on negative parental models, and the like.

Even less frequently studied, but as noted by Plomin likely even more important, are the *reactive*, or evocative, genotype–environment correlations. Thus the musically inclined child might elicit reactions from parents, teachers, and peers that encourage these talents. In other words, children evoke environments correlated with their genetic endowment. Thus in the case of offspring of parents with affective disorders, the child's tendencies toward whatever might be the building blocks of depression—say affective dysregulation or dysphoria—might elicit parental and peer reactions that are relatively negative. The sensitive, or even irritable, child might elicit rejection from others, or might be ignored and overlooked, and the responses of others might contribute further to feelings of low self-regard, sensitivity, withdrawal, and the like. As the child grows older, emotional and behavioral dysfunctions are likely to interfere increasingly with interpersonal and scholastic success, and frustration and failure in these domains contribute to the display of symptoms that further elicit negative responses from the environment.

Finally, the *active* genotype–environment correlations subsume conditions in which the child actively seeks environments that are correlated with her or his genetic endowments. The musically inclined child seeks musical experiences; in the same way, children inclined toward depression might seek experiences consistent with their predispositions. Current research cannot be sure of what this means, but it may imply that children's depression tendencies lead to at least selective interpretations of environments to be consistent with their views. As Plomin says, the worriers will find things to worry about no matter how smoothly things seem to be going. In parallel to our own sample, depressed children may interpret their environments in a distorted fashion that emphasizes failure, rejection, and worthlessness. And if their skill acquisition had already been limited and dysfunctional in the ways noted, they might indeed find it difficult to succeed and easy to fail. Certainly, the self-concept and skill deficits of depressive children are likely to impair their academic and social success and to *cause* stressors to occur as described earlier.

These variants of gene–environment associations make it clear that the quest for simple relationships between a few variables is misguided. Our attempts to proceed with integrative models must therefore be seen as approximations, or as working models, rather than attempts at completely capturing the pathways between parental disorder and child outcome. Nevertheless, it seems clear that a strong case can be made for gene–environment correlations and that children appear to "inherit" some biological qualities that may later eventuate in depression as well as environments that shape and pull their experiences (and biological processes) in ways that lead to depression.

Implications for an Intergenerational Transmission Perspective on Depression

The diverse results of the present study, and the psychosocial interactional perspective that they imply, suggest the need for a complex model capturing the transactive, historical, environmental, and interpersonal qualities that have thus far been separately linked to children's outcomes. In Chapter 7 a statistical structural equation model was presented (Hammen, Burge, & Stansbury, 1990), with maternal characteristics and child characteristics mutually influencing each other and both causally linked with subsequent outcomes in the children. Structural equation modeling is one useful technique for attempting to sort out the relationships between overlapping, nonorthogonal factors in samples where random assignment of characteristics is impossible, as in natural clinical samples. We now attempt to expand this model, to include three features leading to the prediction of offspring outcomes: three generations of influence, the construct of "stress generation," and a unique specificity test for depression (Hammen, Burge, Brown, & Stansbury 1990.)

The three generations of influence we include are mother's family of origin, mother, and children. And it is implied that the children at risk who have depressive outcomes may themselves become depressed parents with depressed children, in a self-perpetuating cycle.

While family–genetic studies have clearly demonstrated the intergenerational transmission of affective disorders, implying a genetic diathesis, we emphasize a nongenetic, environmental transmission mechanism. Women who were raised in dysfunctional families where their own parents (and siblings) had psychiatric disorders are likely to have impaired parenting skills. Such deficits can arise from various sources: disturbances in their own parents' caretaking, impairing adaptive learning and attachment; adverse conditions either caused by or consequences of parental psychopathology that disrupted learning of skills; and possibly their own early symptomatology arising under conditions that might have impaired their acquisition of appropriate interpersonal skills relating to social problem solving, conflict resolution, and attachment-intimacy.

Previous support for this hypothesis can be found in studies of retrospective reports of depressed adults' child-rearing and observations of depressed mothers interacting with their children (see Chapter 6). Additionally, several British studies have shown that depressed mothers with children reported difficulties with their own mothers (e.g., Mills et al., 1985; Murray, 1988). And daughters of psychiatrically disturbed women who themselves had disorders (mostly depression) reported significantly higher rates of both maternal and paternal neglect and abuse (Andrews, Brown, & Creasey, 1990). Earlier, Brown and colleagues reported that depressed community women with children tended to have had more adverse childhood parenting experiences (e.g., Harris, Brown, & Bifulco, 1986), and Birtchnell, Evans, and Kennard (1988) found that women with neurotic symptomatology had had negative experiences with their own mothers and tended to have poor marital relationships and more emotional and behavioral problems in their children. Taken together, these pieces of information suggest that women's adverse childhood experiences with their own parents (possibly associated with parental pathology) predict maternal distress/depression and child caretaking difficulties and psychopathology with their own children.

Figure 9.1 and Table 9.1 present the elements of the model. In our model, we posit a latent factor of "maternal background" causally linked to "maternal parenting." The *maternal background* variable is jointly comprised of presence of diagnosable psychopathology in the woman's parents and siblings along with her own history of episodes of depression and treatment. It is predicted to be causally linked to self-reported and observed *parenting* behaviors with her child.

A second major feature of the model is inclusion of the construct of "stress generation." Depressed persons can be viewed as individuals whose symptoms, characteristics, and behaviors contribute to the environments in which they live; they are not simply victims of their environments. The relative contributions of symptoms, skill deficits, consequences of chronic impairment, and the like, to the generation of stressors (or to the failure to adequately resolve typical stressful circumstances) remain to be seen. Nevertheless, we speculate that depressed individuals—both adults and children—contribute to stress occurrence; in turn, stressful conditions and events contribute to further depression.

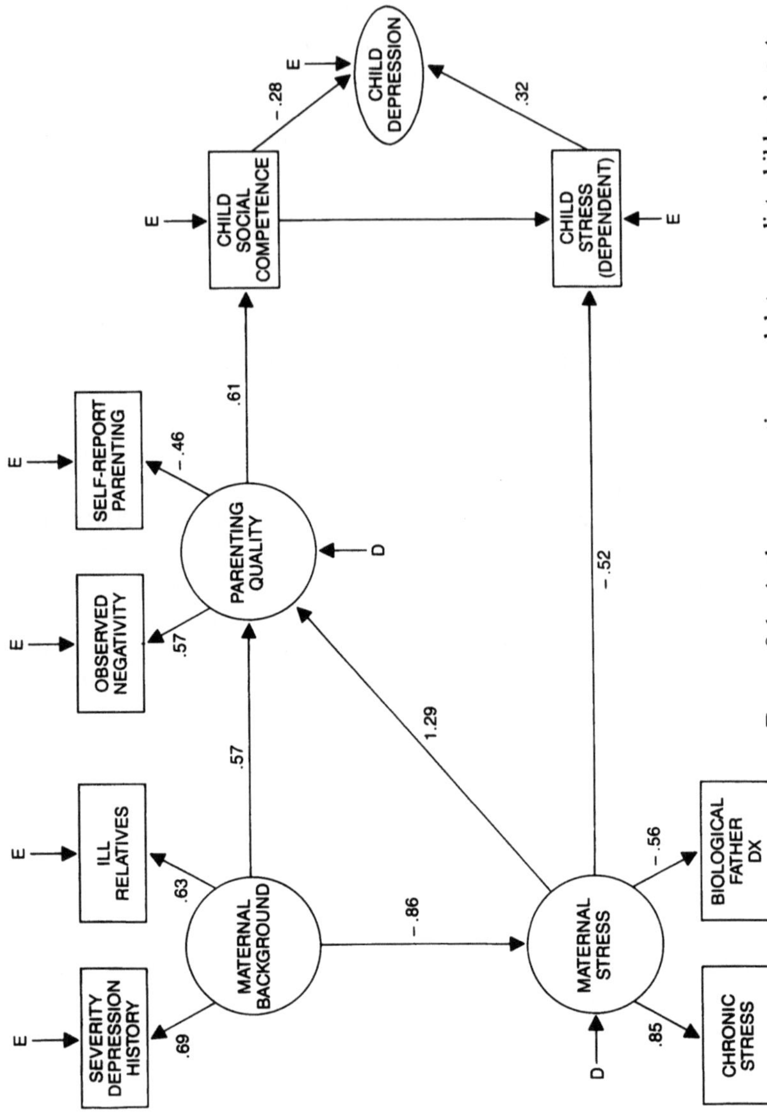

FIGURE 9.1. A three-generation model to predict children's outcomes in a high risk sample. From Hammen, Burge, Brown, and Stansbury (1990). Under review.

TABLE 9.1. Variables included in the structural equation model.

Maternal background	
	Severity of depression rating scale (7-point scale of previous episodes/hospitalizations)
	Number of ill maternal relatives (parents, siblings)
Maternal stress	
	Chronic stress total from five areas (omits relationships with children)[a]
	Severity of diagnosis of child's biological father
Parenting quality	
	Conflict Discussion task proportion of negative minus positive comments
	Social Adjustment Scale self-reported parenting subscale
Child social competence	
	Child Behavior Check List Social Competence score[a]
Child stress	
	Six-month follow-up total objective impact score for "dependent" events
Child outcome diagnostic scores	
	1. Depression: mean diagnostic rating across follow-ups for affective disorders
	2. Nondepression: mean diagnostic rating across follow-ups for disorders besides depression
	3. Any diagnosis: mean diagnostic rating across follow-ups for any disorders

[a] Higher scores indicate better or more adaptive functioning; for all other variables, higher values indicate more negative or impaired behavior.

As noted in Chapter 5, we found that maternal episodic stress was higher in unipolar depressed women than normal women and that the former were significantly more likely than all other groups to have negative interpersonal events to which they contributed. Others have certainly speculated about depression causing stressors (e.g., Barnett & Gotlib, 1988; Coyne et al., 1990; Depue & Monroe, 1986). We go further than the demonstration of increased exposure to "dependent" episodic events: We predict that a woman's chronic stress level will be influenced by her "background," both parental psychopathology and prior psychiatric history. Moreover, an additional aspect of stress generation is *assortative mating*. Women don't have dysfunctional husbands thrust upon them; they select them. Thus stress generation also includes the likelihood that women from backgrounds of parental psychopathology and personal psychiatric history marry men with diagnosable disorders (or have early pregnancies with men whom they do not stay with). In any case, the outcome is likely to be high rates of marital distress and early divorce.

There is clear research evidence to support the idea of assortative mating and high rates of marital conflict in women with affective disorders (see Chapter 5–7; Barnett & Gotlib, 1988). Recently, also, British studies have suggested a link between adverse childhood parenting experiences and adult depression, as mediated through their effects on premarital pregnancy and unsupportive marital relations (e.g., Andrews & Brown, 1988; Bifulco et al., 1987; Harris, Brown, & Bifulco, 1987). One intriguing study has in fact found that first-degree relative of depressed adults not only had the expected elevated rates of depression themselves, but they also had significantly higher rates of stressful life events than did community members (McGuffin, Katz, & Bebbington, 1988). The investigators suggested that both liability to depression and propensity to experience life events are familial.

In our model, we posit a direct link betweeen the latent variable "maternal background" and the latent variable "maternal stress." Maternal stress is comprised of chronic, ongoing conditions (excluding relationships with children), and assortative mating is defined as severity of psychopathology in the biological father of the child. The model further predicts a causal path between maternal stress and "parenting quality." In other words, parenting behaviors by the mother (indexed by self-reported parenting on the Social Adjustment Scale and by direct observations in the Conflict Discussion task) are a direct consequence of her family pathology and previous psychiatric history and indirectly mediated by background factors causing chronic stressful conditions and assortative mating.

Stress generation in the children is also predicted. One outcome of quality of parenting is social competence in the child (as noted in Chapter 8), and we hypothesize that this set of characteristics contributes to the likelihood that adverse events will occur. Thus the Achenbach Social Competence score of the child is predicted to be an outcome of parenting quality and a predictor of the amount of stress the child experiences that was rated to be at least partly dependent on the child's behaviors or characteristics. We also expect that children's dependent life stress is predicted by maternal chronic stress and paternal psychopathology, so that the model reflects two paths to children's dependent stress totals.

A third unique aspect of the model is the test of the specificity of depression as the outcome of the predicted interrelated variables. It is unclear whether the patterns are unique to depression, or whether they represent *any* psychopathology, or even whether they best capture nondepressive disorders. Certainly many of the features of this model are not dissimilar from those related to other forms of child psychopathology, such as conduct disorder (e.g., see Patterson, De Barsyshe, & Ramsey, 1989), or possibly alcohol/substance abuse. This is an area largely unexplored, but the first step is at least to test whether the present model holds for depression, and whether it also predicts children's other diagnostic outcomes.

Children's outcomes are measured longitudinally, taking advantage of the prospective design of the study to examine the contributions of preexisting conditions to subsequent outcomes. Although the problem of "nonorthogonal risk factors" remains a thorny one in which causal interrelationships cannot be clearly specified in a naturalistic study, the temporal precedence of conditions antedating children's outcomes increases our confidence in making causal inferences.

Additional elements of the model as implied in Figure 9.1 are deficits in social and interactional behaviors, in both mothers and children, that impair their relationships with others. For mothers this refers to parenting (and implicitly, marital interactions), and for children it is incorporated as a factor (such as social competence) that influences the occurrence of stress.

The model was tested statistically using the structural equation procedures of Bentler (1985), called EQS. To evaluate depressive outcomes in the child, the model was fit to the data, yielding a nonsignificant chi-square indicating statistical similarity between the hypothesized and actual data (χ^2 [23] = 30.5, p = .14). Fit indices indicate the extent to which the model is an improvement over the prediction of independent associations between variables, and they range from 0 to 1.0. The Bentler–Bonett Normed Fit Index (NFI; Bentler & Bonett, 1980) is .83. Recently, however, Bentler (1990) noted that the NFI is affected by sample size and may be reduced in small samples even when the model is correct. Therefore, a newly developed Comparative Fit Index (Bentler, 1990) was computed and yielded a value of .95, which indicates excellent fit of the model. Figure 8.1 presents the standardized weights, and with a single exception all are significant at least at $p < .025$, one-tailed. The direct link between maternal background and parenting quality was only marginally significant.

Additionally, the predicted model was tested for nondepressed diagnoses and for presence of any diagnoses. The model also fit children's nondepressed diagnoses, χ^2 (23) = 25.9, p = .31, with the Normed Fit Index at .85 and a Comparative Fit Index of .98. Not surprisingly, therefore, the model also fits for prediction of any diagnoses, χ^2 (23) = 30.9, p = .12, NFI = .84, CFI = .95. Thus it appears that the model is not specific to depression but also predicts any diagnostic outcomes in the present sample.

Limitations of the Model

The model is an attempt to predict depressive outcomes in children of depressed mothers, and as such, is not directly generalizable to all instances of depression. It might be expected, however, that this pathway to depression is an especially pernicious one, and that many chronically or recurrently depressed adults come from dysfunctional families (with high rates of affective disorder), following the patterns described.

The model is, of course, limited by its reliance on the data that were available to test it. Thus important qualifiers and mediators may have been omitted, and future finer-grained studies are needed to fill in such gaps. Several of these areas are discussed later in more detail, concerning questions about specific aspects of the transactions between mothers and children, aspects of maternal depression that have specific consequences, children's social skills and problem-solving behaviors that arise in such contexts, and the like. The model tested and supported here is certainly not the only possible pattern of linkages between variables and outcomes. It was selected to include variables available and theoretically determined pathways; however, other models may also be valid.

A key gap in the present model was the lack of reciprocal influences, such as those between mother and child. As indicated in previous chapters, such mutual influences are clearly operative, and we found support for them in other analyses. However, the present statistical procedure had to be constrained in certain ways owing to limited sample size, which restricts the numbers of variables and paths that can reliably be tested.

One might also wonder where dysfunctional cognitions fit in. These are not directly included in the model, but they play an important role, in that they are believed to index representations of the self, the world, and social relationships and exert important influences on the ways in which events are construed and behavioral actions selected and performed. Thus, for instance, cognitions about self-worth and competence probably figure into the prediction of mate selection, how women interpret their children's behaviors, how children interpret and select their peer relationships and other behaviors, and they may determine the specific kinds of stressful events that are likely to produce depression. In future work, more fine-grained assessments of such cognitive representations of the self and the world and others might shed significant light on sources of vulnerability to dysfunction.

Other limitations of the model must be acknowledged: Although this is an environmental transmission model of family antecedents of risk for depression, we cannot rule out biological contributions. Indeed, developments in genetics and greater precision in neurochemical theories will be most welcome in helping to further elaborate the interactions among complex factors. Additional pathways might be relevant but were not included, such as a direct pathway from paternal pathology to child characteristics, or from grandparent pathology to child outcomes. Much larger samples would be needed to test more elaborate models. The present study is a balance between empirical and theoretical considerations on the one hand and practical limitations of sample size and variables on the other. Thus it is intended to represent an example of the kinds of models that ought to be constructed to represent complex, historical, interpersonal, and environmental ingredients in depression—but it is not likely to be the "final" such model. In short, it is a working model whose success might be evaluated in terms of its ability to provoke further tests, elaborations, and improvements.

Limitations of the Study and Suggestions for Future Research

Generalizability

Results of the present investigation can be generalized to families with mothers who have affective disorders that are recurrent in nature. The unipolar sample, by selection, included women with multiple episodes and early onset (before the child's birth). Since unipolar depression (major depressive episodes or dysthymia) is a very broad term including relatively mild, one-time conditions as well as recurring episodes, the results may not generalize to other outpatient samples. Nevertheless, we think that the women in the study are typical of true affective disorders. Although relatively more impaired than many women outpatients treated for depression, there is the possibility that the most severely ill women were excluded. For instance, those who had lost custody of their youngsters because of their illness were not included. In any case, future studies of offspring adjustment should include a wide array of level of disorder.

It is also the case that the results may generalize only to families of ill mothers, since we did not include families of ill fathers, and of course only women with children.

All offspring high risk studies are limited in generalizability, in the sense that psychopathology in the children may be unrepresentative of children's disorders in general. That is, children who are depressed in this sample may not represent childhood depression that arises in other circumstances—or, for that matter, adult depressions that arise later in life. On the other hand, more and more studies of depression in children find that a parent is also depressed (e.g., Kovacs et al., 1989), so that the children in this study who evidenced major depression may not be dissimilar from other children so affected. Nonetheless, extensions of conclusions to non–high risk populations must be limited.

A common limitation of high risk studies is that children's outcomes may be due not to parental psychopathology as such but to some third variable. In the present study, of course, a variety of such factors were indeed explored and found to have significant associations with children's outcomes.

Methodological Shortcomings

The samples of the individual disorders represented by the mothers were relatively small. Aggregating across the entire group and comparing different kinds of high risk groups improved the precision and sensitivity of the tests of hypotheses. Nevertheless, much larger samples would have been desirable to improve confidence in the reliability of findings. The original design called for larger samples, but it proved to be enormously difficult to find appropriate subjects. Subjects had to be women, with children in the right age ranges, with recurrent disorder, who were willing to participate for up to 3 years. We discovered that only a minority of affective disorders patients were women with children living at home, in the right age ranges. Large numbers of women patients did not have families, or were too old or too young to have children in the age range of the study, or did not have recurrent episodes, or did not have early onsets. Nearly all available women who were asked to participate agreed to do so, however.

Both divorce and the 8 to 16 age range contributed unwanted variability to the sample. It would have been virtually impossible within a reasonable period to include only married women, or to include children of a narrower age range. As Downey and Coyne (1990) and others (e.g., Keller et al. 1986; Rutter & Quinton, 1984) have noted, divorce or family conflict plays a large role in what happens to offspring of depressed parents. Unable to control in our sampling for this variability, we attempted to analyze for it in several ways, including chronic stressful conditions, father absence or presence, and father psychopathology. Nevertheless, several specific models suggested by Coyne and Downey (1990) ought to be tested in appropriately large samples varying in marital status.

Further research with psychopathology comparison groups would be desirable; as noted later, issues concerning specificity of childeren's outcomes are of great interest. It woud be useful to determine how children of depressed mothers differ from those with anxiety disorders, substance abuse disorders, and the like. Unfortunately, our original goal to include such a comparison fell by the wayside when it became apparent that most such women also had significant histories of, or current experiences with, depression. It will be of enormous theoretical interest to determine how specific disorders eventuate in particular behaviors that affect children's risk for negative outcomes.

Also, significant developmental differences in the processes accounting for children's adjustment need to be explored. In general, we did not find age differences in outcomes by group, and since the samples were evenly distributed by children's ages, the results were not apparently skewed by age differences. Nevertheless, future studies will be able to draw much more precise conclusions about age-related outcomes and mechanisms by restricting the samples to more homogeneous ages.

Another apparent limitation was the reliance on telephone interviewing for the follow-up contacts. This was a necessary, practical solution to the problem of retaining the sample, and in general we were satisfied that interviews of both mothers and children yielded accurate and complete information, supplemented by therapist and school reports. However, it is possible that such interviewing constrained the reports of significant information. Maybe the life circumstances and clinical outcomes were even worse than we knew, but we don't think bias occurred in the opposite direction.

When we review procedures that we wish we had included or done differently, it is easy to see that our direct observation task of mother–child interaction was a very limited sample. The reality is that it would have been difficult to have the pairs discuss a conflict for *more* than 5 minutes. For many pairs the task was so aversive that they had trouble doing it even for a brief while, so that it is unclear that extending it would have been better. Nevertheless, sampling of other interactions, or even home observations, would have been desirable.

In an ideal study, we would have liked to have interviewed all the first-degree family members, all the children in the family, and the biological fathers. We had to rely on maternal reports for information about such individuals; although we attempted to use very behaviorally specific information in judging relatives' psychopathology, it is possible that direct interviews would have yielded different information.

Closing Conceptual Gaps

The present study accumulated an enormous amount of information and painted a coherent and consistent picture of potential risk factors, their interrelations, and children's outcomes. Yet every door that was opened seemed to reveal a nearly endless corridor lined with doors to the many rooms still to be explored. Not only is there a vast array of topics to be pursued, many at microanalytic levels of complex processes, but also we have a sense of an enormous gap left to be filled. Simply put, we know a lot about children's symptoms and about the qualities of their lives and the events that happened to them—but we know relatively little about what the children were *doing*.

Further Studies of Children's Competence and Social Functioning

A strong candidate for further investigation is children's competence behaviors. Emotion regulation, social cognition, social skills, problem solving, and coping with adverse events are all areas of competent behavior that are essential to adaptation and healthy functioning. (Some of these topics were reviewed in Chapter 8.) Diagnostic evaluations of children tell us that something has gone wrong with these skills but do not provide information on what the skills are, how they are related to family functioning, and how they might be disrupted by symptomatology. Depressed children, for instance, show significant impairment in social and educational functioning but, as Kovacs (1989) reminds us, we need to know more about the social skill deficits that seem to persist after symptom remission, and to understand how social, cognitive, and performance difficulties affect the course of the disorder. Also, depressive disorders appear to interfere with acquisition of intellectual, social, and behavioral skills, but this process has rarely been studied. The NIMH Laboratory of Developmental Psychology has undertaken important analyses of social competence in young offspring of women with affective disorders, finding evidence of impairment (e.g., Denham & Zahn-Waxler, 1989), and such work needs to be pursued and expanded by other investigators (see also Goodman & Brumley, 1990). This work would likely encompass cognitive factors as well, including schemas representing the self that guide actions, how they are shaped and how they further shape affect and behavior. Studies of the effects of, and consequences to, children's competence will also extend research on resilience in children and the individual differences (including nonshared environmental factors) that differentiate between children's outcomes when exposed to parental depression (e.g., Dodge, 1990; Forehand et al., 1987; Rutter, 1990).

Further Studies of Attachment and Competence Development

Not only do we need to know considerably more about what depressed children do that may affect both their subsequent development and future depression, but the processes linking family conditions and aspects of competent performance also need to be studied. As Hartup (1989) noted, children's effectiveness in dealing with the social world emerges from their experiences in close relationships, with both their caretakers and their peers. Thus disruptions in secure attachment to the mother seem to interfere with emotion regulation, self-regard, peer relationships, effective problem solving and cognitive development, school performance, and even IQ. Developmental psychologists and developmental psychopathologists are attacking some of these research problems—starting with infant–mother interactions. This is exciting work, and exactly the kind that is needed to fill in the many gaps in our understanding of how maternal depression may exact its severe toll on children. Such work will also help to clarify those aspects of parental depressions (or even whether the effects are due to depression or to some correlated factors) that have specific effects on children's outcomes. For example, sadness, withdrawal, helplessness, irritability, low energy and lack of involvement, or enmeshment, may be distinct processes with different outcomes (e.g., Downey & Coyne, 1990; Rutter, 1990).

Further Studies of Family Process in Depressed Families

Coyne's ideas about the mutually aversive, downward slide of interactions with depressed persons (e.g., Coyne et al., 1990) remind us of the numerous unresolved questions about such interactions and raise questions about how these ideas can be extended to mother–child pairs where one or both are depressed. Perhaps depressive communication styles have a pattern, a coercive process, of their own, involving avoidance, aborted problem solving, and conflict. Such processes may overwhelm even good coping skills—or cause depression in those who are ill-equipped to escape their aversive impact. Very little research has been done on how depressed mothers and their children experience interactions with a depressed (or irritable) family member. This level of analysis would further the exploration of the family process of depression, just as Patterson's work contributed to understanding the coercive family process of aggressive children (e.g., Patterson, 1982). Not only is the mutual effect of depressed persons on each other worthy of further study, but there is considerable room for specific investigation of the behaviors and skills of depressed and stressed parents and the reciprocal impact of children on parents (e.g., Blechman & Tryon, in press; Forehand et al., 1987; Rutter, 1990).

Further Research on the Specificity of Children's Disorders

How can we understand why one child develops depression while another displays conduct disorder? The present study does not shed much light on the question of specific outcomes. In common with most studies of depression in children (e.g., Kovacs, Feinberg, Crouse-Novak, Palauskas, & Finkelstein, 1984), the depressed children in the present sample were frequently likely to have co-occurring disorders. Does this mean that there are some nonspecific psychopathological processes that develop into more coherent forms over time? That children experience separate biological and psychosocial risk factors for one or both? Is this an artifact of a diagnostic system that does not operate in dimensional terms? Clearly, this is an intriguing area with major theoretical implications that should propel investigators to tackle the matter. Not only might such pursuits involve further studies of risk factors and their operation, but they would also require longitudinal studies into adulthood to explore the temporal consistency and specificity of the disorders. There are also potential integrations with biological and genetic predispositions (e.g., Dodge, 1990; Rutter, 1990).

On this note, it is time to look ahead not only to future research programs but also to the future of the children of women with affective disorders.

Depressed Children: What Happens Next?

Although relatively few studies have followed children and adolescents into adulthood to examine the relationship between previous depression and later depression, there is highly suggestive evidence of a pernicious, continuing negative course. The current study indicated significant rates of academic and social maladjustment that portend poorly for adult competence. Also, if our stress-generation model is apt, the children at risk in this study will continue to engage in behaviors and display attributes that create ongoing difficulties that may tax their limited coping capabilities.

Most longitudinal studies that followed children of parents with depression into adulthood are relatively small-scale case studies, but there are several follow-ups of *depressed children*.

Two studies followed youngsters into adulthood. A longitudinal study of high school students reexamined them 9 years later when they averaged 24 years old. Results directly implicate prior depression as a predictor of young adult depression and various psychosocial difficulties (Kandel & Davies, 1986). For instance, dysphoric feelings in adolescence were a significant predictor of dysphoric feelings 9 years later. Women who had reported more depressive symptoms as adolescents were more likely to have been treated by mental health professionals and to have sought their help at an earlier age than nondepressed adolescent women. Both men and women who were previously dysphoric in high school were more likely to have dropped out of school than nondysphoric individuals. The depressed women compared to the nondepressed, were more likely to report later marital disruption and divorce; the depressed men were likely to report later difficulty is sustaining employment. Both depressed adolescent men and women were likely to report that they later engaged in deviant and delinquent activities and used more psychoactive drugs than the nondepressed. The area of social functioning was especially noteworthy. Youngsters who reported depressive symptoms as teenagers were found to report less intimacy and involvement with their spouse or partners as adults, and this commonly mirrored their adolescent reports of their relationships with their parents. In other words, teenagers who had reported depressive symptoms in their youth compared to the nondepressed, reported less close and satisfying relationships with their parents, especially the opposite-sex parent. Family history of psychiatric problems was also predictive of early adult depressive symptoms. Finally, it is noteworthy that more of the previously depressed young women had children than did their nondepressed counterparts. Kandel and Davies (1986) speculates that having children may be an attempt by dysphoric young women to "increase their sense of connectedness to and intimacy with others in their social network." This intriguing possibility needs to be explored, but it clearly brings up the possibility of cycles of family psychopathology continuing.

The second longitudinal study of youth followed depressed children who had been clinically treated, compared with a matched control group of psychiatrically disturbed but not depressed youngsters. Harrington, Fudge, Rutter, Pickles, and Hill (1990) studied the individuals an average of 18 years since treatment and assessed their subsequent psychiatric status. They found that the formerly depressed children had high rates of relapse, with 60% experiencing at least one recurrence of major depressive episodes. The depressed group of children had elevated rates of other diagnoses as well, and they differed from the psychiatric control group only in affective disorders. Such rates of comorbidity suggest that co-occurring diagnoses may be stable and observable in adulthood, just as they are in childhood.

Lewinsohn and colleagues, both in retrospective analyses and in longitudinal follow-ups, reported an especially high rate of relapse of major depression for young women who had earlier (often adolescent) episodes (e.g., Lewinsohn, Hoberman, & Rosenbaum, 1989). Numerous clinical studies have also found that previous depression predicts future depression, but the ages of previous depression are not commonly reported in such studies so that it is unclear how many followed childhood onsets.

Finally, several studies of depressed children followed them for a few years, finding that early onset predicts a longer time to recovery (e.g., Kovacs et al., 1984) and that childhood onset of depression predicts likelihood of recurrence of major depression (Kovacs, Feinberg, Crouse-Novak, Paulauskas, Pollock & Finkelstein, 1984). Such results are generally consistent with adult studies that report early onset is associated with a more pernicious adult course of disorder (reviewed in Hammen, in press-b). Thus it is not difficult to predict future depression in the lives of clinically depressed children in this study, and it is probably also likely that concurrent disorders that the children experienced will cause adult difficulties as well. This includes conduct, substance abuse, and anxiety disorders.

Finally, if Kandel and Davies (1986) are right about the consequences of dysphoria, we might also expect the youngsters in our study to form unsatisfying attachments and possibly to have children of their own at early ages. This may bring the cycle around again, to future generations of children of depressed parents. Let us hope that before much more time passes, even greater amounts of effort will be spent to develop effective preventive and treatment programs for such dysfunctional families than have been spent on verifying their risk for disorder. Although the present research has painted a grim picture of the psychological factors predicting dysfunction in the offspring of depressed women, at least they are factors that may lend themselves to treatment. It is to be hoped that some of the conditions that were studied and clarified in this work will useful to those who are in a position to provide assistance to the children and parents in need.

References

Abramson, L.Y., Alloy, L.B., & Metalsky, G.I. (1988). The cognitive diathesis-stress theories of depression: Toward an adequate evaluation of the theories' validities. In L.B. Alloy (Ed.), *Cognitive processes in depression* (pp. 3–30). New York: Guilford Press.

Abramson, L.Y., Seligman, M.E.P., & Teasdale, J.D. (1978). Learned helplessness in humans: Critique and reformulation. *Journal of Abnormal Psychology, 87*, 49–74.

Achenbach, T.M. (1978). The child behavior profile: I. Boys 6–11. *Journal of Consulting and Clinical Psychology, 46*, 478–488.

Achenbach, T.M., & Edelbrock, C.S. (1983). *Manual for the Child Behavior Checklist Behavior Profile.* Burlington, VT: Thomas M. Achenbach, Department of Psychiatry, University of Vermont.

Achenbach, T.M., McConaughy, S.H., & Howell, C.T. (1987). Child/adolescent behavioral and emotional problems: Implications of cross-informant correlations for situational specificity. *Psychological Bulletin, 101*, 213–232.

Adrian, C. (1988). *Stress processes and psychological disorder in children of parents with affective psychopathology: A review of the literature on psychosocial risk factors and on children's stress.* Unpublished manuscript, University of California, Los Angeles.

Adrian, C. (1990). *Differential vulnerability to stress in children of mothers with affective disorders and mothers without history of major psychopathology.* Unpublished doctoral dissertation, University of California, Los Angeles.

Adrian, C., & Hammen, C. (1990). Children of depressed mothers: Stress exposure and responses to stressful life events. Manuscript in preparation.

Akiskal, H.S., Bitar, A.H., Puzantian, V.R., Rosenthal, T.L., & Walker, P.W. (1978). The nosological status of neurotic depression: A prospective three- to four-year follow-up examination in light of the primary–secondary and unipolar–bipolar dichotomies. *Archives of General Psychiatry, 35*, 756–766.

Akiskal, H.S., Downs, J., Jordon, P., Watson, S., Dougherty, D, & Pruitt, D.B. (1985). Affective disorders in referred children and younger siblings of manic depressives. *Archives of General Psychiatry, 42*, 996–1003.

Akiskal, H.S., King, D., Rosenthal, T.L., Robinson, D., & Scott-Strauss, A. (1981). Chronic depression. *Journal of Affective Disorders, 3*, 297–315.

Alloy, L.B. (1988). *Cognitive processes in depression.* New York: Guilford Press.

Altmann, E.O., & Gotlib, I.H. (1988). The social behavior of depressed children: An observational study. *Journal of Abnormal Child Psychology, 16*, 29–44.

Ambelas, A. (1979). Psychologically stressful events in the precipitation of manic episodes. *British Journal of Psychiatry, 135*, 15–21.

Anderson, C.A., & Hammen, C. (1990a). *Psychosocial functioning in children at risk for depression: Longitudinal follow-up*. Unpublished manuscript.

Anderson, C.A., & Hammen, C. (1990b). *Disturbed and nondisturbed siblings in high risk families: Correlates of vulnerability*. Unpublished manuscript.

Andreasen, N.C. (in press). The genetics of affective disorders: An overview. In B. Bloom & K. Schlesinger (Eds.), *The First Boulder Symposium on Clinical Psychology: Depression*. Hillsdale, NJ: Lawrence Erlbaum Associates.

Andrews, B. & Brown, G. (1988). Marital violence in the community: A biographical approach. *British Journal of Psychiatry, 153*, 305–312.

Andrews, B., Brown, G., & Creasey, L. (1990). Intergenerational links between psychiatric disorder in mothers and daughters: The role of parenting experience. *Journal of Child Psychology and Psychiatry, 31*, 1115–1129.

Angst, J. (1973). The course of monopolar depression and bipolar psychoses. *Psychiatrie, Neurologie et Neurochirurgie, 76*, 489–500.

Angst, J. (1984, April). *A prospective study on the course of affective disorders*. Paper presented at the National Institute of Mental Health Consensus Development Conference, Washington, DC.

Anthony, E.J. (1974). The syndrome of the psychologically invulnerable child. In A.E. Koupernic (Ed.), *The child in his family: Children at psychiatric risk*. New York: Wiley.

Anthony, E.J. (1983). An overview of the effects of maternal depression on the infant and child. In H.L. Morrison (Ed.), *Children of depressed parents* (pp. 1–6). New York: Grune & Stratton.

Anthony, E.J. (1987a). Children at high risk for psychosis growing up successfully. In E.J. Anthony & B.J. Cohler (Eds.), *The invulnerable child* (pp. 147–184). New York: Guilford Press.

Anthony, E.J. (1987b). Risk, vulnerability, and resilience: An overview. In E.J. Anthony & B.J. Cohler (Eds.), *The invulnerable child* (pp. 3–48). New York: Guilford Press.

Arieti, S., & Bemporad, J. (1980). The psychological organization of depression. *American Journal of Psychiatry, 137*, 1360–1365.

Asarnow, J.R. (1988). Peer status and social competence in child psychiatric inpatients: A comparison of children with depressive, externalizing, and concurrent depressive and externalizing disorders. *Journal of Abnormal Child Psychology, 16*, 151–162.

Asarnow, J.R., & Bates, S. (1988). Depression in child psychiatric inpatients: Cognitive and attributional patterns. *Journal of Abnormal Child Psychology, 16*, 601–615.

Asarnow, J.R., Carlson, G.A., & Guthrie, D. (1987). Coping strategies, self-perceptions, hopelessness, and perceived family environments in depressed and suicidal children. *Journal of Consulting and Clinical Psychology, 55*, 361–366.

Bandura, A. (1982). Self-efficacy mechanism in human agency. *American Psychologist, 37*, 122–147.

Barnett, P.A., & Gotlib, I.H. (1988). Psychosocial functioning and depression:

Distinguishing among antecedents, concomitants, and consequences. *Psychological Bulletin, 104*, 97–126.

Barocas, R., Seifer, R., & Sameroff, A.J. (1985). Defining environmental risk: Multiple dimensions of psychological vulnerability. *American Journal of Community Psychology, 13*, 433–447.

Baron, M., Risch, N., Hamburger, R., Mandel, B., Kushner, S., Newman, M., Drumer, D., & Belmaker, R. (1987). Genetic linkage between X-chromosome markers and affective illness. *Nature, 326*, 289–292.

Beardslee, W.R., Bemporad, J., Keller, M.B., & Klerman, G.L. (1983). Children with parents with major affective disorder: A review. *American Journal of Psychiatry, 140*, 825–832.

Beardslee, W.R., Keller, M.B., & Klerman, G.L. (1985). Children of parents with affective disorder. *International Journal of Family Psychiatry, 6*, 283–299.

Beardslee, W.R., & Podorefsky, D. (1988). Resilient adolescents whose parents have serious affective and other psychiatric disorders: Importance of self-understanding and relationships. *American Journal of Psychiatry, 145*, 63–69.

Beardslee, W.R., Schultz, L.H., & Selman, R.L. (1987). Level of social-cognitive development, adaptive functioning, and DSM-III diagnoses in adolescent offspring of parents with affective disorders: Implications of the development of the capacity for mutuality. *Developmental Psychology, 23*(6), 807–815.

Beck, A.T. (1967). *Depression: Clinical, experimental, and theoretical aspects*. New York: Harper & Row.

Beck, A.T. (1976). *Cognitive therapy and the emotional disorders*. New York: International Universities Press.

Beck. A.T. (1982). Cognitive therapy of depression: New perspectives. In P. Clayton & J. Barret (Eds.), *Treatment of depression: Old controversies and new approaches* (pp. 265–290). New York: Raven Press.

Beck, A.T., Steer, R.A., & Garbin, M.G. (1988). Psychometric properties of the Beck Depression Inventory: Twenty-five years of evaluation. *Clinical Psychology Review, 8*, 77–100.

Beck, A.T., Ward, C., Mendelson, M., Mock, J. & Erbaugh, J. (1961). An inventory for measuring depression. *Archives of General Psychiatry, 4*, 53–63.

Becker, J. (1979). Vulnerable self-esteem as a predisposing factor in depressive disorders. In R.E. Depue (Ed.), *The psychobiology of the depressive disorders: Implications for the effects of stress* (pp. 317–334). New York: Academic Press.

Benassi, V.A., Sweeney, P.D., & Dufour, C.L. (1988). Is there a relation between locus of control orientation and depression? *Journal of Abnormal Psychology, 97*, 357–367.

Benfield, C.Y., Palmer, D.J., Pfefferbaum, B., & Stowe, M.L. (1988). A comparison of depressed and nondepressed disturbed children on measures of attributional style, hopelessness, life stress, and temperament. *Journal of Abnormal Child Psychology, 16*, 397–410.

Bentler, P. (1985). *Theory and implementation of EQS: A structural equation program*. Los Angeles: BMDP Statistical Software.

Bentler, P.M. (1989). *EQS Structural equations program manual*. Los Angeles: BMDP Statistical Software.

Bentler, P.M. (1990). Comparative fit indexes in structural models. *Psychological Bulletin, 107*, 238–246.

Bentler, P.M., & Bonett, D. (1980). Significance tests and goodness of fit in the analysis of covariance structures. *Psychological Bulletin*, *88*, 588–606.

Bettes, B. (1988). Maternal depression and motherese: Temporal and intonational features. *Child Development*, *59*, 1089–1096.

Bibring, E. (1953). Mechanisms in depression. In P. Greenacre (Ed.), *Affective disorders: Psychoanalytic contributions to their study*. New York: International Universities Press.

Bidzinska, E. (1984). Stress factors in affective diseases. *British Journal of Psychiatry*, *144*, 161–166.

Bifulco, A.T., Brown, G.W., & Harris, T.O. (1987). Childhood loss of parent, lack of adequate parental care and adult depression: A replication. *Journal of Affective Disorders*, *12*, 115–128.

Billings, A.G., Cronkite, R., & Moos, R. (1983). Social-environmental factors in unipolar depression: Comparisons of depressed patients and nondepressed controls. *Journal of Abnormal Psychology*, *92*, 119–133.

Billings, A.G., & Moos, R.H. (1982). Psychosocial theory and research on depression: An integrative framework and review. *Clinical Psychology Review*, *2*, 213–217.

Billings, A.G., & Moos, R.H. (1983). Comparisons of children of depressed and nondepressed parents: A social-environmental perspective, *Journal of Abnormal Child Psychology*, *11*, 463–485.

Billings, A.G., & Moos, R.H. (1984). Coping, stress, and social resources among adults with unipolar depression. *Journal of Personality and Social Psychology*, *46*, 877–891.

Billings, A.G., & Moos, R.H. (1985a). Children of parents with unipolar depression: A controlled 1-year follow-up. *Journal of Abnormal Child Psychology*, *14*, 149–166.

Billings, A.G., & Moos, R.H. (1985b). Psychosocial processes of remission in unipolar depression: Comparing depressed patients with matched community controls. *Journal of Consulting and Clinical Psychology*, *53*, 314–325.

Birtchnell, J., Evans, C., & Kennard, J. (1988). Life history factors associated with neurotic symptomatology in a rural community sample of 40–49-year-old women. *Journal of Affective Disorders*, *14*, 271–285.

Black, D.W., Bell, S., Hulbert, J., & Nasrallah, A. (1988). The importance of Axis II in patients with major depression: A controlled study. *Journal of Affective Disorders*, *14*, 115–122.

Bland, R.C., Newman, S.C., & Orn, H. (1986). Recurrent and nonrecurrent depression: A family study. *Archives of General Psychiatry*, *43*(11), 1085–1089.

Blatt, S., Quinlan, D., Chevron, E., McDonald, C., & Zuroff, D. (1982). Dependency and self-criticism: Psychological dimensions for depression. *Journal of Consulting and Clinical Psychology*, *50*, 113–124.

Blechman, E.A., McEnroe, M.J., Carella, E.T., & Audette, D.P. (1986). Childhood competence and depression. *Journal of Abnormal Psychology*, *95*, 223–227.

Blechman, E.A., & Tryon, A.S. (in press). Familial origins of competence and depression. In B. Bloom & K. Schlesinger (Eds.), *The First Boulder Symposium on Clinical Psychology: Depression*. Hillsdale, NJ: Lawrence Erlbaum Associates.

Blehar, M.C., Weissman, M.M., Gershon, E.S., & Hirschfeld, R.M.A. (1988). Family and genetic studies of affective disorders. *Archives of General Psychiatry*, *45*, 289–292.

Blumberg, S.H., & Izard, C.E. (1985). Affective and cognitive characteristics of depression in 10- and 11-year-old children. *Journal of Personality and Social Psychology*, *49*, 194–202.

Bowlby, J. (1980). *Loss: Sadness and depression*. New York: Basic Books.

Boyd, J.H., & Weissman, M.M. (1981). Epidemiology of affective disorders. *Archives of General Psychiatry*, *38*, 1039–1046.

Breier, A., Kelsoe, J., Kirwin, P., Beller, S., Wolkowitz, O., & Pickar, D. (1988). Early parental loss and development of adult psychopathology. *Archives of General Psychiatry*, *45*, 987–993.

Breslau, N., Davis, G.C., & Prabucki, K. (1988). Depressed mothers as informants in family history research: Are they accurate? *Psychiatry Research*, *24*, 345–359.

Breznitz, Z., & Sherman, T. (1987). Speech patterning of natural discourse of well and depressed mothers and their young children. *Child Development*, *58*, 395–400.

Brody, G.H., & Forehand, R. (1986). Maternal perceptions of child maladjustment as a function of the combined influence of child behavior and maternal depression. *Journal of Consulting and Clinical Psychology*, *54*, 237–240.

Brown, G., Bifulco, A., & Harris, T.O. (1987). Life events, vulnerability and onset of depression: Some refinements. *British Journal of Psychiatry*, *150*, 30–42.

Brown, G., Bifulco, A., Harris, T., & Bridge, L. (1986). Life stress, chronic subclinical symptoms and vulnerability to clinical depression. *Journal of Affective Disorders*, *11*, 1–19.

Brown, G.W., & Harris, T. (1978). *Social origins of depression*. London: Free Press.

Burbach, D.J., & Borduin, C.M. (1986). Parent–child relations and the etiology of depression: A review of methods and findings. *Clinical Psychology Review*, *6*, 133–135.

Burge, D. (1990). *Sequential analysis of the interaction of depressed mothers and their children*. Unpublished doctoral dissertation. University of California, Los Angeles.

Burge, D., & Hammen, C. (in press). Maternal communication: A predictor of children's outcomes at follow-up in a high risk sample. *Journal of Abnormal Psychology*.

Bugenthal, D.B., & Shennum, W.A. (1984). "Difficult" children as elicitors and targets of adult communication patterns: An attributional behavioral transactional analysis. *Monographs of the Society for Research in Child Development*, *49* (1, Serial No. 205).

Campbell-Goymer, N.R., & Allgood, W.C. (1984, March). *Cognitive correlates of childhood depression*. Paper presented at the annual conference of the Southeastern Psychological Association, New Orleans, LA.

Caplan, G. (1980). An approach to preventive intervention in child psychiatry. *Canadian Journal of Psychiatry*, *25*, 671–682.

Carey, W.B. (1986). Clinical interactions of temperament: Transitions from infancy to childhood. In R. Plomin & J. Dunn (Eds.), *The study of temperament:*

Changes, continuities, and challenges (pp. 151–162). Hillsdale, NJ: Lawrence Erlbaum Associates.

Chambers, W., Puig-Antich, J., Hirsch, M., Paez, P., Ambrosini, P., Tabrizi, M., & Davies, M. (1985). The assessment of affective disorders in children and adolescents by semi-structured interview. *Archives of General Psychiatry, 42*, 696–702.

Cicchetti, D., & Schneider-Rosen, K. (1986). An organizational approach to childhood depression. In M. Rutter, C.E. Izard, & P.E. Read (Eds.), *Depression in young people* (pp. 71–134). New York: Guilford Press.

Clayton, P.J. (1984, April). *Overview of recurrent mood disorders: Definitions and natural course*. Paper presented at the National Institute of Mental Health Consensus Development Conference, Washington, DC.

Cohen, L.H., Burt, C.E., & Bjork, J.P. (1987). Effects of life events experienced by young adolescents and their parents. *Developmental Psychology, 23*, 583–592.

Cohler, B.J, Grunebaum, H.U., Weiss, J.L., Hartmen, C.R., & Gallant, D.H. (1977). Child care attitudes and adaptation to the maternal role among mentally ill and well mothers. *American Journal of Orthopsychiatry, 46*, 123–133.

Cohn, J.F., Campbell, S.B., Matias, R., & Hopkins, J. (1990). Face-to-face interactions of postpartum depressed and nondepressed mother–infant pairs at 2 months. *Developmental Psychology, 26*, 15–23.

Cohn, J., Matias, R., Tronick, E., Connell, D., & Lyons-Ruth, K. (1986). Face-to-face interactions of depressed mothers and their infants. In E. Tronick & T. Field (Eds.), *Maternal depression and infant disturbance*. (New Directions for Child Development, No. *34*, pp. 31–46). San Francisco: Jossey-Bass.

Cohn, J.F., & Tronick, E.Z. (1983). Three-month-old infants' reaction to simulated maternal depression. *Child Development, 54*, 185–193.

Cole, D.A. (in press). The relation of social and academic competence to depressive symptoms in childhood. *Journal of Abnormal Psychology*.

Cole, D.A., & Rehm, L.P. (1986). Family interaction patterns and childhood depression. *Journal of Abnormal Child Psychology, 14*(2), 297–314.

Compas, B.E. (1987). Stress and life events during childhood and adolescence. *Clinical Psychology Review, 77*, 275–302.

Compas, B.E. (1987). Coping with stress during childhood and adolescence. *Psychological Bulletin, 101*, 393–403.

Compas, B.E., Howell, D.C., Phares, V., Williams, R.A., & Giunta, C.T. (1989). Risk factors for emotional/behavioral problems in young adolescents: A prospective analysis of adolescent and parental stress and symptoms. *Journal of Consulting and Clinical Psychology, 57*, 732–740.

Compas, B.E., Howell, D.C., Phares, V., Williams, R.A., & Ledoux, N. (1989). Parent and child stress and symptoms: An integrative analysis. *Developmental Psychology, 25*(4), 550–559.

Compas, B., Wagner, B., Slavin, L., & Vannatta, K. (1986). A prospective study of life events, social support, and psychological symptomatology during the transition from high school to college. *American Journal of Community Psychology, 14*, 241–257.

Conners, C. (1969). A teacher rating scale for use in drug studies with children. *American Journal of Psychiatry, 126*(6), 152–156.

Conners, C.K., Himmelhock, J., Goyette, C.H., Ulrich, R., & Neil, J.F. (1979). Children of parents with affective illness. *Journal of the American Academy of Child Psychiatry, 18*, 600–607.

Conrad, M., & Hammen, C. (1989). Role of maternal depression in perceptions of child maladjustment. *Journal of Consulting and Clinical Psychology, 57*, 663–667.

Cooper, S.F., Leach, C., Storer, D., & Tonge, W.L. (1977). The children of psychiatric patients: Clinical findings. *British Journal of Psychiatry, 131*, 514–522.

Coyne, J.C. (1976). Toward an interactional description of depression. *Psychiatry, 39*, 28–40.

Coyne, J.C., Burchill, S.A.L., & Stiles, W.B. (1990). An interactional perspective on depression. In C.R. Snyder & D.O. Forsyth (Eds.), *Handbook of social and clinical psychology: The health perspective*. New York: Pergamon Press.

Coyne, J.C., & Gotlib, I.H. (1983). The role of cognition in depression: A critical appraisal. *Psychological Bulletin, 94*, 472–505.

Coyne, J.C., Kahn, J., & Gotlib, I.H. (1987). Depression. In T. Jacob (Ed.), *Family interaction and psychopathology* (pp. 509–533). New York: Plenum.

Coyne, J.C., Kessler, R.C., Tal, M., Turnbull, J., Wortman, C.B., & Greden, J. (1987). Living with a depressed person. *Journal of Consulting and Clinical Psychology, 55*, 347–352.

Coyne, J.C., Wortman, C., & Lehman, D. (1985, August). *When support fails: Miscarried helping processes*. Paper presented at the annual convention of the American Psychological Association, Los Angeles, CA.

Cutrona, C. (1983). Causal attributions and perinatal depression. *Journal of Abnormal Psychology, 92*, 161–172.

Cytryn, L., McKnew, D.H., Bartko, J.J., Lamour, M., & Hamovit, J. (1982). Offspring of patients with affective disorders: II. *Journal of the American Academy of Child Psychiatry, 21*, 389–391.

Daniels, D., Moos, R.H., Billings, A.G., & Miller, J.J., III. (1987). Psychosocial risk and resistance factors among children with chronic illness, healthy siblings, and healthy controls. *Journal of Abnormal Child Psychology, 15*(2), 295–308.

Davenport, Y.B., Zahn-Waxler, C., Adland, M.L., & Mayfield, A. (1984). Early child-rearing practices in families with a manic-depressive parent. *American Journal of Psychiatry, 141*(2), 230–235.

Dean, A., Lin, N., & Ensel, W.M. (1981). The epidemiological significance of social support systems in depression. *Research in Community and Mental Health, 2*, 77–109.

Decina, P., Kestenbaum, C.J., Farber, S., Kron, L., Gargan, M., Sackheim, H.A., & Fieve, R.R. (1983). Clinical and psychological assessment of children of bipolar probands. *American Journal of Psychiatry, 140*, 548–553.

Denham, S.A., & Zahn-Waxler, C. (1989). *Social competence in young preschoolers: Continuity and change from two to five years*. Presented at the biennial meetings of the Society for Research in Child Development, Kansas City, MO.

Dent, J., & Teasdale, J.D. (1988). Negative cognition and the persistence of depression. *Journal of Abnormal Psychology, 97*, 29–34.

Depue, R.A., & Monroe, S.M. (1986). Conceptualization and measurement of human disorder and life stress research: The problem of chronic disturbance. *Psychological Bulletin, 99*, 36–51.

Depue, R.A., Slater, J., Wolfstetter-Kausch, H., Klein, D., Gopelrud, E., & Farr, D. (1981). A behavioral paradigm for identifying persons at risk for bipolar depressive disorder: A conceptual framework and five validation studies. *Journal of Abnormal Psychology*, *90*, 381–439.

Derogatis, L., Lipman, R., Rickels, K., Uhlenhuth, E., & Covi, L. (1974). The Hopkins Symptom Checklist (HSCL): A self-report symptom inventory. *Behavioral Science*, *19*, 1–15.

Derry, P., & Kuiper, N. (1981). Schematic processing and self-reference in clinical depression. *Journal of Abnormal Psychology*, *90*, 286–297.

Digdon, N., & Gotlib, I.H. (1985). Developmental considerations in the study of childhood depression. *Developmental Review*, *5*, 162–199.

Dobson, K.S., & Shaw, B.F. (1987). Specificity and stability of self-referent encoding in clinical depression. *Journal of Abnormal Psychology*, *96*, 34–40.

Dodge, K,A. (1990). Developmental psychopathology in children of depressed mothers. *Developmental Psychology*, *26*, 3–6.

Downey, G., & Coyne, J.C. (1990). Children of depressed parents: An integrative review. *Psychological Bulletin*, *108*, 50–76.

Downey, G., & Walker, E. (1988). Social cognition and adjustment in children at risk for psychopathology. *Developmental Psychology*, *25*, 835–845.

Dunn, L.M., & Dunn, L.M. (1981). Peabody Picture Vocabulary Test–Revised. American Guidance Service, Circle Pines, MN.

Edelbrock, C., & Achenbach, T. (1984). The teacher version of the Child Behavior Profile: I. Boys aged 6–11. *Journal of Consulting and Clinical Psychology*, *52*, 207–217.

Edelbrock, C., Greenbaum, R., & Conover, N.C. (1985). Reliability and concurrent relations between the Teacher version of the Child Behavior Profile and Conners' Revised Teacher Rating Scale. *Journal of Abnormal Psychology*, *13*, 295–304.

Egeland, J.A., Gerhard, D.S., Pauls, D.L., Sussex, J.N., Kidd, K.K., Allen, C.R., Hostetter, A.M., & Housman, D.A. (1987). Bipolar affective disorders linked to DNA markers on chromsome 11. *Nature*, *325*, 783–787.

El-Guebaly, N., Offord, D.R., Sullivan, K.T., & Lynch, G.W. (1978). Psychosocial adjustment of the offspring of psychiatric inpatients: The effect of alcoholic, depressive and schizophrenic parentage. *Canadian Psychiatric Association Journal*, *23*, 281–289.

Ellicott, A., Hammen, C., Gitlin, M., Brown, G., & Jamison, K. (1990). Life events and bipolar disorder over a longitudinal course. *American Journal of Psychiatry*, *147*, 1194–1198.

Endicott, J., & Spitzer, R.L. (1979). Use of Research Diagnostic Criteria and the Schedule for Affective Disorders and Schizophrenia to study affective disorders. *American Journal of Psychiatry*, *136*, 52–56.

Felner, R.D., Gillespie, J.F., & Smith, R. (1985). Risk and vulnerability in childhood: A reappraisal. *Journal of Clinical Child Psychology*, *14*(1), 2–4.

Fendrich, M., Warner, V., & Weissman, M.M. (1990). Family risk factors, parental depression and psychopathology in offspring. *Developmental Psychology*, *26*, 40–50.

Fergusson, D.M., Horwood, L.J., Gretton, M.E., & Shannon, F.T. (1985). Family life events, maternal depression, and maternal and teacher descriptions of child behavior. *Pediatrics*, 75(1), 30–35.

Field, T. (1984). Early interactions between infants and their postpartum depressed mothers. *Infant Behavior and Development, 7*, 517–522.

Field, T., Healy, B., Goldstein, S., & Guthertz, M. (1990). Behavior–state matching and synchrony in mother–infant interactions of nondepressed versus depressed dyads. *Development Psychology, 26*, 7–14.

Field, T., Healy, B., Goldstein, S., Perry, S., Bendell, D., Schanberg, S., Zimmerman, E.A., & Kuhn, C. (1988). Infants of depressed mothers show "depressed" behavior even with nondepressed adults. *Child Development, 59*, 1569–1579.

Field, T., Sandberg, D., Garcia, R., Vega-Lahr, N., Goldstein, S., & Guy, L. (1985). Pregnancy problems, postpartum depression and early mother–infant interactions. *Developmental Psychology, 21*, 1152–1156.

Fischler, G.L., & Kendall, P.C. (1988). Social cognitive problem solving and childhood adjustment: Qualitative and topological analyses. *Cognitive Therapy and Research, 12*, 133–153.

Fisher, L., & Kokes, R.F. (1983). Assessing the relationship between parental behavior and child functioning. In H.L. Morrison (Ed.), *Children of depressed parents* (pp. 47–64). New York: Grune & Stratton.

Fisher, L., Kokes, R.F., Cole, R.E., Perkins, P.M., & Wynne, L.C. (1987). Competent children at risk: A study of well-functioning offspring of disturbed parents. In E.J. Anthony & B.J. Cohler (Eds.), *The invulnerable child* (pp. 211–228). New York: Guilford Press.

Fleming, A., Ruble, D., Flett, G., & Shaul, D. (1988). Postpartum adjustment in first-time mothers: Relations betweeen mood, maternal attitudes, and mother–infant interactions. *Developmental Psychology, 24*, 71–81.

Forehand, R., McCombs, A., & Brody, G.H. (1987). The relationship between parental depressive mood states and child functioning. *Advances in Behavior Research and Therapy, 9*, 1–20.

Forehand, R., Wells, K., McMahon, R., Griest, D., & Rogers, T. (1982). Maternal perception of maladjustment in the clinic-referred children: An extension of earlier research. *Journal of Behavioral Assessment, 4*, 145–151.

Friedmann, M.S. (1989). *The effect of children's perceptions of maternal depression on their own functioning and subsequent risk of developing a psychological disorder*. Unpublished undergraduate honors thesis, University of California, Los Angeles.

Gaensbauer, T.J., Harmon, R.J., Cytryn, L., & McKnew, D.H. (1984). Social and affective development in infants with a manic–depressive parent. *American Journal of psychiatry, 141*, 223–229.

Gamer, E., Gallant, D., Grunebaum, H.U., & Cohler, B.J. (1977). Children of psychotic mothers. *Archives of General Psychiatry, 34*, 592–597.

Garmezy, N. (1985). Stress-resistant children: The search for protective factors. In J.E. Stevenson (Ed.), *Aspects of current child psychiatry research* (Journal of Child Psychology and Psychiatry Book Suppl. No. 4, pp. 213–223). Oxford, England: Pergamon Press.

Garmezy, N., & Devine, V. (1984). Project competence: The Minnesota studies of children vulnerable to psychopathology. In N. Watt, E.J. Anthony, L. Wynne, & J. Rolf (Eds.), *Children at risk for schizophrenia* (pp. 289–303). New York: Cambridge University Press.

Garmezy, N., & Rutter, M. (1983). *Stress, coping, and development in children*. New York: McGraw-Hill.

Garrison, W.T., & Earls, F.J. (1987). *Temperament and child psychopathology*. Newbury Park, CA: Sage.

Gelfand, D.M., & Teti, D.M. (1990). *The effects of maternal depression on children*. *Clinical Psychology Review*, *10*, 329–354.

Gershon, E.S. (1990). Genetics. In F.K. Goodwin & K.R. Jamison (Eds.), *Manic-depressive illness* (pp. 373–401). New York: Oxford University Press.

Gershon, E.S., Hamovit, J., Guroff, J.J., Dibble, E., Leckman, J.F., Sceery, W., Targum, S.D., Nurnberger, J.I., Goldin, L.R., & Bunney, W.E. (1982). A family study of schizoaffective, bipolar I, biopolar II, unipolar, and normal control probands. *Archives of General Psychiatry*, *39*, 1157–1167.

Gershon, E.S., Hamovit, J.H., Guroff, J.J., & Nurnberger, J.I. (1987). Birth-cohort changes in manic and depressive disorders in relatives of bipolar and schizoaffective patients. *Archives of General Psychiatry*, *44*, 314–319.

Gershon, E.S., McKnew, D., Cytryn, L., Hamovit, J., Schreiber, J., Hibbs, E., & Pelligrini, D. (1985). Diagnoses in school-age children of bipolar affective disorder patients and normal controls. *Journal of Affective Disorders*, *8*, 283–291.

Gold, P.W., Goodwin, F.K., & Chrousos, G.P. (1988). Clinical and biochemical manifestations of depression: Relation to the neurobiology of stress. *New England Journal of Medicine*, *319*, 413–420.

Goldin, L.R., & Gershon, E.S. (1988). The genetic epidemiology of major depressive illness. In A.J. Frances & R.E. Hales (Eds.), *Review of Psychiatry* (Vol. 7, pp. 149–167). Washington, DC: American Psychiatric Press.

Goodman, S.H., & Brumley, H.E. (1990). Schizophrenic and depressed mothers: Relational deficits in parenting. *Developmental Psychology*, *26*(1), 31–39.

Goodwin, F., & Jamison, K.R. (1984). The natural course of manic-depressive illness. In R. Post & J. Ballenger (Eds.), *Neurobiology of mood disorders* (pp. 20–37). Baltimore, MD: Williams & Wilkins.

Goplerud, E., & Depue, R.A. (1985). Behavioral response to naturally-occurring stress in cyclothymes, dysthymes, and controls. *Journal of Abnormal Psychology*, *94*, 128–139.

Gordon, D., Burge, D., Hammen, C., Adrian, C., Jaenicke, C., & Hiroto, D. (1989). Observations of interactions of depressed women with their children. *American Journal of Psychiatry*, *146*, 50–55.

Gotlib, I.H., & Cane, D.B. (1987). Construct accessibility and clinical depression: A longitudinal investigation. *Journal of Abnormal Psychology*, *96*, 199–204.

Gotlib, I.H., & Colby, C.A. (1987). *Treatment of depression: An interpersonal systems approach*. New York: Pergamon Press.

Gotlib, I.H. & Lee, C.M. (1990). Children of depressed parents: A review and directions for future research. In C.D. McCann, & N.S. Endler (Eds.), *Depression: New directions in research, theory and practice*. Toronto: Wall & Thompson.

Greenhill, L.L., & Shopsin, B. (1979). Survey of mental disorders in the children of patients with affective disorders. In J. Mendlewicz & B. Shopsin (Eds.), *Genetic aspects of affective illness*. New York: Spectrum Publications (Eds.), (pp. 75–92).

Greenhill, L.L., Shopsin, B., & Temple, H. (1980). Children of affectively ill parents: Psychiatric status determined by structured interview. *Psychopharmacology Bulletin*, *16*, 23–24.

Griest, D., Forehand, R., Wells, K., & McMahon, R. (1980). An examination of differences between nonclinic and behavior-problem clinic-referred children and their mothers. *Journal of Abnormal Psychology*, *89*, 497–500.

Griest, D., Wells, K., & Forehand, R. (1979). An examination of predictors of maternal perceptions of maladjustment in clinic-referred children. *Journal of Abnormal Psychology*, *88*, 277–281.

Haley, G.M., Fine, S., Marriage, K., Moretti, M.M., & Freeman, R.J. (1985). Cognitive bias and depression in psychiatrically disturbed children and adolescents. *Journal of Consulting and Clinical Psychology*, *53*, 535–537.

Hamilton, E. W., & Abramson, L.Y. (1983). Cognitive patterns and major depressive disorder: A longitudinal study in a hospital setting. *Journal of Abnormal Psychology*, *92*, 173–184.

Hammen, C. (1985). Predicting depression: A cognitive-behavioral perspective. In P. Kendall (Ed.), *Advances in cognitive-behavioral research and therapy* (Vol. 4) (pp. 30–74). New York: Academic Press.

Hammen, C. (1988a). Depression and cognitions about stressful life events. In L. Alloy (Ed.), *Cognitive processes in depression*. (pp. 77–108). New York: Guilford Press.

Hammen. C. (1988b). Self-cognitions, stressful events, and the prediction of depression in children of depressed mothers. *Journal of Abnormal Child Psychology*, *16*, 347–360.

Hammen, C. (1990-a). Cognitive approaches to depression in children: Current findings and new directions. In B. Lahey and A. Kazdin (Eds.), *Advances in Clinical Child Psychology*, Vol. 13. New York: Plenum.

Hammen, C. (1990-b). Vulnerability to depression: Personal, situational, and family aspects. In R. Ingram (Ed.), *Contemporary approaches to depression: Treatment, research, and theory*. New York: Plenum.

Hammen, C. (in press-a). The generation of stress in the course of unipolar depression. *Journal of Abnormal Psychology*.

Hammen, C. (in press-b). Mood disorders (unipolar depression). In M. Hersen & S. Turner (Eds.), *Adult psychopathology and diagnosis* (2 edn.). New York: Wiley.

Hammen, C. (in press-c). Psychological vulnerability to depression: A cognitive-environmental perspective. In B. Bloom & K. Schlesinger (Eds.), *The First Boulder Symposium on Clinical Psychology: Depression*. Hillsdale, NJ: Lawrence Erlbaum Associates.

Hammen, C., Adrian, C., Gordon, D., Burge, D., Jaenicke, C., & Hiroto, D. (1987). Children of depressed mothers: Maternal strain and symptom predictors of dysfunction. *Journal of Abnormal Psychology*, *96*, 190–198.

Hammen, C., Adrian, C., & Hiroto, D. (1988). A longitudinal test of the attributional vulnerability model in children at risk for depression. *British Journal of Clinical Psychology*, *27*, 37–46.

Hammen, C., & Anderson, C. (1990). *Longitudinal study of children of depressed mothers: Unipolar vs. bipolar comparisons*. Unpublished manuscript.

Hammen, C., Burge, D., & Adrian, C., (in press). The relationship between mother and child episodes in a longitudinal study of risk for depression. *Journal of Consulting and Clinical Psychology.*

Hammen, C., Burge, D., Brown, G., & Stansbury, K. (1990). A three generation family context model of depression in children at risk. Ms. under review.

Hammen, C., Burge, D., Burney, E., & Adrian, C. (1990). Longitudinal study of diagnoses in children of women with unipolar and bipolar affective disorder. *Archives of General Psychiatry*, *47*, 1112–1120.

Hammen, C., Burge, D., & Stansbury, K. (1990). Relationship of mother and child variables to child outcomes in a high risk sample: A causal modeling analysis. *Developmental Psychology*, *26*, 24–30.

Hammen, C., Davila, J., Brown, G., Gitlin, M. & Ellicott, A. (1991). Stress as a mediator of the effects of psychiatric history on severity of unipolar depression. Manuscript under review.

Hammen, C., Ellicott, A., Gitlin, M., & Jamison, K.R. (1989). Sociotropy/autonomy and vulnerability to specific life events in unipolar and bipolar patients. *Journal of Abnormal Psychology*, *98*, 154–160.

Hammen, C., & Goodman-Brown, T. (1990). Self-schemas and vulnerability to specific life stress in children at risk for depression. *Cognitive Therapy and Research*, *14*, 215–227.

Hammen, C., Gordon, D., Burge, D., Adrian, C., Jaenicke, C., & Hiroto, D. (1987). Maternal affective disorders, illness, and stress: Risk for children's psychopathology. *American Journal of Psychiatry*, *144*, 736–741.

Hammen, C., & Krantz, S. (1985). Measures of psychological processes in depression. In E.E. Beckham & W.R. Leber (Eds.), *Handbook of depression: Treatment, assessment, and research* (pp. 408–444). Homewood, IL: Dorsey Press.

Hammen, C., Marks, T., deMayo, R., & Mayol, A. (1985). Self-schemas and risk for depression: A prospective study. *Journal of Personality and Social Psychology*, *49*, 1147–1159.

Hammen, C., Marks, T., Mayol, A., & deMayo, R. (1985). Depressive self-schemas, life stress, and vulnerability to depression. *Journal of Abnormal Psychology*, *94*, 308–319.

Hammen, C., Mayol, A., deMayo, R., & Marks, T. (1986). Initial symptom levels and the life event–depression relationship. *Journal of Abnormal Psychology*, *95*, 114–122.

Hammen, C., Miklowitz, D.J., & Dyck, D.G. (1986). Stability and severity parameters of depressive self-schema responding. *Journal of Social and Clinical Psychology*, *4*, 23–45.

Hammen, C., & Peters, S.D. (1978). Interpersonal consequences of depression: Responses to men and women enacting a depressed role. *Journal of Abnormal Psychology*, *87*, 322–332.

Hammen, C., & Zupan, B.A. (1984). Self-schemas, depression, and the processing of personal information in children. *Journal of Experimental Child Psychology*, *37*, 598–608.

Harder, D.W., Kokes, R.F., Fisher, L., & Strauss, J.S. (1980). Child competence and psychiatric risk: IV. Relationships of parent diagnostic classifications and parent psychopathology severity to child functioning. *Journal of Nervous and Mental Disease*, *168*(6), 343–347.

Harrington, R., Fudge, H., Rutter, M., Pickles, A., & Hill, J. (1990). Adult outcomes of childhood and adolescent depression. *Archives of General Psychiatry*, *47*, 465–473.

Harris, T., Brown, G.W., & Bifulco, A. (1986). Loss of parent in childhood and adult psychiatric disorder: The role of parental care. *Psychological Medicine*, *16*, 641–659.

Harris, T., Brown, G.W., & Bifulco, A. (1987). Loss of parent in childhood and adult psychiatric disorder: The role of social class position and premarital pregnancy. *Psychological Medicine*, *17*, 163–183.

Hart, D., & Damon, W. (1986). Developmental trends in self-understanding. *Social Cognition*, *4*, 388–407.

Harter, S. (1983). Children's understanding of multiple emotions: A cognitive-developmental approach. In W.F. Overton (Ed.), *The relationship between social and cognitive development* (pp. 147–194). Hillsdale, NJ: Lawrence Erlbaum Associates.

Harter, S. (1986). Cognitive-developmental processes in the integration of concepts about emotions and the self. *Social Cognition*, *4*, 119–151.

Hartup, W. (1983). The peer system. In E.M. Hetherington (Ed.), *Handbook of child psychology: Vol 4. Socialization, personality, and social development* (pp. 103–196). New York: Wiley.

Hartup, W.W. (1989). Social relationships and their developmental significance. *American Psychologist*, *44*, 120–126.

Hazzard, A., Christensen, A., & Margolin, G. (1983). Children's perceptions of parental behaviors. *Journal of Abnormal Child Psychology*, *11*, 49–59.

Herjanic, B., & Reich, W. (1982). Development of a structured psychiatric interview for children: Agreement between child and parent on individual symptoms. *Journal of Abnormal Child Psychology*, *10*, 307–324.

Hetherington, E., & Martin, B. (1986). Family interaction. In H. Quay & J. Werry (Eds.), *Psychopathological disorders of childhood* (2nd ed.) New York: Wiley.

Hirsch, B.J., Moos, R.H., & Reischl, T.M. (1985). Psychosocial adjustment of adolescent children of a depressed, arthritic, or normal parent. *Journal of Abnormal Psychology*, *94*, 154–164.

Hodges, K.K. (1983). *The Child Assessment Schedule*. Unpublished manuscript, University of Missouri.

Hodges, K., McKnew, D., Cytryn, L. (1982). The Child Assessment Schedule (CAS) diagnostic interview: A report on reliability and validity. *Journal of the American Academy of Child Psychiatry*, *21*, 468–473.

Holahan, C. J., & Moos, R.H. (1987). Risk, resistance, and psychological distress: A longitudinal analysis with adults and children. *Journal of Abnormal Psychology*, *96*(1), 3–13.

Hollon, S.D., Kendall, P.C., & Lumry, A. (1986). Specificity of depressotypic cognitions in clinical depression. *Journal of Abnormal Psychology*, *95*, 52–59.

Holmes, S.J., & Robins, L.N. (1987). The influence of childhood disciplinary experience on the development of alcoholism and depression. *Journal of Child Psychology and Psychiatry*, *28*(3), 399–415.

Hooley, J., Orley, J., & Teasdale, J. (1986). Levels of expressed emotion and relapse in depressed patients. *British Journal of Psychiatry*, *148*, 642–647.

Hooley, J.M., & Teasdale, J.D. (1989). Predictors of relapse in unipolar

depressives: Expressed emotion, marital distress, and perceived criticism. *Journal of Abnormal Psychology*, *98*(3), 229–235.
Hops, H., Biglan, A. Sherman, L., Arthur, J., Friedman, L., & Osteen, V. (1987). Home observations of family interactions of depressed women. *Journal of Consulting and Clinical Psychology*, *55*(3), 341–346.
Howes, C. (1987a). Peer interaction of young children. *Monographs of the Society for Research in Child Development*, *53*(1, Serial No. 217).
Howes, C. (1987b). Social competence with peers in young children: Developmental sequences. *Developmental Review*, *7*, 252–272.
Jaenicke, C., Hammen, C., Zupan, B., Hiroto, D., Gordon, D., Adrian, C., & Burge, D. (1987). Cognitive vulnerability in children at risk for depression. *Journal of Abnormal Child Psychology*, *15*, 559–572.
Jouriles, E.N., Murphy, C.M., & O'Leary, K.D. (1989). Effects of maternal mood on mother–son interaction patterns. *Journal of Abnormal Child Psychology*, *17*(5), 513–525.
Jouriles, E.N., & O'Leary, K.D. (1990). Influences of parental mood on parent behavior. In E.A. Blechman & M.J. McEnroe (Eds.), *Emotion and the family*. Hillsdale, NJ: Lawrence Erlbaum Associates.
Kagan, J., Reznick, J.S., & Snidman, N. (1987). The physiology and psychology of behavioral inhibition in children. *Child Development*, *58*, 1459–1473.
Kandel, D.B., & Davies, M. (1986). Adult sequelae of adolescent depressive symptoms. *Archives of General Psychiatry*, *43*, 255–262.
Kanfer, F. (1970). Self-regulation: Research issues and speculations. In C. Neuringer & J.L. Michael (Eds.), *Behavior modification in clinical psychology* (pp. 178–220). New York: Appleton-Century-Crofts.
Karno, M., Hough, R.L., Burnam, A., Escobar, J.I., Timbers, D.M., Santana, F., & Boyd, J.H. (1987). Lifetime prevalence of specific psychiatric disorders among Mexican Americans and non-Hispanic whites in Los Angeles. *Archives of General Psychiatry*, *44*, 695–701.
Kaslow, N.J., Rehm, L.P., Pollack, S.L., & Siegel, A.W. (1988). Attributional style and self-control behavior in depressed and nondepressed children and their parents. *Journal of Abnormal Child Psychology*, *16*, 163–175.
Kaslow, N.J., Rehm, L.P., & Siegel, A.W. (1984). Social-cognitive and cognitive correlates of depression in children. *Journal of Abnormal Child Psychology*, *12*, 605–620.
Kauffman, C., Grunebaum, H., Cohler, B., & Gamer, E. (1979). Superkids: Competent children of psychotic mothers. *American Journal of Psychiatry*, *136*, 1398–1402.
Kazdin, A.E., Esveldt-Dawson, K., Sherick, R.B., & Colbus, D. (1985). Assessment of overt behavior and childhood depression among psychiatrically disturbed children. *Journal of Consulting and Clinical Psychology*, *53*, 201–210.
Kazdin, A.E., French, N.H., Unis, A.S., Esveldt-Dawson, K., & Sherick, R.B. (1983). Hopelessness, depression, and suicidal intent among psychiatrically disturbed inpatient children. *Journal of Consulting and Clinical Psychology*, *51*, 504–510.
Kazdin, A.E., & Petti, T.A. (1982). Self-report and interview measures of childhood and adolescent depression. *Journal of Child Psychology and Psychiatry*, *23*, 437–457.

Kazdin, A.E., Rodgers, A., & Colbus, D. (1986). The Hopelessness Scale for Children: Psychometric characteristics and concurrent validity. *Journal of Consulting and Clinical Psychology*, *54*, 241–245.

Keller, M.B. (1985). Chronic and recurrent affective disorders: Incidence, course, and influencing factors. In D. Kemali & G. Recagni (Eds.), *Chronic treatments in neuropsychiatry*. New York: Raven Press.

Keller, M.B. (1988). Diagnostic issues and clinical course of unipolar illness. In A.J. Frances & R.E. Hales (Eds.), *Review of psychiatry* (pp. 188–212). Washington, DC: American Psychiatric Press.

Keller, M.B., Beardslee, W.R., Dorer, D.J., Lavori, P.W., Samuelson, H., & Klerman, G.R. (1986). Impact of severity and chronicity of parental affective illness on adaptive functioning and psychopathology in children. *Archives of General Psychiatry*, *43*, 930–937.

Keller, M.B., Lavori, P.W., Endicott, J., Coryell, W., & Klerman, G.L. (1983). "Double depression:" Two-year follow-up. *American Journal of psychiatry*, *140*, 689–694.

Kennedy, S., Thompson, R., Stancer, H.C., Roy, A., & Persad, E. (1983). Life events precipitating mania. *British Journal of Psychiatry*, *142*, 398–403.

Klein, D.N., Clark, D.C., Dansky, L., & Margolis, E.T. (1988). Dysthymia in offspring of parents with primary unipolar affective disorder. *Journal of Abnormal Psychology*, *97*, 265–274.

Klein, D.N., Depue, R.A., & Slater, J.F. (1985). Cyclothymia in the adolescent offspring of parents with bipolar affective disorder. *Journal of Abnormal Psychology*, *94*, 115–127.

Klerman, G.L., Lavori, P.W., Rice, J., Reich, T., Endicott, J., Andreason, N. C., Keller, M.C., & Hirshfeld, R.M.A. (1985). Birth-cohort trends in rates of major depressive disorder among relatives of patients with affective disorder. *Archives of General Psychiatry*, *42*, 689–695.

Klerman, G.L., & Weissman, M.M. (1989). Increasing rates of depression. *Journal of the American Medical Association*, *261*, 2229–2235.

Kochanska, G., Kuczynski, L., Radke-Yarrow, M., & Welsh, J.D. (1987). Resolutions of control episodes between well and affectively ill mothers and their young children. *Journal of Abnormal Child Psychology*, *15*(3), 441–456.

Koenig, L.J. (1988). Self-image of emotionally disturbed adolescents. *Journal of Abnormal Child Psychology*, *16*, 111–126.

Kovacs, M. (1981). Rating scales to assess depression in school children. *Acta Paedopsychiatrica*, *46*, 305–315.

Kovacs, M. (1989). Affective disorders in children and adolescents. *American Psychologist*, *44*, 209–215.

Kovacs, M., Feinberg, T.L., Crouse-Novak, M.A., Paulauskas, S.L., & Finkelstein, R. (1984). Depressive disorders in childhood: I. A longitudinal prospective study of characteristics and recovery. *Archives of General Psychiatry*, *41*, 229–237.

Kovacs, M., Feinberg, T.L., Crouse-Novak, M.A., Paulauskas, S.L., Pollock, M., & Finkelstein, R. (1984). Depressive disorders in childhood: II. A longitudinal study of the risk for a subsequent major depression. *Archives of General Psychiatry*, *41*, 643–649.

Kovacs, M., Gatsonis, C., Paulauskas, S.L., & Richards, C. (1989). Depressive

disorders in childhood: IV. A longitudinal study of comorbidity with and risk for anxiety disorders. *Archives of General Psychiatry*, *46*, 776–782.
Kuiper, N., & Derry, P. (1982). Depressed and nondepressed content in self-reference in mild depressives. *Journal of Personality*, *50*, 62–74.
Kuyler, P.L., Rosenthal, L., Igel, G., Dunner, D.L., & Fieve, R.R. (1980). Psychopathology among children of manic-depressive patients. *Biological Psychiatry*, *15*, 589–597.
Lazarus, R.S., & Folkman, S. (1984). *Stress, appraisal, and coping*. New York: Springer.
Leahy, R.L. (1985a). The costs of development: Clinical implications. In R.L. Leahy (Ed.), *The development of the self* (pp. 267–294). Orlando, FL: Academic Press.
Leahy, R.L. (Ed.). (1985b). *The development of the self*. Orlando, FL: Academic Press.
Leahy, R.L., & Shirk, S.R. (1985). Social cognition and the development of the self. In R.L. Leahy (Ed.), *The development of the self* (pp. 123–150). Orlando, FL: Academic Press.
Leckman, J.F., Weissman, M.M., Merikangas, K.R., Pauls, D.L., & Prusoff, B.A. (1983). Panic disorder and major depression: Increased risk of depression, alcoholism, panic, and phobic disorders in families of depressed probands with panic disorder. *Archives of General Psychiatry*, *40*, 1055–1060.
Lee, C.M., & Gotlib, I.H. (1989a). Clinical status and emotional adjustment of children of depressed mothers. *American Journal of Psychiatry*, *146*, 478–483.
Lee, C.M., & Gotlib, I.H. (1989b). Maternal depression and child adjustment: A longitudinal analysis. *Journal of Abnormal Psychology*, *98*, 78–85.
Lefkowitz, M.M., & Tesiny, E.P. (1980). Assessment of childhood depression. *Journal of Consulting and Clinical Psychology*, *48*, 43–50.
Leitenberg, H., Yost, L.W., & Carroll-Wilson, M. (1986). Negative cognitive errors in children: Questionnaire development, normative data, and comparisons between children with and without self-reported symptoms of depression, low self-esteem, and evaluation anxiety. *Journal of Consulting and Clinical Psychology*, *54*, 528–536.
Leon, G.R., Kendall, P.C., & Garber, J. (1980). Depression in children: Parent, teacher, and child perspectives. *Journal of Abnormal Child Psychology*, *8*, 221–235.
Lewinsohn, P.M. (1974). A behavioral approach to depression. In R.J. Friedman & M.M. Katz (Eds.), *The psychology of depression: Contemporary theory and research*. (pp. 157–178). Washington, DC: Winston/Wiley.
Lewinsohn, P.M., Hoberman, H.M., & Rosenbaum, M. (1988). A prospective study of risk factors for unipolar depression. *Journal of Abnormal Psychology*, *97*(3), 251–264.
Lewinsohn, P.M., Hops, H., Roberts, R., & Seeley, J.R. (1988, November). *Adolescent depression: Prevalence and psychosocial aspects*. Paper presented at the American Public Health Association's Annual Meeting, Boston, MA.
Lewinsohn, P.M., & Rosenbaum, M. (1987). Recall of parental behavior by acute depressives, remitted depressives, and non-depressives. *Journal of Personality and Social Psychology*, *52*(3), 611–619.
Lewinsohn, P.M., Steinmetz, J., Larson, D., & Franklin, J. (1981). Depression-

related cognitions: Antecedent or consequence? *Journal of Abnormal Psychology*, *90*, 213–219.

Lewinsohn, P.M., Zeiss, A.M., & Duncan, E.M. (1989). Probability of relapse after recovery from an episode of depression. *Journal of Abnormal Psychology*, *98*(2), 107–116.

Lewis, R.J., Dlugokinski, E.L., Caputo, L.M., & Griffin, R.B. (1988). Children at risk for emotional disorders: Risk and resource dimensions. *Clinical Psychology Review*, *8*, 417–440.

Linville, P.W. (1987). Self-complexity as a cognitive buffer against stress-related illness and depression. *Journal of Personality and Social Psychology*, *52*, 663–676.

Livingood, A.B., Daen, P., & Smith, B.D. (1983). The depressed mother as a source of stimulation for her infant. *Journal of Clinical Psychology*, *39*, 369–375.

Lloyd, C. (1980). Life events and depressive disorders reviewed: 2. Events as precipitating factors. *Archives of General Psychiatry*, *37*, 541–548.

Longfellow, C., & Belle, D. (1984). Stressful environments and their impact on children. In J. Humphrey (Ed.), *Stress in childhood* (pp. 63–78). New York: AMS.

Lyons-Ruth, K., Zoll, D., Connell, D., & Grunebaum, H.U. (1986). The depressed mother and her one-year-old infant: Environment, interaction, attachment, and infant development. In E. Tronick & T. Field (Eds.), *Maternal depression and infant disturbance*, New Directions for Child Development, No *34*, (pp. 31–46). San Francisco: Jossey-Bass.

Maccoby, E.A., & Martin, B. (1983). Socialization in the context of the family: Parent–child interaction. In E.M. Hetherington (Ed.), *Handbook of child psychology, Vol. 4. Socialization, personality, and social development* (pp. xx–xx). New York: Wiley.

Markus, H. (1977). Self-schemata and processing information about self. *Journal of Personality and Social Psychology*, *35*, 63–78.

Masten, A.S., & Garmezy, N. (1985). Risk, vulnerability, and protective factors in developmental psychopathology. In B.B. Lahey and A.E. Kazdin (Eds.), *Advances in clinical child psychology* (Vol. 8, pp. 1–52). New York: Plenum.

Masten, A.S., Garmezy, N., Tellegen, A., Pellegrini, D.S., Larkin, K., & Larsen, A. (1988). Competence and stress in school children: The moderating effects of individual and family qualities. *Journal of Child Psychology and Psychiatry*, *29*, 745–764.

Mayo, J.A., O'Connell, R.A., & O'Brien, J.D. (1979). Families of manic-depressive patients: Effect of treatment. *American Journal of Psychiatry*, *136*, 1535–1539.

McCauley, E., Mitchell, J., Burke, P., & Moss, S. (1988). Cognitive attributes of depression in children and adolescents. *Journal of Consulting and Clinical Psychology*, *56*, 903–908.

McCranie, E., & Bass, J. (1984). Childhood family antecedents of dependency and self-criticism: Implications for depression. *Journal of Abnormal Psychology*, *93*, 3–8.

McGee, R., Anderson, J., Williams, S., & Silva, P.A. (1986). Cognitive correlates of depressive symptoms in 11-year-old children. *Journal of Abnormal Child Psychology*, *14*, 517–524.

McGuffin, P., Katz, R., & Bebbington, P. (1988). The Camberwell Collaborative

Depression Study: III. Depression and adversity in the relatives of depressed probands. *British Journal of Psychiatry*, *152*, 775–782.

McKnew, D.H., Jr., & Cytryn, L. (1973). Historical background in children with affective disorders. *American Journal of Psychiatry*, *130*, 1278–1280.

McKnew, D.H., Cytryn, L., Efron, A.M., Gershon, E.S., & Bunney, W.E., Jr. (1979). Offspring of patients with affective disorders. *British Journal of Psychiatry*, *134*, 148–152.

Merikangas, K.R., Prusoff, B.A., & Weissman, M.M. (1988). Parental concordance for affective disorders: Psychopathology in offspring. *Journal of Affective Disorders*, *15*, 279–290.

Merikangas, K.R., Weissman, M.M., Prusoff, B.A., & John, K. (1988). Assortative mating and affective disorders: Psychopathology in offspring. *Psychiatry*, *51*, 48–57.

Miklowitz, D., Goldstein, M., Nuechterlein, K., Snyder, K., & Mintz, J. (1988). Family factors and the course of bipolar affective disorder. *Archives of General Psychiatry*, *45*, 225–231.

Miller, I., & Norman, W. (1986). Persistence of depressive cognitions within a subgroup of depressed inpatients. *Cognitive Therapy and Research*, *10*, 211–224.

Mills, M., Puckering, C., Pound, A., & Cox, A. (1985). What is it about depressed mothers that influences their children's functioning? In J.E. Stevenson (Ed.), *Recent research in developmental psychopathology* (pp. 11–17). Oxford, England: Pergamon Press.

Moos, R., & Moos, B. (1981). *Family Environment Scale manuel.* Palo Alto, CA: Consulting Psychologists Press.

Morrison, H.L. (Ed.) (1983). *Children of depressed mothers: Risk, identification, and intervention*. New York: Grune & Stratton.

Murray, L. (1988). The Cambridge study of postnatal depression and infant development. Presented at the Round Table Meeting of the Royal Society, London, England, Feb. 26, 1988: Childbirth as a life event.

Nolen-Hoeksema, S. (1987). Sex differences in unipolar depression: Evidence and theory. *Psychological Bulletin*, *101*, 259–282.

Nolen-Hoeksema, S., Girgus, J.S., & Seligman, M.E.P. (1986). Learned helplessness in children: A longitudinal study of depression, achievement, and explanatory style. *Journal of Personality and Social Psychology*, *51*, 435–442.

Nurnberger, J.I., Hamovit, J., Hibbs, E.D., Pelligrini, D., Guroff, J.J., Maxwell, M.E., Smith, A., & Gershon, E.S. (1988). A high-risk study of primary affective disorder: Selection of subjects, initial assessment, and 1- to 2-year follow-up. In D.L. Dunner, E.S. Gershon, & J.E. Barrett (Eds.), *Relatives at risk for mental disorder* (pp. 161–177). New York: Raven Press.

Oliver, J., Handal, P., Finn, T., & Herdy, S. (1987). Depressed and nondepressed students and their siblings in frequent contact with their families: Depression and perceptions of the family. *Cognitive Therapy and Research*, *11*, 501–515.

Orvaschel, H., Puig-Antich, J., Chambers, W., Tabrizi, M., & Johnson, R. (1982). Retrospective assessment of prepubertal major depression with the Kiddie-SADS-E. *Journal of the American Academy of Child Psychiatry*, *21*, 392–397.

Orvaschel, H., Walsh-Allis, G., & Ye, W. (1988). Psychopathology in children of parents with recurrent depression. *Journal of Abnormal Child Psychology*, *16*, 17–28.

Orvaschel, H., Weissman, M.M., & Kidd, K.K. (1980). Children and depression. *Journal of Affective Disorders*, *2*, 1–16.

Overall, J.E., Higgins, W., & DeSchweinitz, A. (1976). Comparison of differential diagnostic discrimination for abbreviated and standard MMPI. *Journal of Clinical Psychology*, *32*, 237–245.

Palermo, D.S. (1989). *Coping with uncertainty: Behavioral and developmental perspectives*. Hillsdale, NJ: Lawrence Erlbaum Associates.

Panaccione, V.F., & Wahler, R.G. (1986). Child behavior, maternal depression, and social coercion as factors in the quality of child care. *Journal of Abnormal Child Psychology*, *14*(2), 263–278.

Parker, G. (1981). Parental reports of depressives. *Journal of Affective Disorders*, *3*, 131–140.

Patterson, G. (1982). *A social learning approach: 3. Coercive family process*. Eugene, OR: Castalia.

Patterson, G.R., DeBaryshe, B.D., & Ramsey E. (1989). A developmental perspective on antisocial behavior. *American Psychologist*, *44*, 329–335.

Paulson, A., Crowe, R., Noyes, R., & Pfohl, B. (1988). Reliability of the telephone interview in diagnosing anxiety disorders. *Archives of General Psychiatry*, *45*, 62–63.

Paykel, E.S. (1979). Recent life events in the development of the depressive disorder. In R.A. Depue (Ed.), *The psychobiology of the depressive disorders: Implications for the effects of stress* (pp. 245–262). New York: Academic Press.

Pearlin, L., Menaghan, E., Lieberman, M., & Mullan, J. (1981). The stress process. *Journal of Health and Social Behavior*, *22*, 337–356.

Pellegrini, D., Kosisky, S., Nackman, D., Cytryn, L., McKnew, D.H., Gershon, E., Hamovit, J., & Cammuso, K. (1986). Personal and social resources in children of patients with bipolar affective disorder and children of normal control subjects. *American Journal of Psychiatry*, *143*, 856–861.

Perris, C., Arrindell, W.A., Perris, H., Eisemann, M., Van Der Ende, J., & Von Knorring, L. (1986). Perceived depriving parental rearing and depression. *British Journal of Psychiatry*, *148*, 170–175.

Peterson, C., & Seligman, M.E.P. (1984). Causal explanations as a risk factor for depression: Theory and evidence. *Psychological Review*, *91*, 347–374.

Peterson, L., Mori, L., & Carter, P. (1985). The role of the family in children's responses to stressful medical procedures. *Journal of Clinical Child Psychology*, *14*(2), 98–104.

Peterson, L., Mullins, L.L., & Ridley-Johnson, R. (1985). Childhood depression: Peer reactions to depression and life stress. *Journal of Abnormal Child Psychology*, *13*, 597–609.

Pettit, G.S., Dodge, K.A., & Brown, M.M. (1988). Early family experience, social problem solving patterns, and children's social competence. *Child Development*, *59*, 107–120.

Piers, E. (1977). *The Piers-Harris Children's Self-Concept Test: Research Monograph 1*. Nashville, TN: Counselor Recordings and Tests.

Piers, E., & Harris, D. (1969). *The Piers-Harris Children's Self-Concept Scale*. Nashville, TN: Counselor Recordings and Tests.

Plomin, R. (1986). *Development, genetics, and psychology*. Hillsdale, NJ: Lawrence Erlbaum Associates.

Plomin, R., & Daniels, D. (1987). Why are children in the same family so different from one another? *Behavioral and Brain Sciences, 10,* 1–15.

Post, R.M., Rubinow, D.R., & Ballenger, J.C. (1984). Conditioning, sensitization, and kindling: Implications for the course of affective illness. In R. Post & J. Ballenger (Eds.), *Neurobiology of mood disorders* (pp. 432–466). Baltimore, MD: Williams & Wilkins.

Pound, A., Cox, A., Puckering, C., & Mills, M. (1985). The impact of maternal depression on young children. In J.E. Stevenson (Ed.), *Recent research in developmental psychopathology* (pp. 3–10). Oxford, England: Pergamon Press.

Poznanski, E.O., Krahenbuhl, V., & Zrull, J.P. (1976). Childhood depression. A longitudinal perspective. *Journal of the American Academy of Child Psychiatry, 15,* 491–501.

Puig-Antich, J., Chambers, W., & Tabrizi, M.A. (1983). The clinical assessment of current depressive episodes in children and adolescents: Interviews with parents and children. In B.P. Cantwell & G.A. Carlson (Eds.), *Affective disorders in childhood and adolescence* (pp. 157–180). New York: SP Medical and Scientific Books.

Puig-Antich, J., Goetz, D., Davies, M., Kaplan, T., Davies, S., Ostrow, L., Asnis, L., Twomey, J., Iyengar, S., & Ryan, N.D. (1989). A controlled family history study of prepubertal major depressive disorder. *Archives of General Psychiatry, 46,* 406–418.

Puig-Antich, J., Lukens, E., Davies, M., Goetz, D., Brennon-Quattrock, J., & Todak, G. (1985a). Psychosocial functioning in prepubertal major depressive disorders: I. Interpersonal relationships during the depressive episode. *Archives of General Psychiatry, 42,* 500–507.

Puig-Antich, J., Lukens, E., Davies, M., Goetz, D., Brennon-Quattrock, J., & Todak, G. (1985b). Psychosocial functioning in prepubertal major depressive disorders: II. Interpersonal relationships after sustained recovery from affective episodes. *Archives of General Psychiatry, 42,* 511–517.

Putallaz, M. (1987). Maternal behavior and children's sociometric status. *Child Development, 58,* 324–340.

Radke-Yarrow, M., Cummings, E.M., Kuczynski, L., & Chapman, M. (1985). Patterns of attachment in two- and three-year olds in normal families and families with parental depression. *Child Development, 36,* 884–893.

Radke-Yarrow, M., Richters, J., & Wilson, W.E. (1988). Child development in the network of relationships. In R.A. Hinde & J. Stevenson-Hinde (Eds.), *Relationships within families: Mutual influences* (pp. 48–67). Oxford, England: Clarendon Press.

Radke-Yarrow, M., & Sherman, T. (1990). Hard growing: Children who survive. In J. Rolf, A. Masten, D. Cicchetti, K. Nuechterlein, & S. Weintraub (Eds.), *Risk and protective factors in the development of psychopathology.* Cambridge, England: Cambridge University Press.

Rehm, L.P. (1977). A self-control model of depression. *Behavior Therapy, 8,* 787–804.

Rehm, L.P. (1988). Self-management and cognitive processes in depression. In L.B. Alloy (Ed.), *Cognitive processes in depression* (pp. 143–176). New York: Guilford Press.

Rehm, L.P., & Naus, M.J. (1990). A memory model of emotion. In R. Ingram

(Ed.), *Contemporary psychological approaches to depression: Treatment, research, and theory*. New York: Plenum.

Rice, J., Reich, T., Andreasen, N.C., Endicott, J., Van Eerdewegh, M., Fishman, R., Hirschfeld, R.M.A., & Klerman, G.L. (1987). The familial transmission of bipolar illness. *Archives of General Psychiatry*, *44*, 441–447.

Richters, J.E. (1987). Chronic versus episodic stress and the adjustment of high-risk offspring. In K. Hahlweg & M.J. Goldstein (Eds.), *Understanding major mental disorder: The contribution of family interaction research* (pp. 74–90). New York: Family Process Press.

Roback-Moyal, B. (1977). Locus of control, self-esteem, stimulus appraisal, and depressive symptoms in children. *Journal of Consulting and Clinical Psychology*, *45*, 951–952.

Roback-Moyal, B. (1981). The identification of depressive children. Unpublished manuscript.

Robins, L. N., Helzer, J.E., Croughan, J., & Ratcliff, K.S. (1981). National Institute of Mental Health Diagnostic Interview Schedule. *Archives of General Psychiatry*, *38*, 381.

Robins, L.N., Helzer, J.E., Weissman, M.M., Orvaschel, H., Gruenberg, E., Burke, J.D., Jr., & Regier, D.A. (1984). Lifetime prevalence of specific psychiatric disorders in three sites. *Archives of General Psychiatry*, *41*, 949–958.

Rolf, J. (1972). The social and academic competence of children vulnerable to schizophrenia and other behavior pathologies. *Journal of Abnormal Psychology*, *80*, 225–243.

Rosenbaum, J.F., Biederman, J., Gersten, M., Hirshfeld, D.R., Meminger, S.R., Herman, J.B., Kagan, J., Reznick, J.S., & Snidman, N. (1988). Behavioral inhibition in children of parents with panic disorder and agoraphobia. *Archives of General Psychiatry*, *45*, 463–470.

Rosenberg, M. (1965). *Society and the adolescent self-image*. Princeton, NJ: Princeton University Press.

Rutter, M. (1966). The children of sick parents: Environmental and psychiatric studies. *Maudsley Monograph, No. 16*. London: Oxford University Press.

Rutter, M. (1978). Early sources of security and competence. In B. J. Garton (Ed.), *Human growth and development*. New York: Oxford University Press.

Rutter, M. (1985). Resilience in the face of adversity: Protective factors and resistence to psychiatric disorder. *British Journal of Psychiatry*, *147*, 598–611.

Rutter, M. (1989). Intergenerational continuities and discontinuities in serious parenting difficulties. In D. Cicchetti & V. Carlson (Eds.), *Research on the consequences of child maltreatment* (pp. 317–348). New York: Cambridge University Press.

Rutter, M. (1990). Commentary: Some focus and process considerations regarding effects of parental depression on children. *Developmental Psychology*, *26*, 60–67.

Rutter, M., & Quinton, P. (1984). Parental psychiatric disorder: Effects on children. *Psychological Medicine*, *14*, 853–880.

Sameroff, A.J., Barocas, R., & Seifer, R. (1984). The early development of children born to mentally ill women. In N. Watt, E.J. Anthony, L. Wynne, & J. Rolf (Eds.), *Children at risk for schizophrenia* (pp. 482–514). New York: Cambridge University Press.

Sameroff, A.J., Seifer, R., & Zax, M. (1982). Early development of children at risk for emotional disorder. *Monographs of the Society for Research in Child Development, 47*, (7, Serial No. 199).

Saylor, C.F., Finch, A.J., Jr., Baskin, C.H., Furey, W., & Kelly, M.M. (1984). Construct validity for measures of childhood depression: Application of multitrait-multimethod methodology. *Journal of Consulting and Clinical Psychology, 52*, 977–985.

Saylor, C.F., Finch, A.J., Jr., Spirito, A., & Bennett, B. (1984). The Children's Depression Inventory: A systematic evaluation of psychometric properties. *Journal of Consulting and Clinical Psychology, 52*, 955–967.

Segal, Z.V. (1988). Appraisal of the self-schema construct in cognitive models of depression. *Psychological Bulletin, 103*, 147–162.

Seifer, R., & Sameroff, A.J. (1987). Multiple determinants of risk and invulnerability. In E.J. Anthony & B.J. Cohler (Eds.), *The Invulnerable child* (pp. 51–69). New York: Guilford Press.

Seligman, M.E.P. (1975). *Helplessness*. San Francisco: Freeman.

Seligman, M.E.P., Abramson, L.Y., Semmel, A., & von Baeyer, C. (1979). Depressive attributional style. *Journal of Abnormal Psychology, 88*, 242–247.

Seligman, M.E.P., Peterson, C., Kaslow, N.J., Tenenbaum, R.L., Alloy, L.B., & Abramson, L.Y. (1984). Attributional style and depressive symptoms among children. *Journal of Abnormal Psychology, 93*, 235–241.

Selman, R.L., Beardslee, W., Schultz, L.H., Krupa, M., & Podorefsky, D. (1986). Assessing adolescent interpersonal negotiation strategies: Toward the integration of structural and functional models. *Developmental Psychology, 22*, 450–459.

Shea, M.T., Glass, D.R., Pilkonis, P.A., Watkins, J., & Docherty, J.P. (1987). Frequency and implications of personality disorders in a sample of depressed outpatients. *Journal of Personality Disorders, 1*, 27–42.

Slavin, L.A., & Compas, B.E. (1989). The problem of confounding social support and depressive symptoms: A brief report on a college sample. *American Journal of Community Psychology, 17*(1), 57–65.

Spiegel, D., & Wissler, T. (1986). Family environment as a predictor of psychiatric rehospitalization. *American Journal of Psychiatry, 143*, 56–60.

Strauss, C.C., Lahey, B.B., Frick, P., Frame, C., & Hynd, G.W. (1988). Peer social status of children with anxiety disorders. *Journal of Consulting and Clinical Psychology, 56*, 137–141.

Strober, M., Morell, W., Burroughs, J., Lampert, C., Danforth, H., & Freeman, R. (1988). A family study of bipolar I disorder in adolescence: Early onset of symptoms linked to increased familial loading and lithium resistance. *Journal of Affective Disorders, 15*, 255–268.

Swearingen, E., & Cohen, L. (1985). Measurement of adolescents' life events: The Junior High School Life Experiences Survey. *American Journal of Community Psychology, 13*, 69–85.

Sweeney, P.D., Anderson, K., & Bailey, S. (1986). Attributional style in depression: A meta-analytic review. *Journal of Personality and Social Psychology, 50*, 974–991.

Teasdale, J.D. (1983). Negative thinking in depression: Cause, effect, or reciprocal relationship? *Advances in Behavior Research and Therapy, 5*, 3–25.

Teasdale, J.D., & Dent, J. (1987). Cognitive vulnerability to depression: An investigation of two hypotheses. *British Journal of Clinical Psychology, 26*, 113–126.

Tesiny, E.P., & Lefkowitz, M.M. (1982). Childhood depression: A six-month follow-up study. *Journal of Consulting and Clinical Psychology, 50*, 778–780.

Thoits, P.A. (1983). Dimensions of life events that influence psychological distress: An evaluation and synthesis of the literature. In H.B. Kaplan (Ed.), *Psychosocial stress: Trends in theory and research* (pp. 33–103). New York: Academic Press.

Thomson, B., & Vaux, A. (1986). The importation, transmission, and moderation of stress in the family system. *American Journal of Community Psychology, 14*(1), 39–57.

Turner, S.M., Beidel, D.C., & Costello, A. (1987). Psychopathology in the offspring of anxiety disorders patients. *Journal of Consulting and Clinical Psychology, 55*, 229–235.

Wagner, B., Compas, B., & Howell, D. (1988). Daily and major life events: A test of an integrative model of psychosocial stress. *American Journal of Community Psychology, 16*, 189–205.

Walker, E., Downey, G., & Nightingale, N. (1989). The nonorthogonal nature of risk factors: Implications for research on the causes of maladjustment. *Journal of Primary Prevention, 9*(3), 143–163.

Waters, B., Marchenko, I., & Smiley, D. (1983). Affective disorder, paranatal and educational factors in the offspring of bipolar manic-depressive. *Canadian Journal of Psychiatry, 28*, 527–531.

Watt, N., Anthony, E.J., Wynne, L., & Rolf, J. (1984). *Children at risk for schizophrenia*. New York: Cambridge University Press.

Webster-Stratton, C., & Hammond, M. (1988). Maternal depression and its relationship to life stress, perceptions of child behavior problems, parenting behaviors, and child conduct problems. *Journal of Abnormal Child Psychology, 16*(3), 299–315.

Weintraub, S. (1987). Risk factors in schizophrenia: The Stony Brook high-risk project. *Schizophrenia Bulletin, 13*(3), 439–450.

Weintraub, S., & Neale, J.M. (1984). Social behavior of children at risk for schizophrenia. In N. Watt, E.J. Anthony, L.C. Wynne, & J.E. Rolf (Eds.), *Children at risk for schizophrenia* (pp. 279–286). Cambridge, England: Cambridge University Press.

Weintraub, S., Winters, K.C., & Neale, J.M. (1986). Competence and vulnerability in children with an affectively disordered parent. In M. Rutter, C. Izard, & P. Read (Eds.), *Depression in young people: Developmental and clinical perspectives* (pp. 205–220). New York: Guilford Press.

Weissman, M.M. (1988). Psychopathology in the children of depressed parents: Direct interview studies. In D.L. Dunner, E.S. Gershon, & J.E. Barett (Eds.), *Relatives at risk for mental disorders*. New York: Raven Press.

Weissman, M.M., & Bothwell, S. (1976). The assessment of social adjustment by patient self-report. *Archives of General Psychiatry, 33*, 1111–1115.

Weissman, M.M., Gammon, G.D., John, K. Merikangas, K.R., Warner, V., Prusoff, B.A., & Sholomkas, D. (1987). Children of depressed parents: Increased psychopathology and early onset of major depression. *Archives of General Psychiatry, 44*, 847–853.

Weissman, M.M., Gershon, E.S., Kidd, K.K., Prusoff, B.A., Leckman, J.F., Dibbie, E., Hamovit, J., Thompson, W.D., Pauls, D.L., & Guroff, J.J. (1984). Psychiatric disorders in the relatives of probands with affective disorders: The Yale–NIMH collaborative family study. *Archives of General Psychiatry*, *41*, 13–41.

Weissman, M.M., John, K., Merikangas, K.R., Prusoff, B.A., Wickramaratne, P., & Gammon, G.D. (1986). Depressed parents and their children: General health, social, and psychiatric problems. *American Journal of Diseases in Children*, *140*, 801–805.

Weissman, M.M., Kidd, K.K., & Prusoff, B.A. (1982). Variability in rates of affective disorders in relatives of depressed and normal probands. *Archives of General Psychiatry*, *39*, 1397–1403.

Weissman, M.M., Leckman, J.F., Merikangas, K.R., Gammon, G.D., & Prusoff, B.A. (1984). Depression and anxiety disorders in parents and children: Results form the Yale Family Study. *Archives of General Psychiatry*, *41*, 845–852.

Weissman, M.M., Merikangas, K.R., Wickramaratne, P., Kidd, K.K., Prusoff, B.A., Leckman, J.F., & Pauls, D.L. (1986). Understanding the clinical heterogeneity of major depression using family data. *Archives of General Psychiatry*, *43*, 430–434.

Weissman, M.M., & Paykel, E.S. (1974). *The depressed woman: A study of social relationships*. Chicago: University of Chicago Press.

Weissman, M.M., Paykel, E.S., & Klerman, G.L. (1972). The depressed woman as a mother. *Social Psychiatry*, *7*, 98–108.

Weissman, M.M., Prusoff, B.A., Gammon, G.D., Merikangas, K.R., Leckman, J.F., & Kidd, K.K. (1984). Psychopathology in the children (age 6–10) of depressed and normal parents. *Journal of the American Academy of Child Psychiatry*, *23*, 78–84.

Weissman, M.M., Sholomkas, D., & John, K. (1981). The assessment of social adjustment: An update. *Archives of General Psychiatry*, *38*, 1250–1258.

Weissman, M.M., Wickramaratne, P., Warner, V., John, K., Prusoff, B.A., Merikangas, K.R., & Gammon, G.D. (1987). Assessing psychiatric disorders in children: Discrepancies between mothers' and children's reports. *Archives of General Psychiatry*, *44*, 747–753.

Wells, K.B., Stewart, A., Hays, R.D., Burnam, A., Rogers, W., Daniels, M., Berry, S., Greenfield, S., & Ware, J. (1989). The functioning and well-being of depressed patients: Results from the Medical Outcomes Study. *Journal of the American Medical Association*, *262*, 914–919.

Welner, Z., & Garrison, W.T. (1985). Blind high-risk study of depressives' offspring: Preliminary data. *International Journal of Family Psychiatry*, *6*, 301–314.

Welner, Z., Welner, A., McCrary, M.D., & Leonard, M.A. (1977). Psychopathology in children of inpatients with depression: A controlled study. *Journal of Nervous and Mental Disorders*, *164*, 408–413.

West, M.O., & Prinz, R.J. (1987). Parental alcoholism and childhood psychopathology. *Psychological Bulletin*, *102*, 204–218.

Whalen, C., Henker, B., Collins, B., McAuliffe, S. & Vaux, A. (1979). Peer interaction in a structured communication task: Comparisons of normal and hyperactive boys and of methylphenidate (Ritalin) and placebo effects. *Child Development*, *50*, 388–401.

Whiffen, V.E., & Gotlib, I.H. (1989). Infants of postpartum depressed mothers: Temperament and cognitive status. *Journal of Abnormal Psychology*, *98*(3), 274–279.

Williams, H., & Carmichael, A. (1985). Depression in mothers in a multi-ethnic urban industrial municipality in Melbourne. Aetiological factors and effects on infants and preschool children. *Journal of Child Psychology and Psychiatry*, *26*(2), 277–288.

Winokur, G. (1979), Familial (genetic) subtypes of pure depressive disease. *American Journal of Psychiatry*, *136*, 911–913.

Winters, K.C., Stone, A.A., Weintraub, S., & Neale, J.M. (1981). Cognitive and attentional deficits in children vulnerable to psychopathology. *Journal of Abnormal Child Psychology*, *9*, 435–453.

Worland, J., Janes, C., Anthony, E., McGinniss, M., & Cass, L. (1984). St. Louis Risk Research Project: Comprehensive progress report of experimental studies. In N.F. Watt, E.J., Anthony, L., Wynne, & J. Rolf (Eds.), *Children at risk for schizophrenia* (pp. 105–147). New York: Cambridge University Press.

Worland, J., Weeks, D.G., & Janes, C.L. (1987). Predicting mental health in children at risk. In E.J. Anthony & B.J. Cohler (Eds.), *The invulnerable child* (pp. 185–210). New York: Guilford Press.

Wyman, P.A., Cowen, E.L., Hightower, A.D., & Pedro-Carroll, J.L. (1985). Perceived competence, self-esteem, and anxiety in latency-aged children of divorce. *Journal of Clinical Child Psychology*, *14*(1), 20–26.

Wynne, L., Cole, R., & Perkins, P. (1987). University of Rochester Child and Family Study: Risk research in progress. *Schizophrenia Bulletin*, *13*, 403–476.

Zahn-Waxler, C., Cummings, E.M., Iannotti, R.J., & Radke-Yarrow, M. (1984). Young children of depressed parents: A population at risk for affective problems. In D. Cicchetti (Ed.), *Childhood depression*. (pp. 81–105). San Francisco: Jossey-Bass.

Zahn-Waxler, C., Cummings, E.M., McKnew, D., & Radke-Yarrow, M. (1984). Altruism, aggression, and social interaction in young children with a manic-depressive parent. *Child Development*, *55*, 112–122.

Zahn-Waxler, C., Kochanska, G., Krupnick, J., & McKnew, D. (1990). Patterns of guilt in children of depressed and well mothers. *Developmental Psychology*, *26*(1), 51–59.

Zahn-Waxler, C., Mayfield, A., Radke-Yarrow, M., McKnew, D.H., Cytryn, L., & Davenport, Y.B. (1988). A follow-up investigation of offspring of parents with bipolar disorder. *American Journal of Psychiatry*, *145*, 506–509.

Zahn-Waxler, C., McKnew, D.H., Cummings, E.M., Davenport, Y.B., & Radke-Yarrow, M. (1984). Problem behaviors and peer interactions of young children with a manic-depressive parent. *American Journal of Psychiatry*, *141*, 236–240.

Zimmerman, M., Coryell, W., & Pfohl, B. (1986). Validity of familial subtypes of primary unipolar depression. *Archives of General Psychiatry*, *43*(11), 1090–1096.

Zimmerman, M., Coryell, W., Stangl, D., & Pfohl, B. (1987). Validity of an operational definition for neurotic unipolar major depression. *Journal of Affective Disorders*, *12*, 29–40.

Zis, A.P., & Goodwin, F.K. (1979). Major affective disorder as a recurrent illness: A clinical review. *Archives of General Psychiatry*, *36*, 835–839.

Zuckerman, M. (1971). Abbreviated Manual with Scoring Keys and Norms for

Form V of the Sensation Seeking Scale. Available from the author, Department of Psychology, University of Delaware, Newark, DE 19711.
Zupan, B.A., Hammen, C., & Jaenicke, C. (1987). The effects of current mood and prior depressive history on self-schematic processing in children. *Journal of Experimental Child Psychology*, *43*, 149–158.

MIX
Papier aus verantwortungsvollen Quellen
Paper from responsible sources
FSC® C105338
www.fsc.org

If you have any concerns about our products,
you can contact us on
ProductSafety@springernature.com

In case Publisher is established outside the EU,
the EU authorized representative is:
Springer Nature Customer Service Center GmbH
Europaplatz 3, 69115 Heidelberg, Germany

Printed by Libri Plureos GmbH
in Hamburg, Germany